Annals of Information Systems

AF761839

Series Editors
Ramesh Sharda
Oklahoma State University
Stillwater, OK, USA

Stefan Voß
University of Hamburg
Hamburg, Germany

For further volumes:
http://www.springer.com/series/7573

Athina Lazakidou
Editor

Web-Based Applications in Healthcare and Biomedicine

Springer

Editor
Athina Lazakidou
Department of Nursing
University of Peloponnese
231 00 Sparta
Sparta General Hospital Bldg.
Greece
lazakid@uop.gr

ISSN 1934-3221 e-ISSN 1934-3213
ISBN 978-1-4419-1273-2 e-ISBN 978-1-4419-1274-9
DOI 10.1007/978-1-4419-1274-9
Springer New York Dordrecht Heidelberg London

Library of Congress Control Number: 2009937782

© Springer Science+Business Media, LLC 2010
All rights reserved. This work may not be translated or copied in whole or in part without the written permission of the publisher (Springer Science+Business Media, LLC, 233 Spring Street, New York, NY 10013, USA), except for brief excerpts in connection with reviews or scholarly analysis. Use in connection with any form of information storage and retrieval, electronic adaptation, computer software, or by similar or dissimilar methodology now known or hereafter developed is forbidden.
The use in this publication of trade names, trademarks, service marks, and similar terms, even if they are not identified as such, is not to be taken as an expression of opinion as to whether or not they are subject to proprietary rights.

Printed on acid-free paper

Springer is part of Springer Science+Business Media (www.springer.com)

Preface

Web-based applications provide the power of desktop and server applications with the flexibility and accessibility of the web. Using web browsers, users can securely access applications from anywhere within the reach of the company intranet or extranet. The special issue strives to explore the advanced web-based information systems and database applications in healthcare area.

Healthcare organizations are undergoing major reorganizations and adjustments to meet the increasing demands of improved healthcare access and quality, as well as lowered costs. As the use of information technology to process medical data increases, much of the critical information necessary to meet these challenges is being stored in digital format. Web-enabled information technologies can provide the means for greater access and more effective integration of healthcare information from disparate computer applications and other information resources.

This book presents studies from leading researchers and practitioners focusing on the current challenges, directions, trends, and opportunities associated with healthcare organizations and their strategic use of web-enabled technologies. Managing healthcare information systems with web-enabled technologies is an excellent vehicle for understanding current and potential uses of Internet technology in the broad areas of healthcare and medical applications.

The covered topics include semantic web applications, workflow management systems, process management and workflow management systems, content management and portal technology, location-aware systems and mobile technology, prototypes of web-based information systems, data and web mining, access control and security in web-based information systems, web-based information systems and databases, transaction management over the web and tools for the implementation of web-based information systems.

This handbook is an excellent source of comprehensive knowledge and literature on the topic of distributed health and e-health applications.

All of us who worked on the book hope that readers will find it useful.

Athina A. Lazakidou, Ph.D.

Contents

Contributors

Beatriz Sainz Abajo Department of Signal Theory and Communications, University of Valladolid, Campus Miguel Delibes, s/n, 47011 – Valladolid, Spain, beasai@tel.uva.es

Pantelis Angelidis University of Western Macedonia, Department of Engineering Informatics and Telecommunications, Karamanli and Lygeris, GR-50100 Kozani, Greece, paggelidis@uowm.gr

Ioannis Apostolakis Department of Sciences, Technical University of Crete, Crete, Greece, gapostolakis@nsph.gr

Eleni Christodoulou Computer Science Department, University of Cyprus, CY-1678 Nicosia, Cyprus, cseleni@cs.ucy.ac.cy

Nigel Collier National Institute of Informatics, 2-1-2 Hitotsubashi, Chiyoda-ku, Tokyo, Japan

Mike Conway National Institute of Informatics, 2-1-2 Hitotsubashi, Chiyoda-ku, Tokyo, Japan

Miguel López Coronado Department of Signal Theory and Communications, University of Valladolid, Campus Miguel Delibes, s/n, 47011 – Valladolid, Spain, miglop@tel.uva.es

Son Doan Department of Biomedical Informatics, Vanderbilt University Medical Center, Nashville, TN 37203, USA, doan@nii.ac.jp

D. John Doyle Professor of Anesthesiology, Cleveland Clinic Lerner College of Medicine of Case Western Reserve University, Staff Anesthesiologist, Department of General Anesthesiology, Cleveland Clinic Foundation, 9500 Euclid Avenue, E31 Cleveland, OH 44195, USA, doylej@ccf.org

Lori Frasier MD, Professor of Pediatrics, University of Utah School of Medicine, USA, lori.frasier@ihc.com

Adriana Fodor Institute of Endocrinology, Diabetes and Metabolism, Rambam Medical Center, Haifa, Israel; Diabetes, Nutrition and Metabolic Diseases Center, Cluj-Napoca, Romania, adifodor@yahoo.com

Aikaterini Fountoulaki Industrial Management and Information Systems Lab, MEAD, University of Patras, 26500 Rion-Patras, Greece, fountoul@mech.upatras.gr

María Isabel López Gálvez University Institute of Applied Ophthalmobiology (IOBA), University of Valladolid, Edificio Ciencias de la Salud – Avda. Ramón y Cajal, 7, 47005 – Valladolid, Spain, maribel@ioba.med.uva.es

Dimosthenis Georgiadis Computer Science Department, University of Cyprus, CY-1678 Nicosia, Cyprus, dimos@cs.ucy.ac.cy

Panagiotis Germanakos Computer Science Department, University of Cyprus, CY-1678 Nicosia, Cyprus, pgerman@cs.ucy.ac.cy; Department of Management and MIS, University of Nicosia, 46 Makedonitissas Ave., P.O. Box 24005, 1700 Nicosia, Cyprus, germanakos.p@unic.ac.cy

Patricia Goede VisualShare, Salt Lake City, USA, patricia.goede@hsc.utha.edu

Ralf Herwig Max Planck Institute for Molecular Genetics, Vertebrate Genomics Department, Bioinformatics Group, Ihnestrasse 63-73, D-14195 Berlin, Germany, herwig@molgen.mpg.de

Christina Ilioudi Department of Informatics, University of Piraeus, Karaoli and Dimitriou Str. 80, GR-18534 Piraeus, Greece, cilioudi@yahoo.com

Nikos Karacapilidis Industrial Management and Information Systems Lab, MEAD, University of Patras, 26500 Rion-Patras, Greece, nikos@mech.upatras.gr

George E. Karagiannis Royal Brompton and Harefield NHS Trust, Sydney Street, London SW3 6NP, UK, g.karagiannis@rbht.nhs.uk

Eddy Karnieli Institute of Endocrinology, Diabetes and Metabolism, Rambam Medical Center, Haifa, Israel; Galil Center, Technion–Israel Institute of Technology, Israel

Anastasia N. Kastania Department of Informatics, Athens University of Economics and Business, Patission 76 Str., Athens 10434, Greece, ank@aueb.gr

Harleen Kaur Department of Computer Science, Hamdard University, New Delhi, India, harleen_k1@rediffmail.com

Sophia Kossida Biomedical Research Foundation of the Academy of Athens, 4 Soranou Ephessiou, 115 27 Athens, Greece, skossida@bioacademy.gr

Athina Lazakidou University of Peloponnese, Faculty of Human Movement and Quality of Life Sciences, Dept. of Nursing, Sparti General Hospital Building Complex, GR-23100 Sparti, Greece, lazakid@uop.gr

Georgia Lazakidou Department of Technology Education and Digital Systems, University of Piraeus, Karaoli and Dimitriou Str. 80, GR-18534 Piraeus, Greece, glazak@unipi.gr

Manolis Manatakis Industrial Management and Information Systems Lab, MEAD, University of Patras, 26500 Rion-Patras, Greece, manata@mech.upatras.gr

Marco Masseroli Dipartimento di Elettronica e Informazione, Politecnico di Milano, Milan, Italy, masseroli@elet.polimi.it

Thomas Meinel Max Planck Institute for Molecular Genetics, Vertebrate Genomics Department, Bioinformatics Group, Ihnestrasse 63-73, D-14195 Berlin, Germany, meinel@molgen.mpg.de

Constantinos Mourlas Faculty of Communication and Media Studies, National and Kapodistrian University of Athens, 5 Stadiou Str., GR 105-62, Athens, Greece, mourlas@media.uoa.gr

Michael L. Rigby Royal Brompton and Harefield NHS Trust, Sydney Street, London SW3 6NP, UK, g.karagiannis@rbht.nhs.uk

George Samaras Computer Science Department, University of Cyprus, CY-1678 Nicosia, Cyprus, cssamara@cs.ucy.ac.cy

Roberto Hornero Sánchez Department of Signal Theory and Communications, University of Valladolid, Campus Miguel Delibes, s/n, 47011 – Valladolid, Spain, robhor@tel.uva.es

Konstantinos Siassiakos Military Institute of University Education, Hellenic Naval Academy, Terma, Hatzikyriakou, GR-18539 Piraeus, Greece, siassiakos_k@ideke.edu.gr

Vasileios G. Stamatopoulos Biomedical Research Foundation of the Academy of Athens, 4 Soranou Ephessiou, 115 27 Athens, Greece, vstamatopoulos@bioacademy.gr

Marco Tagliasacchi Dipartimento di Elettronica e Informazione, Politecnico di Milano, Milan, Italy

Iona Thraen Director, Patient Safety Initiative, Utah Department of Health, Salt Lake City, USA, ithraen@utah.gov

Isabel de la Torre Díez Department of Signal Theory and Communications, University of Valladolid, Campus Miguel Delibes, s/n, 47011 – Valladolid, Spain, isator@tel.uva.es

Iraklis Varlamis Department of Informatics and Telematics, Harokopio University of Athens, Athens, Greece, varlamis@hua.gr

Siri Krishan Wasan Department of Mathematics, Jamia Millia Islamia, New Delhi, India, skwasan@yahoo.com

Stelios Zimeras Department of Statistics and Actuarial-Financial Mathematics, University of Aegean, Karlovassi, Samos, Greece, zimste@aegean.gr

About the Editor

Dr. Athina Lazakidou currently works at the University of Peloponnese, Department of Nursing in Greece as Lecturer in Health Informatics, and at the Hellenic Naval Academy as a Visiting Lecturer in Informatics. She worked as a Visiting Lecturer at the Department of Computer Science at the University of Cyprus (2000–2002) and at the Department of Nursing at the University of Athens (2002–2007). She did her undergraduate studies at the Athens University of Economics and Business (Greece) and received her BSc in Computer Science in 1996. In 2000, she received her PhD in Medical Informatics from the Department of Medical Informatics, University Hospital Benjamin Franklin at the Free University of Berlin, Germany. She is also an internationally known expert in the field of computer applications in healthcare and biomedicine, with six books and numerous papers to her credit. She was also Editor of the "*Handbook of Research on Informatics in Healthcare and Biomedicine*" and "*Handbook of Research on Distributed Medical Informatics and E-Health*", the best authoritative reference sources for information on the newest trends and breakthroughs in computer applications applied to healthcare and biomedicine. Her research interests include health informatics, e-learning in medicine, software engineering, graphical user interfaces, (bio)medical databases, clinical decision support systems, hospital and clinical information systems, electronic medical record systems, telematics, and other web-based applications in healthcare and biomedicine.

Chapter 1
Development and Evaluation of a Web-Based Personal Electronic Health Record (pEHR)

Vasileios G. Stamatopoulos, George E. Karagiannis, Michael L. Rigby, and Sophia Kossida

Abstract The objective of personal Electronic Health Record (pEHR) project was to investigate the deployment of an advanced web-based electronic health record service, tailored to the needs of the average European citizen while providing to healthcare professionals the means and the IT tools that will help them to be more effective in daily clinical routine. In this study, a web-based service that authenticates users, provides the personal electronic health record application and enables users to access and/or update their own medical information was developed. The system was evaluated across three different patient groups involving a total of 150 patients suffering from congenital heart disease, Parkinson's disease and diabetes that were recruited from three different European hospitals. The results indicated the pEHR service to be an effective medium for the storage and management of data by different patient groups. Overall, the three patient groups and healthcare professionals considered the service to have comprehensive and valuable content, to be secure and user-friendly and to have a potential for further improvements while they preferred it to be sponsored free.

Keywords: Electronic Health Records · Web-based · Mobile Citizen · Stakeholder Groups

Abbreviations

pEHR	personal Electronic Health Record
EHR	Electronic Health Record

1.1 Introduction

The personal Electronic Health Record (pEHR) for the Mobile Citizen project aims to showcase the concept of an electronic health record (EHR) Internet-based system

V.G. Stamatopoulos (✉)
Biomedical Research Foundation of the Academy of Athens, 4 Soranou Ephessiou, 115 27 Athens, Greece
e-mail: vstamatopoulos@bioacademy.gr

A. Lazakidou (ed.), *Web-Based Applications in Healthcare and Biomedicine*, Annals of Information Systems 7, DOI 10.1007/978-1-4419-1274-9_1,
© Springer Science+Business Media, LLC 2010

that empowers users to create and maintain, at their own responsibility, their pEHR in a user-friendly, interactive and secure way, while providing to the healthcare professionals the information technology tools that will help them to be more effective in their daily clinical routine.

In the past years, the efforts carried out towards the establishment of a common EHR for all citizens within Europe are numerous. However, factual implementation of a common structure and real progress on the area have been achieved mainly in the United States.

Medical information gathering is still done in many cases via paper support, but also there are some local implementations of electronic support. However, the mentioned EHR is neither common to all the practitioners and institutions nor standardized in any way. This means that although there is stored information in electronic format, there is not a common way to communicate it in an easy way among different national healthcare systems if necessary.

1.2 Service Description

1.2.1 Service Model

pEHR services will enable users to create and maintain a personal record in an on-going, user-friendly, interactive and secure way. Given its web-based nature, the proposed EHR will be easily accessible regardless temporal or spatial restrictions [1].

This service addresses the needs of the entire European population. The service users will be able to update their own health record with information regarding their current physical state (e.g. weight), diseases suffered from and relevant treatments (medication, operations, etc.), allergies and health-affecting habits (e.g. smoking or physical exercise). In addition, patients suffering from chronic diseases (e.g. diabetes, cardiovascular diseases, hypertension, etc.) will be able to store important indicators/parameters (i.e. blood glucose level, blood pressure, etc.) related with the state of their disease. Furthermore, the EHR may also contain results of diagnostic examinations in digital format, including diagnostic images such as CT, MRI, X-ray and others. To this end, any hospital or other diagnostic centre willing to provide this additional service to its patients should have an appropriate broadband access to the Internet in order to be able to upload the information to a patient's EHR. Finally, clinicians will be able to record a diagnosis at the patient's request.

The personalized information included in the healthcare record can be communicated, in an interactive way, to authorized healthcare professionals using three different authentication methods: (a) secure login using standard SSL and username and password, (b) a Smartcard and (c) an USB token. Nevertheless, the content of the EHR is the citizen's own responsibility.

This service will be marketed to two different types of customers/patients. On one hand, the service will be available to all European citizens. On the other hand, the service will also be offered to those organizations that could be interested in sponsoring the pEHR services for a specific group of citizens. These entities can be of a different nature, ranging from private companies to regional public healthcare administration, as well as health insurance companies.

1.2.2 Stakeholder Identification and Benefits

Different stakeholder groups are involved in the operation of the pEHR services. In general, the pEHR services will be paid by stakeholders that either have the role of the direct service recipient (that is the citizen/patient) or the intermediate service provider/beneficiary [2].

While pEHR principally targets the individual citizens/patients, other healthcare professional groups/organizations also belong in the potential pEHR users:

- Patient support organizations and self-help groups
- Doctors
- Healthcare organizations
- Insurance companies
- Pharmacies.

Apparently, pEHR enables the citizen/patient to create and update his/her own web-based medical records. Creating a consolidated electronic record, instead of having several local records of different format (e.g. paper or digital) and at different locations that do not communicate with each other, empowers pEHR users to preserve an integrated file that provides, at once, their clinical status and documents the acts of the professionals in a user-friendly, structured and standardized way.

pEHR systems contribute to the availability of medical information to authorized users and empower the patient to build a complete health record, thus enjoying enhanced mobility and autonomy in selecting the appropriate healthcare provider.

The healthcare professionals and service providers share with the patients the need for immediate access to all relevant clinical data necessary for any given situation, irrespective of time and location, especially in cases of emergency.

For the clinical decision to be accurate, the information must be complete and non-corrupted. pEHR enables good clinical practice in a safe manner since it provides access to a consolidated medical record and supplements the already available, yet in most cases incomplete, professional files.

To this end, clinicians can avoid duplication of activities (i.e. repetition of unnecessary diagnostic tests) and minimize medical errors (e.g. avoid prescription of certain drugs in case of allergies, etc.), while maintaining clinical efficacy and containing costs, especially in the case of the publicly funded healthcare. The above holds true for the insurance companies involved in the care-giving process.

Finally, pharmacists may also benefit from the portable patient records introduced by pEHR. They can review existing clinical information, thus avoiding the supply of risky combinations of prescribed and over-the-counter products that may have lethal side effects to the patients/customers.

Given the increasing Internet penetration rates in the European population, the rising rate of healthcare professionals with online presence, the current technological advances and the health policy plans, pEHR has a significant potential on a pan-European level as a complete health record service for subscribed customers.

Within the broader healthcare settings that this service will operate, pEHR can be integrated or can communicate with existing, local health platforms and healthcare networks, as well as serve as the means to update current EHR systems in local settings.

pEHR combined with the European Health Insurance Card will facilitate patient mobility and medical travel. Moreover, pEHR can be linked to any e-Reimbursement, e-Prescribing and e-Booking applications utilized by healthcare providers.

1.3 Technical Implementation

1.3.1 Platform Components and Features

The pEHR platform setup was based on two pre-existing components: the Electronic Document Presentment Platform (EDPP – developed by INFORM) and the Virtual Patient Record (VPR – developed by ICCS).

The two modules offer supplementary functionality:

- Creation and management of parameterized EHR by the VPR
- Registration request management, service administration and security capabilities by the EDPP that is integrated and adjusted easily to specific client requirements.

The pEHR services are delivered over the Internet as a web-based interface. The pEHR platform is highly robust and scalable, mainly because it utilizes state-of-the-art XML and messaging technologies. The built-in infrastructure of the application framework includes a collection of XML-encoded resource files for the semantic interoperability of all application tiers and a set of software libraries for the manipulation of the business objects, messaging services and adaptive user interface construction support. Furthermore, this approach natively incorporates the HL7 standard specification, ensuring interoperability between heterogeneous systems, as well as explicit definition of health domain business processes and objects. The ultimate goal of the application framework is to provide a reliable tool for delivering scalable, highly customizable and robust applications for the healthcare sector, which highly benefit the pEHR service.

The pEHR service software approach natively incorporates the HL7 v. 2.4 standard specifications, ensuring interoperability between heterogeneous systems.

The wide use of XML technologies provides a flexible format for service maintenance and extension. Finally, the availability of the services' medical data as XML-encoded information enables easier integration with a wider range of devices (except web browsers), such as Pocket and Tablet PCs or PDAs, which can provide better mobility to the users. Furthermore, the pEHR platform provides enhanced security features by complying with the most strict security standards, ensuring both user and server sides.

The realization of an information exchange scenario with external organizations and systems such as public EHRs, hospitals, clinics or General Practitioner (GPs) systems could be implemented in the future by the specification and development of a web services interface that will expose an information exchange service to registered service consumers.

Future extension to the pEHR could be the addition of a vital signs monitoring module for the support of telemedicine scenarios. Another potential extension of the system could be the implementation of notification services that would notify a user by email or SMS for actions that have been scheduled in the application, such as a planned visit to a doctor or a medication intake. In addition, it is possible to provide additional specialized information modules in the future customized for specific diseases.

1.4 Evaluation

1.4.1 Methodology

The evaluation is the means for determining the user requirements have been met and implemented correctly, taking under consideration the market requirements. In short, the evaluation is trying to answer the following questions "are we building the system right?" and "are we building the right system?"

In order to fulfil the above-mentioned objectives, the pEHR evaluation process consisted of the following three phases:

- The first internal evaluation dealt with the testing of the pilot components implemented. The technical team assessed the efficiency of the stand-alone components.
- During the second phase, the system and services were thoroughly tested for defects, inconsistencies, missing functionalities and areas of improvement. The system was executed with test data within the consortium and its operational behaviour was observed.
- The third and most important phase refers to the assessment of the system's efficiency, usability, reliability and satisfaction by the two main user groups of the system, namely the patients and health professionals.

The main evaluation criteria for the trial services comprised:

- Functionality and satisfaction
- Reliability
- Safety and trustiness
- Additional functionality
- Willingness to pay/free access.

Our evaluation plan aimed to monitor achievement of the above-mentioned criteria, according to the specific situation of each clinical environment under real-life operational conditions. Our evaluation techniques focused on pointing up requirements for improvement of tested services and suggestions for further enhancements.

The trials for the patients and medical professionals were conducted on an individual basis. Computers with Internet connections were available in the evaluation sites where the trials took place. After an introduction, the user followed testing scenarios. Questions were posed if the users encountered problems and/or unclear screens or functions. Each individual user trial took approximately 1 h. Paper and web-based questionnaires, developed as appropriately, were provided and filled in by the participants following the user trial.

Two main user groups that participated in the evaluation process were:

- Patients
- Healthcare professionals.

Key organizations participating in the pilot were:

(A) The Royal Brompton Hospital, London, UK

- Parents of inpatients at the Department of Paediatric Cardiology
- Healthcare professionals of the same department

(B) The Cardinal Guglielmo Massaia Hospital in Asti, Italy

- Outpatients of the Department of Neurology of the hospital, suffering from Parkinson's disease
- Persons with no specific illness but related to the hospital in some way (workers from provider companies)
- Healthcare professionals, consultant neurologists involved in the treatment of Parkinson's patients as well as other medical doctors and clinical nurses

(C) The University Hospital Puerta de Hierro in Madrid, Spain

- Patients suffering from diabetes
- Healthcare professionals dealing with the treatment of patients, who suffer from diabetes, together with other physicians and clinical nurses

1.4.2 Results and User Comments

The quantitative results of the pEHR evaluation have already been published elsewhere [3]. These results showed significant differences between the three trial sites (a total of 150 patient users). While for the United Kingdom and Spain all Likert scale indices (functionality and satisfaction, reliability, safety and trustiness, additional functionality) were higher than the 50% average with the United Kingdom showing the highest scores, most scores achieved for the Italian population group were below the 50% average.

This was not the case for the comparative results for the healthcare professionals group. Despite the negative results of the Italian patient group, the Italian healthcare professionals group provided significantly higher scores. Spanish healthcare professionals gave the highest index for functionality and satisfaction, with Italy and the United Kingdom to follow.

The willingness to pay score for the patient groups was 34%, significantly under the 50% performance average, while the free access index was at a high 73%. These scores demonstrate a reluctance towards a subscription-based service while the high free access score shows a preference towards free access. The healthcare professionals were also in favour of the free subscription (85%) even though the willingness to pay index was higher than the 50% average (65%).

In order to further validate the user's perception of the pEHR service, several comments were collected throughout the pilot trial phase in all sites. The comments gathered from the users offer a wide range of opinions and hints for the enhancement of the service. The information collected from patients and healthcare professionals during:

- The presentation of the service application to the users
- The in-site training trial phase
- The dedicated fields with open questions in the two questionnaires.

The results showed a difference between patients and healthcare professionals regarding perception of user-friendliness. In fact, the former group showed more difficulties in using the service than the latter. The greater confidence that healthcare professionals have with Internet and web-based services is probably the main reason for this difference between the two user groups. Healthcare professionals more frequently use IT software and web services related to the health sector than patients. On the basis of this existing difficulty, the patients underlined the importance to receive adequate training for the use of the service product.

However, patients valued highly the possibility to use the service from their own home so as to register and upload the information regarding their condition on a daily basis. This condition allows them to feel more comfortable and able to check and update their health information frequently. At the same time, there were also some suggestions from patients for improving the service content, functionality, accessibility and usability. Also the possibility of providing a historical path of the diet can be very interesting for monitoring the patient's health status and the modification in their diet.

Healthcare professionals underlined the importance of having a daily update of the patient's medical status, especially for those suffering from diabetes pathologies. It could really determine, in their perspective, a progress in the direction of a more aware and efficient use of patients' data treatment. In this way, medical prescription could follow a more complete clinical reference framework.

Moreover, doctors as well as local and regional health authorities can benefit from the pEHR service so as to retrieve useful statistical information, specific use case and to find possible communication ways to maintain an uninterrupted information flow with their target medical communities.

Healthcare professionals expressed their concerns on patient's liability to update their own records. This may be, in some cases, a limiting factor for the accuracy of data provided. It depends on the honesty of users registering their data. In the case of healthcare professionals, there is also a risk that the patient's experience will not be considered seriously. Therefore, the question is who determines what is and what is not important, the doctor or the patient?

Finally, two further elements of pEHR which would be useful for both types of users could be:

- Availability of communication channels as a major function of the system. The use of the appropriate communication means will allow the interaction between the two ends of the system, e.g. patients could ask questions or send reports, physicians could provide consultations, change medications intake plans).
- An SMS alarm service was also recommended in order to alert about scheduled appointments.

Following the evaluation phase, an improvement plan was a major task. The nature of any user-driven service makes the improvement of the service and user satisfaction a continuous process. It is expected to be a positive catalyst for changes, providing an opportunity to implement a user focus approach towards any service deployment.

All comments were communicated to the web developers and most of them were incorporated into the platform.

The improvement plan focused on:

- Standardization of information
- User-friendliness, simplicity of interface
- User training
- Communication means
- Increase/improvement of content

1.5 Market Analysis

1.5.1 Healthcare Sector Overview

Overall, the healthcare sector is characterized by different management structures, financing systems, service delivery schemes and models of interaction between the different entities active in the provision of healthcare. It encompasses a complex mix of institutions, businesses, professionals and users, whose role and formats change among countries, according to political, economical, social and cultural factors, as well as technological development. The provision healthcare in Europe is funded mainly by the public sector, although the extent of public–private mix varies considerably. In the United States, the healthcare sector is market-driven. Although the healthcare sector constitutes a large and promising market, it is characterized on a global and European level by discrepancies and fragmentation.

Countries throughout Europe are recognizing the urgent need for better integration among healthcare organizations. Many different stakeholders are now directly involved in patient care, including outpatient clinics, long-term care facilities for the elderly, pharmacies, laboratories, occupational health clinics and home healthcare organizations. Such integration is not just about making it easier to transfer data between a patient's different healthcare settings but also about the need to provide patients with access to healthcare data, to better maintain their health and manage their medical conditions themselves, greatly reducing healthcare spending and improve the well-being of patients.

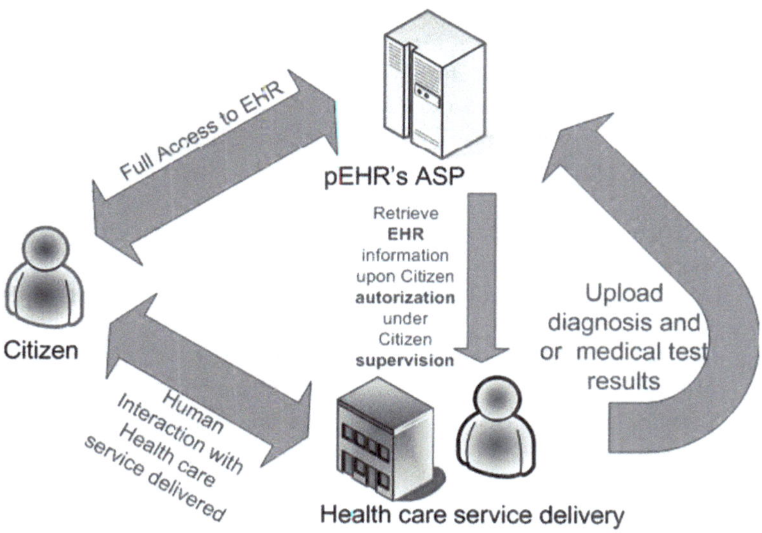

Fig. 1.1 Service model flow chart [1]

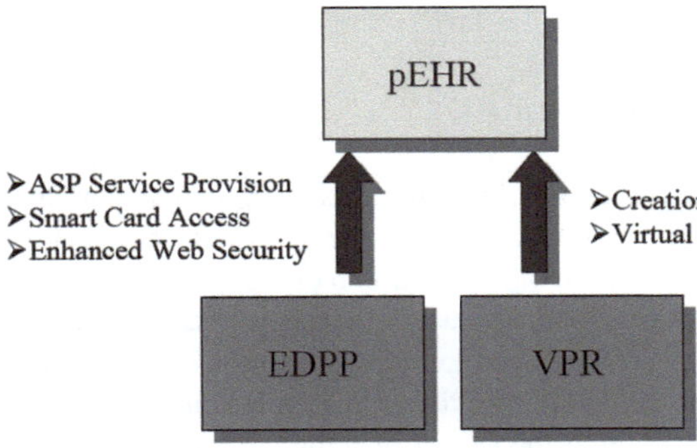

Fig. 1.2 The two basic building blocks for the pEHR platform [3]

Transferring patient data efficiently among different stakeholders may also reduce the likelihood of medical errors, improve patient outcomes, increase administrative efficiency and enhance the patients' overall satisfaction for their healthcare system.

1.5.2 Healthcare Information Society Technology Forecasts

European Community research programmes have been supporting e-Health for the past 15 years approximately. Many research results have now been tested and put into practice. This has made Europe reach a leading position in the use of EHR in primary care and the deployment of health (smart) cards. These developments have contributed to the emergence of e-Health as the third largest industry alongside pharmaceuticals and the medical devices sector in the health sector [4].

Patient clinical data is the most vital piece of information for healthcare providers. EPR solutions is a top information technology investment priority for all healthcare providers in all of the major Western European countries.

Regarding the personal aspect of the EHR, the pEHR is situated on the rise part of the Healthcare Hype Cycle [5] (Fig. 1.3). Gartners' review [6] reveals that an increase in the adoption of consumer-defined health plans will stimulate the adoption of personalized health record in the coming years, because the PHRs provide patients with a sharable and portable medical record; they also improve patient safety and quality through the availability of clinical data at the point of care. This technology is considered in the emerging stage of maturity with a small penetration, which in 2005 was under 1% of the audience and with a high benefit rating [6].

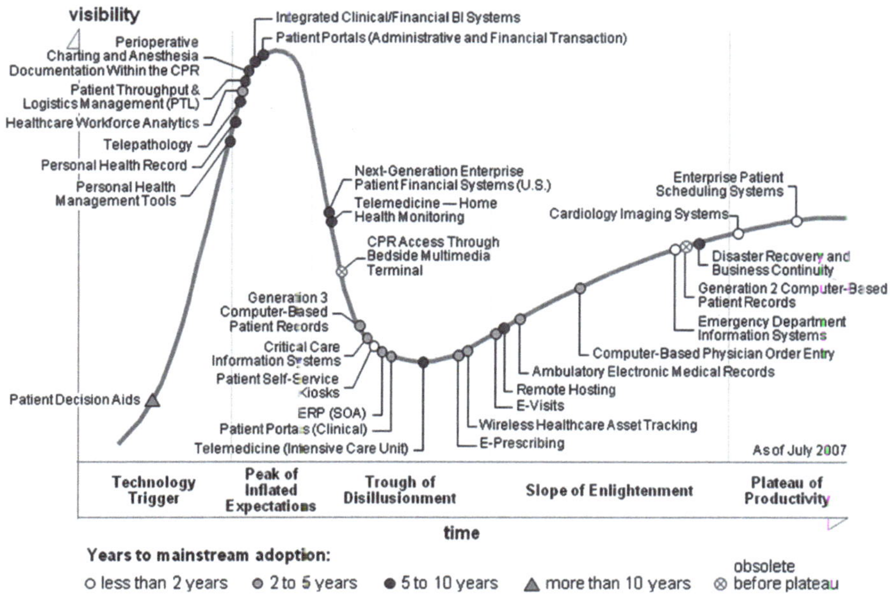

Fig. 1.3 Hype cycle healthcare applications [5]

1.6 Conclusions

The objective of pEHR project was to investigate the deployment of an advanced web-based EHR service, tailored to the needs of the average European citizen while providing to the healthcare professionals the means and the information technology tools that will help them to be more effective in daily clinical routine. This type of service has an added value effect to already operational healthcare information systems, as well as to current and forthcoming telecommunication infrastructures.

Our study has shown that web-based pEHR can have a leading role in establishing the necessary information arrays between patients and healthcare professionals and organizations. From the health services point of view, the implementation of web-based medical records that can be easily maintained by different patient groups can result in the delivery of a better-coordinated care and fast access to patient-generated data.

Our data indicated the pEHR service to be an effective medium for the storage and management of data by different patient groups. Overall, the three patient groups considered the service to have comprehensive and valuable content, to be secure and user-friendly and to have a potential for further improvements while they preferred it to be sponsored free.

The market analysis showed that the market is mature enough and there are prospects for a service such as pEHR. The necessary technologies, Web & USB, are widely available, the technological risks low, and the end-users are becoming more and more Internet-literate. pEHR services can be potentially used by many citizens since the only unique requirement is to have Internet access. Further clinical trials are necessary to prove the impact of the service in the clinical outcomes of the care provided by professionals and institutions to the different patient disease groups.

Acknowledgments The project was cofounded by the European Commission under the eTEN funding scheme. The Consortium that carried out this project consisted of the following partners: Atos Origin S.A., The Grupo de Bioingeniería y Telemedicina (UPM-GBT), Hospital Universitario Puerta de Hierro (HUPH), Inform P. Lykos A.E. (INFORM), A Regional Health Authority of Central Macedonia (A DYPE of CM), Institute of Communication and Computer Systems, (ICCS/NTUA), Data Shop Asti SP.A (DATA SHOP), The Royal Brompton & Harefield NHS Trust (RBH).

References

1. Karagiannis GE, Stamatopoulos VG, Rigby M, Kotis T, Negroni E, Munoz A, Mathes I, Web-based personal health records: the personal electronic health record (pEHR) multicentred trial. J Telemed Telecare 2007;13:32–34.
2. Salama D, Karagiannis G, Stamatopoulos V, Bettoni S, Mathes Y, Hernando Pérez ME, Personal electronic health record services for the mobile citizen. Project Report-Business Plan 2006.
3. Salama D, Personal electronic health record services for the mobile citizen. Final Report 2006.
4. European Commission, e-Health – Making healthcare better for European citizens: an action plan for a European e-Health area 2004.
5. Runyon B, Libman P, Gartner VP sales and marketing: the hype cycle of health care IT, Enterprise Systems Symposium 2008 presentation 2008.
6. Hype cycle for healthcare provider applications and systems, Garner 2005.

Chapter 2
Exploring the Potential of Over-the-Web Psychiatry

Pantelis Angelidis

Abstract Over the past years, the scientific community has witnessed a tremendous growth of applications in healthcare telematics. The adoption rate of web-based practices was not the same for all medical specialties. Some such as cardiology were fast adopters mainly due to the 'electric' nature of the standard diagnostic tools (electro-cardiographer) but others such as psychiatry are still lagging from adopting new methodologies. Now that ubiquitous broadband Internet access is here to stay, the time has come to explore the potential of mental care services that could be offered over the web.

Keywords: Healthcare telematics · Tele-Psychiatry · Video-Conferencing · electronic health records

2.1 History

From the early introduction of voice telephony, patients in distress and frustration used to call their physicians urgently seeking for consultation. These phone calls did not follow any clinical protocol and though efficient in terms of crisis management they did not qualify as a treatment method. Later on, suicides and crises intervention hotlines staffed with trained volunteers provided a more organized form of telephone counselling.

It was back in 1959 when the first tele-psychiatry system was set in operation in Nebraska, USA. Two-way closed circuit microwave television was used to transmit the demonstration of neurologic patients from the State Mental Hospital to Nebraska Psychiatric Institute 112 miles away in Omaha as part of the education of first-year medical students [1].

P. Angelidis (✉)
Department of Engineering Informatics and Telecommunications, University of Western Macedonia, Karamanli and Lygeris, GR-50100 Kozani, Greece
e-mail: paggelidis@uowm.gr

A. Lazakidou (ed.), *Web-Based Applications in Healthcare and Biomedicine*,
Annals of Information Systems 7, DOI 10.1007/978-1-4419-1274-9_2,
© Springer Science+Business Media, LLC 2010

Although tele-psychiatry has a long history, its practical consequences in every day mental healthcare practice have been limited. Development, construction and operation and maintenance costs have been prohibitively high. The majority of 'on-line time' was spent either on medical education as well as on administration purposes.

2.2 Identifying the Beneficiaries of Tele-psychiatry

Tele-medicine is defined as the delivery of healthcare services, where distance is a critical factor, by all healthcare professionals using information and communications technologies for the exchange of valid information for diagnosis, treatment and prevention of disease and injuries, research and evaluation, and for the continuing education of healthcare providers, all in the interest of advancing the health of individuals and their communities [2]. If this definition were explicitly adapted for psychiatry, it abides by the WHO definition on health that it is a state of complete physical, *mental* and *social well-being* and not merely the absence of disease or infirmity [3].

Obvious applications for preserving population's health status include psychiatric care for people living in remote and isolated areas. The uneven distribution of medical practitioners between rural and urban areas is well documented even for the well-developed countries. Tele-psychiatry makes it possible to provide universal access to the same quality level mental healthcare services regardless of the limitations imposed by geographic locations.

However, it is not only the inhabitants of rural areas who are underprivileged regarding the accessibility to these particular services. Certain populations amongst them, the elderly and people with disabilities, find it really hard to cope with public transportation due to general poor health, specific mental condition, e.g. agoraphobia, and deprivation from financial affluence in order to finally visit the appropriate healthcare institution and the specialized psychiatrist. Many are the cases when the mentally ill even lack the required family support and they are left either alone or in the care of the community with the fear of social stigmatization being the rationale behind the abandonment.

Tele-psychiatry could enable patients to be examined, assessed and receive the benefits of specialized psychiatric services in their preferred surroundings and acting complementary to the primary care physician, thus ensuring the continuity of care.

NHS or any form of private care today cannot afford to staff every single hospital or nursing home with specialized psychiatrists. When primary care physicians undergo the critical task of dealing with treatment-resistant patients, they would either deliver suboptimal care or refer the patient to very expensive tertiary hospital care away from his/her family and preferred surroundings, jeopardizing their overall stability and well-being.

It is not only the patients who benefit from the new tools such as remote consultations. The physicians could now have an incentive to remain in rural areas as geographic distance from the sources of knowledge (e.g. prestigious health care institutions) is not synonymous to professional isolation.

2.3 Contemporary Means of Tele-psychiatry

Psychiatry is not a specialty that requires touch during examination of the patient. Sessions are mostly in the form of interviews where interviewer and interviewee have agreed to meet in a predefined location such as a nursing home, hospital, private clinic or even at the patient's home, and physical contact is limited to a mere handshaking at the beginning or the end of the session.

Even duration is not predefined. The sessions could last for as long as the involved parties consider it helpful or efficient. Number of involved people is not standardized either. Group therapies have gained momentum especially when participants form a group sharing experiences and seeking guidance for dealing with issues ranging from substance abuse to mourning and providing care to the chronically ill.

Broadband Internet has made video-conferencing through standard tools such as Windows Live Messenger (MSN), Skype, etc. available to all. Even if the patient cannot configure his or her environment to enable such a facility, social services could cater for such a need at a 'care at home' level. Practically, what video-conferencing offers is a simulation of the consultation session between the psychiatrist and the patient, rendering location insignificant provided that broadband Internet access is established in the concerned region. Multi-party sessions could also be supported simulating group therapeutic consultations.

One of the numerous advantages of tele-psychiatry is that it allows for immediate recordings that could be stored in relevant fields of the patient's electronic health record and reviewed later on by the same physician or sent to another colleague for second opinion and further evaluation. Medical research depends heavily on easy-to-process digitalized data, and these recordings combined with coded history and diagnostics constitute a very promising combination for breakthrough results not only in the field of psychiatry but also in the adjacent field of neurology and its subspecialties, neurobiology and neurophysiology.

An important study by Steffens et al. [4] has demonstrated the added value of the video recordings taken while demented subjects were participating in research interviews. The overall gestalt of the patient in the environment is a very important contributor to diagnostic assessment, which is the basis for an adequate cum effective treatment of the subject's disorder.

Privacy and confidentiality are better addressed in the closed confines of the digital world. There are numerous techniques these days to prohibit eavesdropping on video-conferencing, and data storage from heterogeneous sources is safer than ever through the use of cryptography and smart cards throughout the healthcare network of professionals, thus allowing access to data for only the authorized practitioners.

2.4 Pilot Assessment: The Key to Global Acceptance

Many mental care practitioners insist that tele-psychiatry is just another gimmick. They appear to be reluctant to use a technology considered unproven. Despite its long history, clinical studies establishing accuracy, reliability, ease of use and clinical utility are not that many though their number is fast increasing [5].

A recent study that took place in Greece evaluated the tele-psychiatric process used for assessing and preparing patients who could potentially leave the institution and transferred to boarding homes as part of the national deinstitutionalization program. The study used video-conferencing as the tool to connect University of Athens Psychiatric Clinic and Tripoli's (city of central Peloponnese) Psychiatric hospital [6].

The results of the study were very encouraging. The project has been evaluated through the use of questionnaires given to patients and mental health professionals to fill in. ADSL connection was used and the bandwidth exceeded a lot the sufficient bandwidth for examining and making decisions concerning most mental disorders according to the Telepsychiatry Project of the Consolidated Department of Psychiatry of Harvard medical School (128 kb/s) [7].

The majority of the patients have accepted the new method of examination without problems and the level of satisfaction from the method appears to be high. The health practitioners' acceptance is at the same level and they also claim to have found the video-conference system very easy to use and efficient in their everyday routine.

2.5 Tele-psychiatry: The Experience of the Pilot in Chania, Crete

The Mental Health Center of Chania, Crete in Greece, decided to proceed in the implementation of a tele-psychiatry system, enabling the provision of consultation services in three remote areas. To this end, three rural health units located in the villages of Vamos, Kasteli and Kantanos in the prefectural area of Chania were connected to the Mental Health Center of Chania via a web-based platform in order to conduct on-line sessions with patients, keep electronic psychiatric records for each patient based on international protocols and disease classifications, and monitor patients following hospitalization in mental institutions.

The implementation scenario concerned the conduction of individual sessions over the web between the patient located in the remote rural health unit, who was accompanied by an authorized local social worker, and the psychiatrist expert located in the Psychiatric Clinic of Chania.

The main objective of the pilot implementation was the improvement of the quality of life of patients with mental disorders, following treatment and hospitalization, in order to enable social inclusion and efficient monitoring following hospitalization discharge.

The feasibility study conducted at the end of the pilot period showcased that the implementation of the tele-psychiatry system was cost-effective in the long-term in comparison to the mobile mental health unit that previously served the population at the rural areas under consideration. For example, 154,875 patients can be served via the tele-psychiatry system during a month, whereas on average only 11,932 are being served by the mobile health unit personnel.

Preliminary data also indicate that tele-psychiatry constitutes a sustainable business model in the long run.

2.6 Conclusions

Currently, video-conferencing offered at ADSL connection speed is the main enabler of tele-psychiatry. This technique used in conjunction with a patient's electronic health record can successfully simulate and substitute the in vivo consultation and deliver to the mentally ill the same quality of service regardless of their location.

The burden of dealing with treatment-resisting patients will be lifted from the shoulders of primary health care practitioners since they can afford to electronically refer the patients to a specialized psychiatrist.

The trauma of moving the patients away from their families and familiar surroundings can be avoided and their recovery can take place in an environment in which they feel safe and well adjusted.

References

1. Elizabeth Liebson, MD, Assistant Professor of Psychiatry at Tufts New England Medical Centre in Boston, MA, USA, Telepsychiatry: 35 years' experience by http://www.medscape.com/viewarticle/431064_1.
2. International Society for Telemedicine and eHealth – NGO in Official relation with WHO, Glossary of Telemedical Terms http://www.isft.net/cms/index.php?q_-_z (WHO 1998).
3. Preamble to the Constitution of the World Health Organization as adopted by the International Health Conference, New York, 19–22 June, 1946; signed on 22 July 1946 by the representatives of 61 States (Official Records of the World Health Organization, no. 2, p. 100) and entered into force on 7 April 1948.
4. Steffens DC, Welsh KA, Burke JR, et al. Diagnosis of Alzheimer's disease in epidemiologic studies by staged review of clinical data. Neuropsychiatry Neuropsychol Behav Neurol 2002;9:107–113.
5. Zarate CA, Weinstock L, Cukor P, et al. Applicability of telemedicine for assessing patients with schizophrenia: Acceptance and reliability. J Clin Psychiatry 1997;58:22–25.
6. Zacharopoulou C, Konstantakopoulos G, Tsirika N,Vavourakis P, Lymperaki G, Tempeli A, Valma V, Panagoutsos P, Katsadoros K. Evaluation of a tele-psychiatry pilot project http://www.klimaka.org.gr/newsite/downloads/telepsychiatry.pdf.
7. Baer L, Elford R, Cucor P. Telepsychiatry at forty: what have we learned. Harv Rev Psychiatry 1997;5:7–17.

Chapter 3
An Intelligent Web-Based Healthcare System: The Case of DYMOS

Dimosthenis Georgiadis, Panagiotis Germanakos, George Samaras, Constantinos Mourlas, and Eleni Christodoulou

Abstract Today's information age is accelerating at quantum speed. Advances, such as the Internet and high-speed networks, have propelled the never-ending quest for information. In this regard, eHealth services is a continuously growing sector, driving the need for advances in the dynamic working environment of different medical actors promoting the effective collaboration within the given contextual and technological constraints. Henceforth, this chapter defines and classifies the various virtual communities in the eHealth sector, analyses existing related approaches and identifies current problems, stressing emphasis on the notion of workflow management within the multi/cross-organizational environment. It further proposes an eHealth system, DYMOS, which has been based on a suggested extended collaboration model, with features that tend to tackle the identified weaknesses. Finally, it presents a positive evaluation of the system's efficiency and effectiveness with the implementation of an experimentation phase which has used trials in a real hospital environment.

3.1 Introduction

In recent years, there has been a major reconstruction on healthcare sector due to the diversification of user needs, demands and expectations, within the structure of a modern society [1]. eHealth is the discipline that took over in the past years in the health sector, proving the need for providing a dynamic working environment of different actors (medical ones) promoting effective collaboration among the actors, including the patient, at anytime and any context (place). The needs of mobile users differ significantly from those of desktop users. Getting personalized information 'anytime, anywhere and anyhow' is not an easy task. Researchers and practitioners have to take into account new adaptivity axes based on which personalized interface design of mobile health would be built. Such applications should be

D. Georgiadis (✉)
Computer Science Department, University of Cyprus, CY-1678 Nicosia, Cyprus
e-mail: dimos@cs.ucy.ac.cy

A. Lazakidou (ed.), *Web-Based Applications in Healthcare and Biomedicine*, Annals of Information Systems 7, DOI 10.1007/978-1-4419-1274-9_3,
© Springer Science+Business Media, LLC 2010

characterized by flexibility, accessibility, context awareness, quality and security in a ubiquitous interoperable manner in order to provide the citizens with quality on demand information (services) [2]. User interfaces must now be friendlier enabling active involvement (information acquisition), giving control to the citizen and provide easier means of navigation supported by the small screens of the mobile devices and enable adaptation of hypermedia, multi-media, and multi-modal intelligent and personalized user interfaces.

eHealth services and applications are becoming more and more adopted in today's modern mobile computing society. Some factors that contributed to this end are the tremendous development of the Internet and related technologies, the understanding and exploitation of the business potentials that rest behind this development and the impressive growth of wireless mobile and sensor networks.

So far, workflows are mainly used in business sector, depicting the sequence of operation in order to speed up procedures, better handling of resources and reorganizing energy and information flows. The term workflow is used in computer programming to capture and develop human-to-machine interaction. Workflow applications mainly aim to provide end users with an easier way to orchestrate or describe complex processing of data. Nowadays, users are constantly on the move with their notebooks, personal digital assistants (PDAs) and mobile phones. This trend, where the context of the working environment is constantly changing, spawned the need for dynamic workflows. The benefits of using dynamic workflows are numerous, including dynamic business process restructure, dynamic share of information and dynamic collaboration schemas.

Given the complexity and diversity of the provision of healthcare, in association with critical factors such as quality of care, adaptability, availability, flexibility, confidentiality, security (due to the medical record singularity[1]), expandability and ease of information sharing, the eHealth could be considered as a solid solution for the provision of effective and efficient healthcare, within a more technical-related context (like wireless networks and mobile collaboration).

Mobile devices usually are small with inefficient input methods, small screen, limited battery life and prone to damage and spoilage [3]. These problems should be denoted and handled due to a development of a system in eHealth sector. In addition, specialists wanted efficient help from an eHealth system without re-analysing and restructuring their way of working with the system. After a more thorough examination of these problems, the need for dynamic workflows and the need for time-driven events came to the surface.

Combining the complexity of eHealth with the well-known problems faced in mobile computing (e.g. wireless environment/medium constrains and mobile devices capabilities such as battery, screen) creates a working environment that has not been appropriately addressed till now.

[1] Medical records are intensely personal documents and there are many ethical and legal issues surrounding them such as the degree of third-party access and appropriate storage and disposal.

Our study is focused on the needs for collaboration in the healthcare sector and more specific in the virtual healthcare teams[2] and the creation of dynamic workflows under the same sector. In this chapter our system is presented, which tackles all the pre-mentioned problems of the eHealth sector. All these problems are addressed in more detail in the following sections and a proposed solution is presented along with an evaluation trial of the system using as a case study a local private hospital.

More specifically, in this chapter we define the notion of virtual communities in the eHealth sector, the classification of these communities, the existing systems and the problems that have not been tackled as yet. Additionally, we stress the notion of business processes (aka workflow management) and the lack of dynamic reconstruction due to continuous changes of the organizational needs and stress emphasis on the design and development of personal mobile user interfaces.

The innovation of this work is presented through our system that tackles all the pre-mentioned problems of the eHealth sector. We underpin our decision of our selection of this particular computational model, describe the system components and illustrate some screenshots of the system.

Finally, we assess the system's efficiency and effectiveness through a two-phase evaluation using a trial in a real hospital environment. We present the evaluation methodology and the evaluation results. The impact of the system is that users' support has gradually improved over the past years as they have been increasingly exposed to the system capabilities and have recognized the advantages of the system in their day-to-day work for both administrative and consultation purposes.

3.2 Related Work

It is true that nowadays many eHealth approaches focus on supporting patient/doctor communication, incorporating web-based technologies and employing a particular theoretical collaboration model (see Fig. 3.1) with main influential elements ranging to face-to-face interactions, continuous task, remote interaction and communication and coordination [1]. In this context, a large number of eHealth applications were investigated and analysed with regard to their scope and functionality. Main limitations observed to these approaches as well as to the theoretical model itself were the lack of communication provision among hospital specialists and general practitioners, or among different health provider environments, and the absence of the organization/working environment.

3.2.1 A Comprehensive Review of eHealth Applications

In this section an extensive analysis of eHealth applications is presented based on a basic categorization of their general scope. This classification is divided into the following applications: (i) Support of Users (healthcare specialists and patients), (ii)

[2]Virtual healthcare teams are teams that consist of healthcare professionals who collaborate and share information on patients through digital equipment.

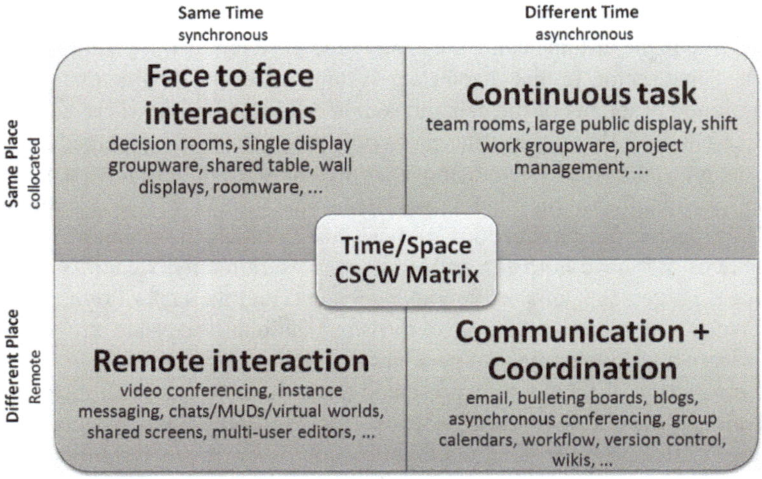

Fig. 3.1 Commonly used collaboration model

eHealth Services (development and utilization), (iii) Monitoring (with the aim of sensors and ICT technologies), (iv) Information Processing (can be communication aid, techniques, algorithms, etc.) and (v) Process Management.

(i) Support of Users

Within the scope of this categorization are the applications that focus on services that aim to support the work of the healthcare providers and also utilize the active participation of the patients, providing a more efficient and effective continuity of care. Such approaches are as follows:

C-CARE [4] aims to develop tools in support of continuity of care by collecting and storing essential, relevant and up-to-date patient health-related information accessible to authorized users, patients included, any time anywhere, e.g. from the patient's home, from a vehicle on the road or from a hospital emergency department. Healthcare professionals will support more effectively the other persons involved in the process of continuous care, including the patients themselves.

HealthMate [5] is a technology innovation project to provide market-oriented wireless solutions to a variety of health problems: care of chronic patients; support of acute patients, including high risk; and tele-assistance applications. The objectives are to develop a portable personal system for health tele-care and tele-consultation based on new generation of wireless communication networks; to integrate advanced, innovative wireless technologies to configure a secure information exchange media between the personal systems and the health service providers; and to assure service continuity at any time and place.

The **HUMAN** [6] project aims at improving the quality and continuity of patient-prisoner care by designing, developing and validating in two different European sites an umbrella of health telemedicine and domotic services, tailored on the inmates' needs, as well as on the requirements of the health professionals operating in the detention centres. Additionally, through a web-based platform it will support distance learning (eLearning) of in-house clinicians, throughout the fruition of e-learning sessions with specialists and general practitioners.

COCOON [7] is an integrated project aimed at supporting healthcare professional in reducing risk management in their daily practices by building knowledge-driven and dynamically adaptive networked communities within European healthcare systems. The risk management for a healthcare professional is completely related to its responsibilities assumption in mainly patient diagnosis and treatment processes.

The **NOESIS** [8] system assists health professionals in the most effective decision-making for prevention, diagnosis and treatment in the complex domain of cardiovascular diseases, allowing a smooth transition from established medical knowledge to personal judgment through an enhanced site seer for medical sciences and a decision support framework capable of producing a preliminary diagnosis.

PIPS [9] is an e-Health integrated project that aims to create novel healthcare delivery models by building an environment for health and knowledge service support. The PIPS project's main goal is to create a new Health and Life Knowledge and Services Support Environment for protecting the health of the Individual. PIPS will provide a set of services for supporting the HC professional to promptly make the best possible decisions regarding prevention, diagnosis and treatment that are tailored to the citizen's personal context, which consider his/her health status and personal preferences.

(ii) eHealth Services

Within this category are applications that focus on providing or developing health services to the users. Some key systems are as follows:

CHS [10] deals with the development of systems and services for the citizen. More specifically, it aims at the development of personal health services that can be used from home that communicate with the rest of the information infrastructure. CHS will develop a new-generation telemedicine service for home care that will improve quality of healthcare and create a large new IT market by involving every single home and every single healthcare provider.

The objective of the **ARTEMIS** [11] project is to develop a semantic web services-based interoperability framework for the healthcare domain. They focus on processes in terms of web services rather than recording and documentation of electronic health records. In other words, their approach allows a standard way of accessing the data since there are very many standards that need to work together.

M-Power [12] is a user-driven research and development project to create a middleware platform supporting rapid development and deployment of services for cognitive disabled and elderly. The platform will be defined within an iterative process including end-user requirements, design, platform development, development of proof-of-concept applications and end-user trials.

(iii) Monitoring

Applications under this category aim to provide monitoring services through the use of vital signal sensors of ICT technologies in general. Some basic research applications are as follows:

MobiHealth [13] aims at developing and trialing new mobile value-added services in the area of healthcare, thus bringing healthcare to the patient. The MobiHealth system allows patients to be fully mobile while undergoing health monitoring. Patients wear a lightweight monitoring system – the MobiHealth BAN (body area network) – which is customized to their individual health needs. Physical measurements such as blood pressure or ECG are measured by the MobiHealth BAN and transmitted wirelessly from the BAN to their doctor, the hospital or their health call centre.

The **TOPCARE** [14] platform was in particular designed for therapy monitoring for home ventilation, for oral coagulation therapies and for PPH patients with infusion therapies, but it is also applicable for therapy monitoring in many chronic diseases. The structure, workflow and organizational procedures for the operation of tele-health centres have been defined. The overall objective of TOPCARE is to develop technical devices and telecommunication structures and to lay the organizational groundwork for bringing cooperative healthcare services into the home of patients.

AUBADE [15] project provides an innovative tool that will lead professionals to a deep study, analysis, understanding, and comprehension of neurological diseases and human emotions. The project has developed an intelligent, multisensor and wearable system for the assessment of the emotional state of humans under special conditions. The project has involved the utilization of innovative technologies such as the recognition of the emotions after the processing of the following biomedical signals: EMG, obtained from the face of the users, ECG, skin conductivity and respiration rate.

The **CLINICIP** [16] system is a low-risk monitoring and control system for metabolic control in critically ill patients. The core of the system is a computer algorithm implemented into an ICU infusion system, which calculates insulin dosage from metabolic parameters to provide decision support for tight glycaemic control. A glucose sensor and a body interface have been integrated to allow for closed-loop insulin infusion.

INTREPID [17] project aims at developing a multisensor wearable system for the treatment of phobias and situational anxiety. INTREPID project actively contributes to the treatment of phobias in an unobtrusive, personalized and intelligent manner. INTREPID will serve to empower community citizens in the management of their individual health, to provide healthcare professionals and facilities with a reliable phobias treatment and decision support tool and to create new opportunities for the medical wearable device industry. INTREPID will build upon the well-documented increasing demand for 'healthy lifestyle' products and services on the consumer side and offer potentially significant returns for those who chose to invest in the project outcome.

MyHeart [18] system is suitable for supporting citizens to fight major cardiovascular diseases (CVD) risk factors and help to avoid heart attack, other acute events by personalized guidelines and giving feedback. It provides the necessary motivation to the new lifestyles. The key challenges for lowering the mortality rate in CVD and their related costs are by successfully guiding, informing and motivating the citizen to adapt to a permanently healthier lifestyle and the early diagnosis of acute events. It is the aim of the MyHeart project to develop innovative, personalized, easy-to-use solutions and tools, which help the citizen to adopt permanent healthier lifestyle.

HealthService24 [19] aims at realizing the mobile health dream. The project partners have developed an innovative mobile healthcare system that supports patients' and health professionals' mobility, increases patients' quality of life and reduces healthcare costs. HealthService24 aims to bridge this gap, offering a viable mobile healthcare service permitting healthcare professionals to remotely assess, diagnose and treat patients while the patients are free to continue with daily life activities. The HealthService24 will allow patients and non-patients to monitor their physical condition and obtain advice and information at any place and moment. Hence the service will enable patients to be fully mobile.

(iv) Information Processing

This category characterizes applications that utilize algorithms, techniques and processes that handle medical data. In addition, this category fits applications that process medical information in order to enhance collaboration between users and systems. Some implementations are as follows:

Mobi-Dev [20] is a European effort which addresses the longstanding and increasingly demanding need of health professionals to effectively, accurately, securely from anywhere, anytime and in user-friendly way communicate with patients' databases located within hospitals, private offices, laboratories or pharmacies. An Internet-based system will be set up to exchange clinical data between the Mobi-Dev portable devices and various kinds of relevant information databases (HIS, GPs personal databases, clinical laboratories and pharmacy databases). Web interfaces with HIS will be realized using standard database interfaces products.

WIDENET [21] proposes dealing with these shortcomings in healthcare, specifically in healthcare records. It aims to continue building a network of national centres following the model of the already successful PROREC Belgium centre, to deal, among others, with the exploitation problem, and also to establish an international European-led organization to coordinate the network on the European scale and strengthen successful suppliers. WIDENET's mission is to promote the adoption and extended use of Standardized Electronic Healthcare Records and the required infrastructure.

BIOPATTERN [22] aims to develop a pan-European, coherent and intelligent analysis of a citizen's bioprofile, to make the analysis of this bio-profile remotely accessible to patients and clinicians, and to exploit bioprofile to combat major diseases such as cancer and brain diseases. BIOPATTERN proposes to provide novel computational intelligent techniques for biopattern analysis and a pan-European integrated, intelligent analysis of an individual's bioprofile. Information from distributed databases will be made available securely over the Internet to provide on-line algorithms, libraries and processing facilities for such analysis.

DICOEMS [23] aims to deliver an eHealth platform that acquires and transfers critical information from the place where a medical emergency occurs to remotely located health specialists for immediate assistance. The system instantiates a portable collaboration environment that brings together the on-the-spot care provider and a network of experts, thus enabling more effective decision support and risk management in primary diagnosis, pre-transfer arrangements and treatment of critical situations.

The main concern of **SemanticMining** [24] has been semantic interoperability, which simply means that meaning is preserved in communication between information systems, a condition which should be natural but has proven to be very hard to achieve, especially so in the complex application area of healthcare. A main concern of SemanticMining has been semantic interoperability in communication between healthcare information systems. The long-term goal of SemanticMining has been the development of generic methods and tools supporting the critical tasks of the field: data mining, knowledge discovery, knowledge representation, abstraction and indexing of information, semantic-based information retrieval in a complex and high-dimensional information space.

(v) Process Management

This category deals with applications that focus on the management of the clinical process. Some key applications are as follows:

The objectives of the **IDEAS** [25] project are the integration, evaluation and demonstration of a universal multi-media distributed and interactive architect, which supports a large set of applications and systems for tele-health, tele-radiology and high-level tele-homecare services, oriented to general medical assistance, to promotion and prevention of health, to render social care to vulnerable groups such as elderly and disabled people. The project will implement the ASP Business Model in the healthcare domain, developing an optimized framework through the integration of standard components and reducing the development costs and time-to-market of tele-health applications.

HEARTFAID [26] aims to make more effective and efficient all the processes related to diagnosis, prognosis and treatment of the heart failure within elderly population. This general goal will be achieved by developing and providing an innovative technological platform that integrates biomedical data within electronic health record systems, for easy and ubiquitous access to heterogeneous patients' data; provides services for healthcare professionals, including patient telemonitoring, signal and image processing, alert and alarm system; supports clinical decision in the heart failure domain, based on pattern recognition in historical data, knowledge discovery analysis and inferences on patients' clinical data.

As Table 3.1 indicates, there is not much research effort on collaboration and workflow support in the existing eHealth applications. Many of these

Table 3.1 eHealth projects' comparison

Project	Area	Collaboration support	Workflow support
C-Care	EHR access through voice	No	No
CHS	Home monitoring	No	No
HEALTHMATE	Tele-care and tele-consultation	No	No
HUMAN	Telemedicine	No	No
IDEAS	Universal multi-media distributed and interactive architect	No	No
MOBIDEV	Integration of eHealth databases	No	No
MOBIHEALTH	Telemedicine	No	No
TOPCARE	Telecommunication	Through cooperative healthcare services	Pre-defined
WIDENET	EHR interconnectivity	No	No
ARTEMIS	Semantic web services	No	No
AUBADE	Analysis of neurological diseases and human emotions	No	No
BIOPATTERN	Citizen's bioprofile	No	No
CLINICIP	Automatic insulin injection	No	No
COCOON	Risk management	Knowledge-driven collaborative practices	No
DICOEMS	Cooperation for critical situation	Portable collaboration environment	No
INTREPID	Intelligent patient treatment with wearable sensors	No	No
MYHEART	Heart failures prevention	No	No
NOESIS	Tools for prevention, diagnosis and treatment support	No	No
SEMANTICMINING	Data mining of medical information	No	No
PIPS	Generic medical database	No	No
HEARTFAID	Diagnose, prognoses and treatment of heart failure	No	No
MPOWER	Middleware platform for rapid development of services	No	No
HEALTHSERVICE24	Mobile healthcare system	No	No

projects utilize gimmicks in order to simulate collaboration, with the exploitation of common/shared EHR and simple messaging techniques. However, we consider that collaboration should include more sophisticated methods like the use of virtual teams and workflows.

3.3 Proposed Theoretical Approach

Given the analysis of the above-mentioned projects and the imminent weaknesses identified, we hereafter propose an extended collaboration model enhancing the existing one with vital modules that could support multi/cross-organization collaboration [27].

3.3.1 The Extended Collaboration Model and Proposed Features Identified

During the user requirements analysis for the development of our proposed system (described below), one fundamental necessity was the support for cross-organization medical teams [27]. A clear classification of the various types and forms of medical teams based on the dimensions of time, place and organization was spawned, identifying eight types of collaboration. Four cases of groups have their members working in the same organization, four cases of groups sharing same labour space and another four cases of groups working simultaneously (Fig. 3.2).

Furthermore, during the same phase of the analysis, a set of features were also identified (Fig. 3.3). These features provide the new dimension of our extended

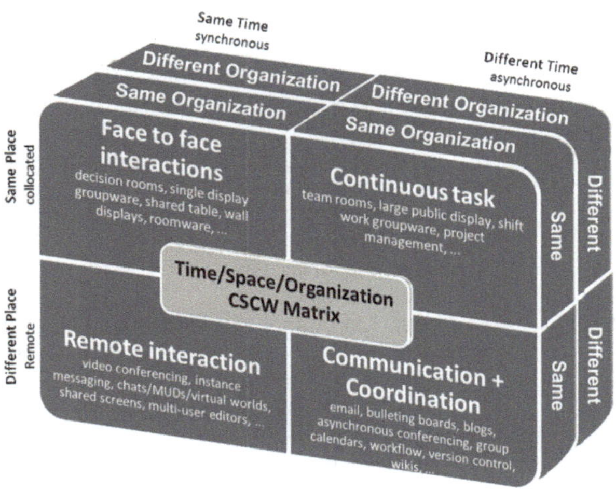

Fig. 3.2 Extended collaboration model

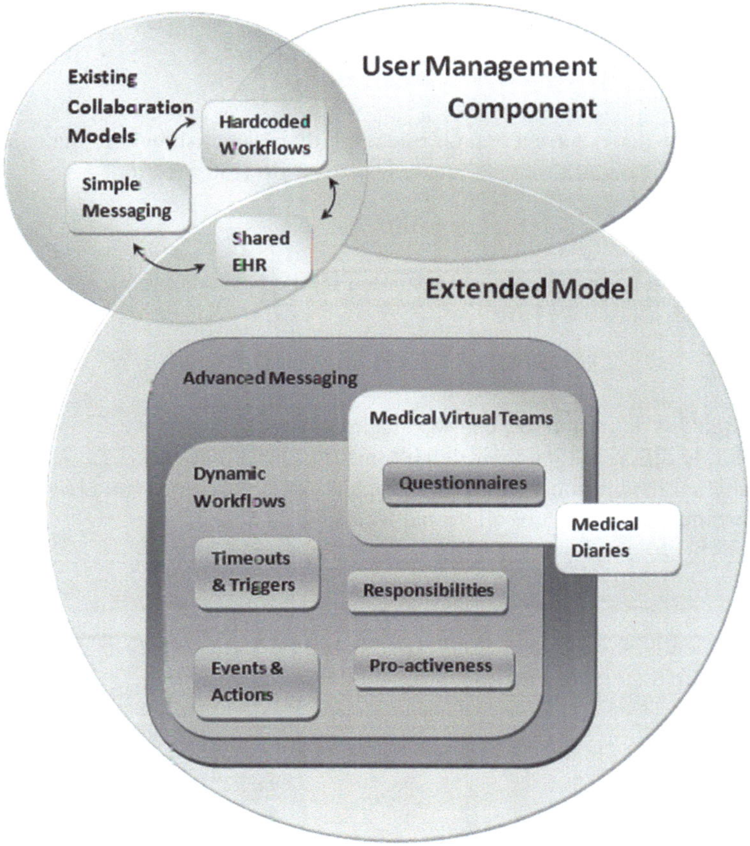

Fig. 3.3 Extended system model

model and a more effective and efficient way of collaborating within the eHealth context. These include (i) medical virtual teams, (ii) dynamic workflows, (iii) events, (iv) actions, (v) timeouts, (vi) triggers, (vii) responsibilities, (viii) questionnaires, (ix) medical diaries and (x) pro-activeness. In the following sections we present these features in more detail.

3.3.2 Medical Virtual Teams

The key elements of our collaboration system are the users, the roles and the virtual teams. By users we denote the set U of the users that are participating in the system.

$$U = \{u_1, u_2, \ldots, u_n\}.$$

By roles we denote the set R of all the available roles that a user can participate in the system.

$$R = \{r_1, r_2, \ldots, r_m\}.$$

Additionally, users have a default role upon their establishment in the collaboration system. This default role is accessed by the following function:

$$dr(u_i) = r_j.$$

The notion of a virtual team T_i is denoted by the Cartesian product of the sets U and R. In other words, we have

$$T_i \subseteq U \times R \Rightarrow T_i = \{(u,r){:}u \in U, r \in R\} \neq \emptyset, i \in N.$$

Through this definition, we can see that the users can participate in a virtual team having a role different than their default one. Furthermore, users can participate in a virtual team having multiple roles and many users participate in a team with the same specific role. The set of all virtual teams VT is defined as

$$\mathrm{VT} = \bigcup_{i=1}^{n} T_i.$$

Consequently, the number of all possible virtual team is $|\mathrm{VT}| = 2|U \times R|$. We can see a graphical representation of the model in Fig. 3.4.

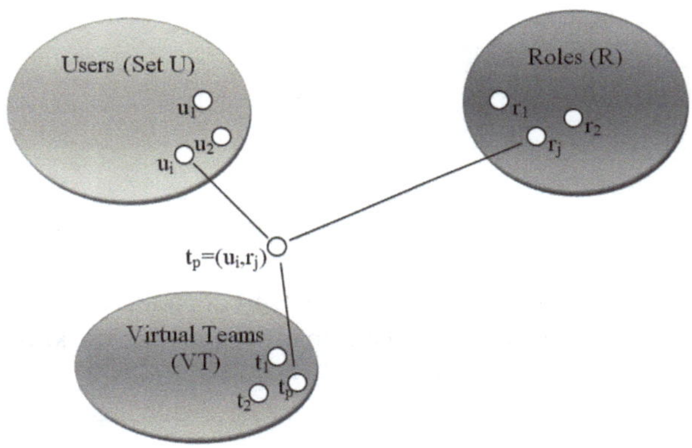

Fig. 3.4 Virtual teams model

3.3.3 Dynamic Questionnaires (Voting)

In this scenario, we demonstrate the dispatch questionnaire and the collection of the answers. Head Nurse (Athena) creates a questionnaire and sends it to the members of a virtual team. The four members of the team receive the questionnaires and answer the questions. The answers are sent back to the Head Nurse (Athena) and she reviews them (Fig. 3.5).

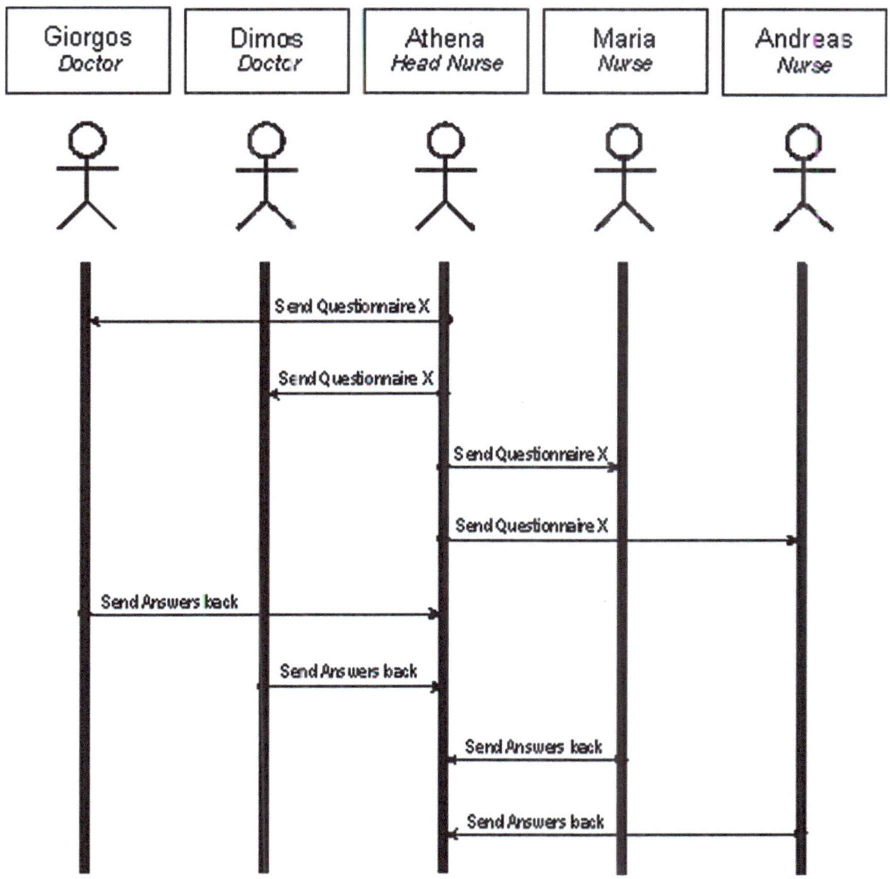

Fig. 3.5 Questionnaires scenario

Questionnaires can be described as a collection of questions. The questionnaires can be sent to individuals in order to be completed. The results are sent back to the sender and gathered in one place, so we can review the results one by one or just have an overall result (voting). This service allows us to create, view, modify, delete and complete questionnaires.

Another key feature of our system is the questionnaires. In order to give a proper definition of what a questionnaire is, we have to define first all the sub-components of a questionnaire. These sub-components are the questions and the answers. Similarly, to the above we have a set of answers.

$$\mathrm{AN} = \{an_1, an_2, \ldots, an_z\}.$$

A question q_i is defined as a set of answers. In other words

$$Q = \{q_1, q_2, \ldots, q_z\}, \text{ where } q_i = \{an : an \in \mathrm{AN}\}.$$

Finally, a questionnaire qu_i is a set of questions.

$$QU = \{qu_1, qu_2, \ldots, qu_z\}, \text{ where } qu_i = \{q : q \in Q\}.$$

In Fig. 3.6 we see the graphical representation of the model.

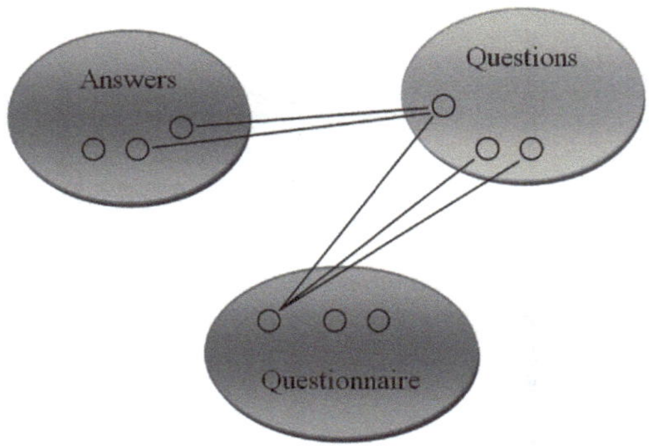

Fig. 3.6 Questionnaires model

3.3.4 Actions

An action is what a person can do. It could be just sending a message or a more complicated act. These messages are predefined and created by the system administrator. The more complicated act is a calling of a stored procedure. This act can encapsulate information that the administrator and/or the users pass. Additionally, an action can call an existing workflow by sending an interactive message:

$$A = \{a_1, a_2, \ldots, a_z\}.$$

3.3.5 Dynamic Workflows (Interactive Message)

One of the scenarios depicts a head nurse that triggers a workflow that requests for a change of medication. An automated message from the workflows is dispatched to the doctor that belongs to the virtual team of the certain patient asking him/her for an approval, since the nurse is not authorized to do so. The doctor responds to the message and the workflow updates the medication and in addition alerts all the corresponding medical team for this important change (Fig. 3.7). Through this workflow, we notice that the head nurse did not have to know the doctor of the patient and the doctor did not have to know the medical team and alert each one of them saving precious time.

Dynamic workflows are sets of actions. They are also called interactive messages because users initiate them by sending a predefined message to another user. These

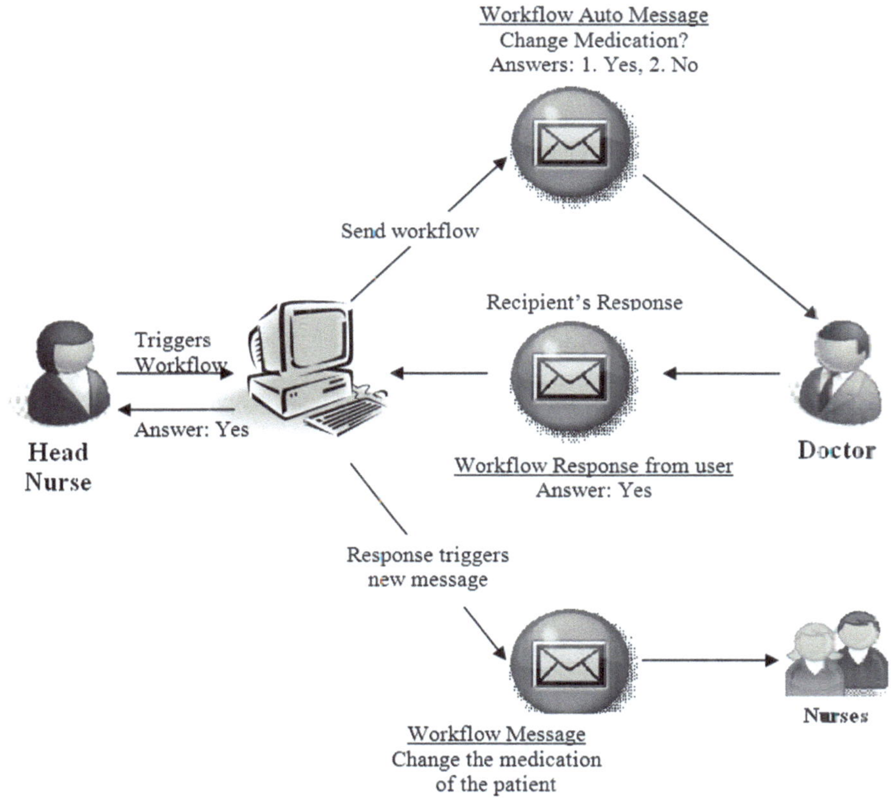

Fig. 3.7 Workflow example

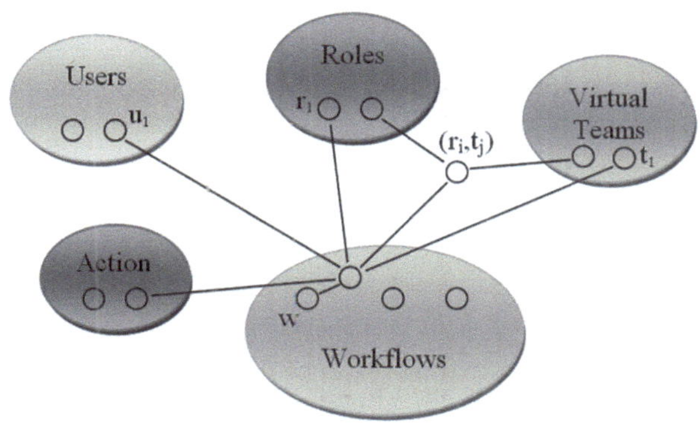

Fig. 3.8 Workflow model

messages are special messages that trigger actions and thus they make the users to interact with each other.

A more complicated notion is the one of the workflows. Workflows are defined as a set of actions connected with users or roles or virtual teams or virtual teams and roles together and with another workflow. For example, we can have the action 'Visit Patient' and send it to

- one user of the system,
- or to every doctor of the system,
- or to the virtual team of the patient,
- or to the doctors of the virtual team.

So, if A is the set of all actions of the system ($A = \{a_1, a_2, \ldots, a_z\}$), then

$$W = \{(x,y)\colon x \in A, y \in U \cup R \cup T \cup R \times T \cup W\}.$$

Under the notion of the pre-mentioned timeouts and triggers, the idea of the events is spawned. Events are the elements e of the set E that triggers a workflow. Such events are the decision-making of a user (complete an action) of it can be a timeout (predefined time expiration of a task). In other words, actions can trigger an event and events can trigger a workflow. So, if the definition of events is

$$E = \{e_1, e_2, \ldots, e_m\},$$

then there is a function g that given an action a, it returns the generated event

$$g(a) = \begin{cases} e & \text{if } a \text{ triggers a new event} \\ \text{NULL} & \text{otherwise} \end{cases}.$$

Similarly, we have a function f that given an event e, it returns the workflow w that it triggers:

$$f(e) = w.$$

In other words, the workflow system is a set of ordered pairs of events e and workflows w (e,w):

$$\text{Dynamic workflows} = \{(e,w)\colon e \in E, w \in W\}.$$

3.3.6 Responsibilities

Some actions are set to be performed by only one user of a certain role. We can notify all users of this role and send them an action to be performed. The first user that will get the action can take the responsibility of completing this task. All other users will be notified that this task is handled by another person. This way we avoid duplication of work. For instance, we can have the scenario that one nurse is asking for a drug prescription from all doctors. We do not want to have more than one doctor to prescribe the same drug. The Responsibility feature solves this problem.

3.3.7 Timeouts and Triggers

In this scenario, Head Nurse (Athena) sends the workflow (ChangeMedication (sameVT)) to the virtual team of a patient (members: Giorgos, Athena, Maria). The workflow automatically sends an action (NewMedication) to the doctors of the team (in this case only to Giorgos). In this workflow there is a 5-min timeout on the action. In case of timeout, a new workflow will be triggered (ChangeMedication(all)). It has the same action (NewMedication), but this time it will be sent to all doctors of the system (Giorgos, Dimos). Next, doctor Dimos takes the responsibility for the action, so an automatic message goes to the other doctors (Giorgos) that doctor Dimos will complete the action. Finally, doctor Dimos sends a message to the Head Nurse (Athena) that she has to change the medication of the patient (Fig. 3.9).

Under the scope of the medical virtual teams, we have assignments of roles to patients. There are times though that certain tasks are of vital significance (urgent tasks) and thus the need for the dimension of time is spawned. We can set a timeout on such crucial action. When the time that we set passes, another action or workflow is trigged. For example, we can have a nurse asking for a doctor's help. Nurse will initially ask help from the doctor of the patient's virtual team. After the timeout

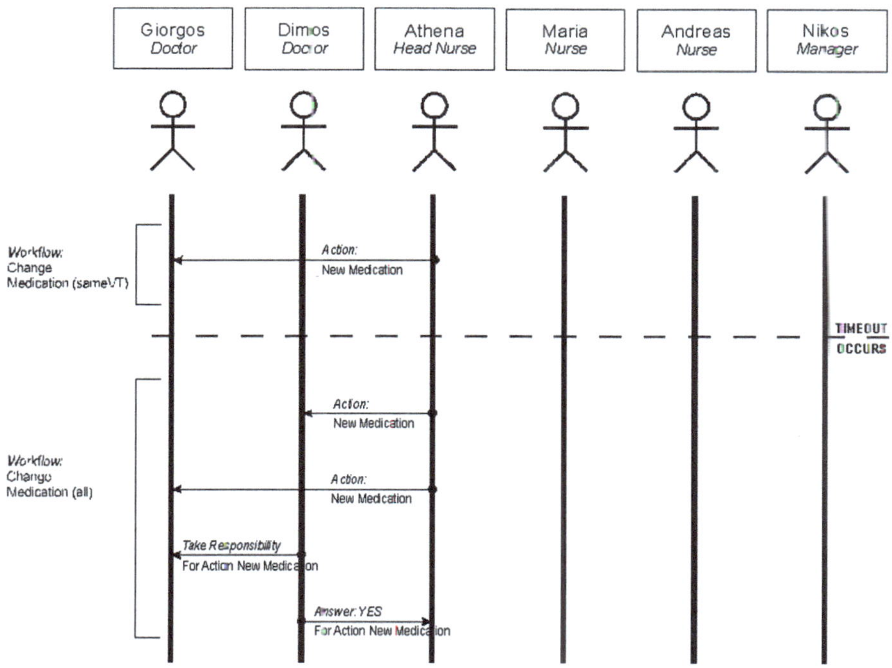

Fig. 3.9 Timeout and responsibility scenario

occurs, another action will be triggered. The new action will be about asking help from any doctor of the system.

3.3.8 Medical Diaries

Medical diaries are an easy self-monitoring method used by patients from any mobile device. During this procedure, patients keep a daily record of their symptoms or pain control ranking the symptom on a scale. It is a very simple procedure, using only clicks and predefined text answers due to the mobile devices limitations. Medical virtual team can review anytime these diaries and suggest or take actions. Additionally, we introduced the notion of the threshold. Threshold is a limit on a diary entry that can be set to trigger a workflow or alert the team. For instance, a patient marks a pain of grade 10 in his pain diary. Then, a message can be send to his/her medical virtual team, notifying them about this event.

3.3.9 Pro-activeness

European Committee is focusing on activity motivation services. The activity motivation services include services that will motivate and encourage persons with chronic conditions to undertake physical and mental exercises and activities, change lifestyle, socialize, etc. Daily tasks assistance will provide patients with direction indications, explanations on how to perform some tasks or even instructions on how to call for human assistance, for example, through the use of the socialization services. Additionally, the system can assist patients by providing them with a type of memory help (reminders, directions indications to a place, memory assistance, etc.).

During the following section, we will present the implementation of the system. For this implementation, we used all the notions and components that are mentioned and presented in this section. The system was implemented into two different applications: the windows-based application that is used from the administrator in order to set up the collaboration rules; and the web-based application that is customized to work on every mobile device and give the ability to the users of using the system 24/7 everywhere and by any means.

3.4 A Proposed System – DYMOS

DYMOS system (**DY**namic **MO**bile Healthcare **S**ystem) supports the extended collaboration model that we presented above. The notions of medical virtual teams, dynamic workflows, questionnaires, actions, events, triggers, timeouts, medical diaries and pro-activeness are implemented along with an administrative console to manage them. An intelligent interface was also adopted in order to provide a more effective and efficient manner of accessing the information.

3.4.1 Architecture

The system architecture is basically divided into five layers. These layers are the application/user, the workflows, the services, the sensors and the database, having the last two as parallel (Fig. 3.10).

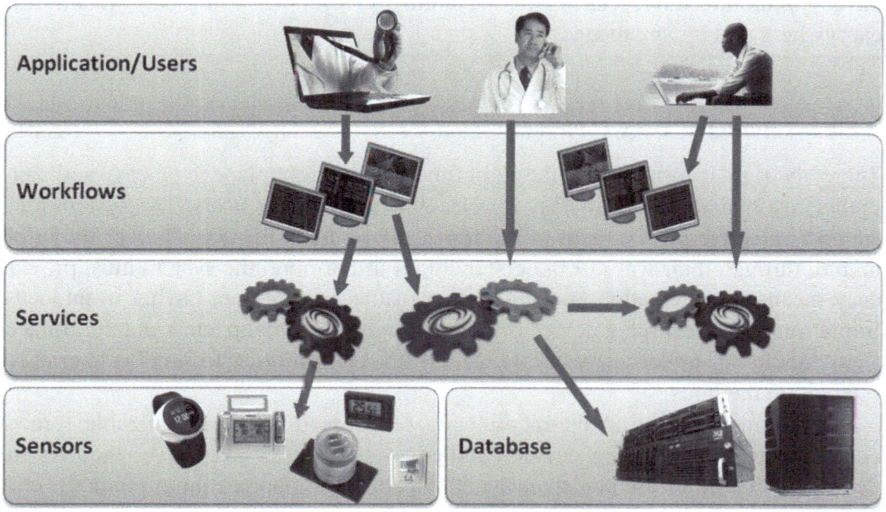

Fig. 3.10 System architecture

The Application/Users layer is the layer that hosts our GUI that provides all the necessary functionality for a flexible, efficient and effective collaboration, covering all the pre-mentioned requirements. This layer can be altered according to the hosting organization's needs, maximizing the added value of the system.

The workflows layer is the layer that hosts the dynamic workflows as described earlier. It resembles the business processes layer in the SOA architecture, having an orchestration and coordination of the basic system services, but in a more dynamic and ad hoc manner.

The services layer hosts the basic services that provide all the functionality of the system such as security, messaging, database access and sensors data access. These services can be called directly from the application or from a workflow, and even more from another workflow.

Finally, the last two layers are the sensor that hosts all the available sensors of the system (temperature, sound, light, vital signals, etc.) and the database layer that hosts the DBMS of the system. This DBMS can store reading from the sensors for future use by the application, all the data for the user management, collaboration features, virtual teams, dynamic workflows, actions, questionnaires, etc.

3.4.2 *Implementation*

For the system's implementation, we have used all the notions and components that are mentioned and presented in the previous sections. The system was implemented as two different but also interrelated applications: the windows-based application that is used from the administrator in order to set up the collaboration rules and the dynamic workflows and the web-based application that is customized to work on every mobile device and give the ability to users of using the system 24/7 everywhere and by any means.

3.4.2.1 Intelligent User Interface

To get the right information at the right time and the right place in an easy and comprehensive manner is not so easy for eHealth application's users. The system must support an active involvement of the users, giving them the control over the information through their ways of understanding. Furthermore, the system must provide easy means for navigation and orientation of the information, having in mind the limitation of the accessing device (mobile phone, PDA, laptop, etc.) and the connectivity medium (wireless network, GSM, GPRS, etc.) in order to support alternative interaction methods.

Having in mind the above-mentioned, we adopted fully customizable screens according to the accessing device handled by the server. The server inquires the device's capabilities (screen size, media capability, supported input methods, etc.) and re-structures the screens in order to meet these capabilities and serves the result. In addition, we minimized the 'clicks' for getting the right information, always considering the users' preferences. Furthermore, menus are customizable per user in order to meet his/her demands. This resulted in serious reduction of time to access a service and the requested information.

3.4.2.2 Windows-Based Application (Administration)

This application is designed to provide the administrator with the ability to coordinate the whole system. Following, we present some screenshots of the implementation of this system.

In Fig. 3.11 we demonstrate the administrators' main menu. The administrator can choose from creating new action, workflows, users, roles and virtual teams, or manage the existing ones. Finally, the administrator can manage the workflow timeouts. The administrator can also view the timeouts, in order to start/stop the existing timeouts monitoring process. Additionally, the administrator can populate lists (that will be used by the end users) manually (list of all possible selections – '|' separated or from database query, e.g. Yes | No | Maybe or 'Select Name, Value From Users') or with the use of plain SQL commands.

The workflows are graphically represented as tree view (Fig. 3.12) for better understanding and error prevention for more complicated workflows. In addition,

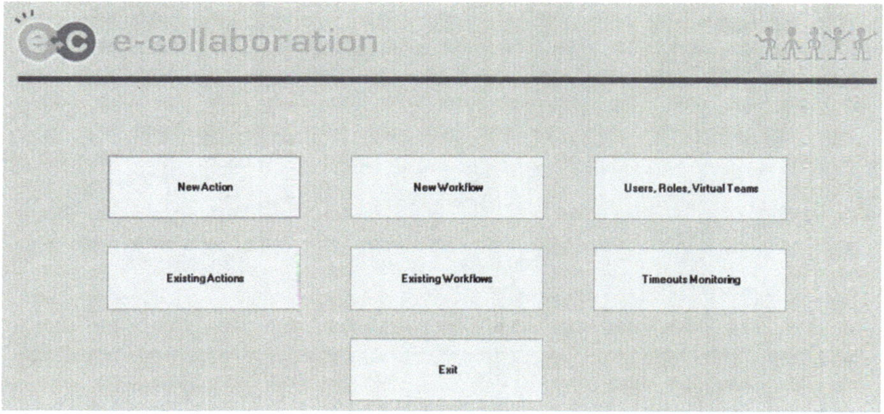

Fig. 3.11 Administrator's interface

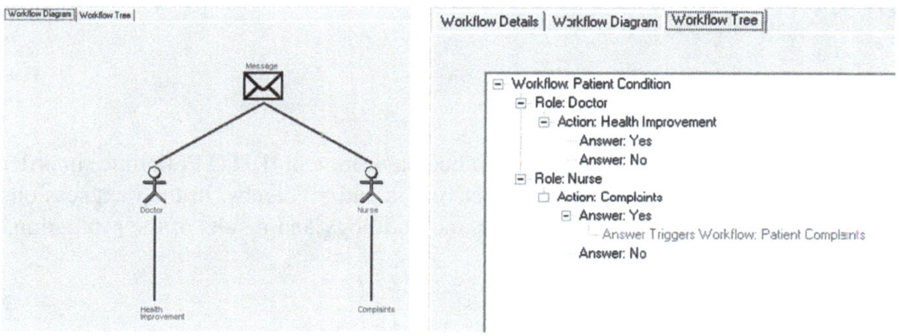

Fig. 3.12 Workflow graphical representation

there is a circle prevention mechanism that prevents the creation of workflows that may result in dead end.

3.4.2.3 Web-Based Application (Users)

Web-based application is used by users in a 24/7 basis through any device (Fig. 3.13). Users have access to their data and can collaborate in innovative ways, using dynamic interactive messages (workflows), questionnaires and virtual teams. In this chapter we present the functionality of the web-based application through the use of a PDA.

Users in the healthcare sector have limited knowledge of mobile devices and the ability to use state-of-the-art technologies such as PDAs and smartphones. Thus, as mentioned above, we adopted screens that are easy to understand and do no need much effort on accessing information by using as much as possible key buttons and minimizing the 'clicks', and consequently we speed up the process.

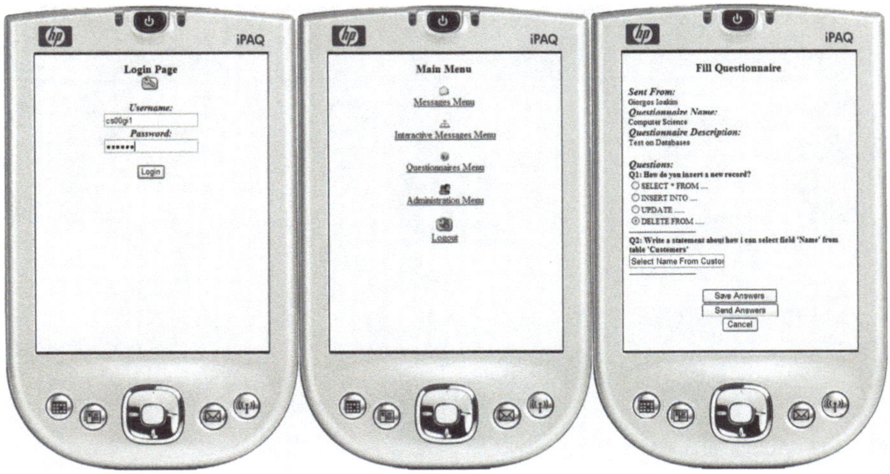

Fig. 3.13 User's interface

3.5 Evaluation

The system evaluation held in a real test bed environment (LITO Policlinic) in order to assess the usability and system effectiveness and efficiency. In the next sessions we present the environment, objectives, methodology and results of the evaluation.

3.5.1 Environment

The evaluation of the system was performed at the premises of LITO Policlinic Paralimniou. Paralimni town is in the Famagusta district that extends for about 900 km^2 with a population of about 100,000, quadrupling during the summer months. LITO Policlinic is a private clinic serving the Famagusta and Larnaca districts, including the tourist triangle of the towns of Paralimni, Ayia Napa and Protaras.

LITO has a good reputation regarding cardiology. It provides apart from hospital care also home care. The provision of home care is regarded as a drive for a more holistic care, aiming for the delivery of better care while reducing the number of visits to health professionals or the need for hospitalization. In general, when a person receives acute medical care in a hospital and reaches a stable phase, the person is in principle ready for discharge. For a person in need of advanced medical and nursing care at home, a referral is made to the home care unit. Cardiac patients referred to this unit are offered continuous care monitoring at home in a way similar to the monitoring they would get at the hospital, implying

- Improved quality of patients' life by providing them better assistance at any time and place. Patients can now enjoy 'optimum' health service with improved quality of life in their own friendly environment,

- Quick access and possibility of continuous communication with the doctor, which makes the patient more comfortable and confident about his/her medical state.

3.5.2 Objectives/Purpose

The objective of the evaluation was to test the DYMOS's services by healthcare professionals (nurse, GP, specialist cardiologist, etc.) in two situations commonly present in cardiac patients:

- Professionals dealing with patients who had an acute episode and have been admitted and stabilized, but need frequent monitoring of the condition and the prescribed drug regime for a further few days.
- Professionals dealing with patients in a suspected acute episode, brought in for examination; a decision needs to be taken whether to keep the patients at the hospital for observation or to discharge them home. In case a patient is discharged and there is a suspicion of an abnormal condition, the professionals should keep frequent monitoring of the patient's state.

The objectives were to

- Assess the shared care model for treating cardiac patients
- Determine professional user's acceptance of DYMOS's services for remote follow-up of patients with cardiac problems
- Assess quality of life, patient compliance and satisfaction with the program and the technology used
- Evaluate the tools for professionals

3.5.3 Methodology

The evaluation was planned as a convenience sample study: patients were included as they become available in the area selected for the study. The evaluation was made by single subject design.

The user groups of the evaluation included

- Five healthcare professionals
- Ten patients with known cardiac problems or patients with suspected cardiac problems
- Three to six months monitoring period for each patient

Any patient, living in the districts of Paralimni and Larnaca area, who had an acute episode and has been admitted and stabilized, but needed frequent monitoring of condition and drug regime for a further few days, or a patient in a suspected acute episode, brought in for examination, was included in the study. With regard to a patient with a suspected acute episode, a decision was taken whether to keep the patients at the hospital for observation or to discharge them home. In case a patient was discharged and there was a suspicion of an abnormal condition, the professionals kept frequent monitoring of the patient's state.

The procedure of the trials was basically divided into two major phases. Phase 1 included 5 healthcare professionals and 10 patients with known cardiac problems or with suspected cardiac problems. The evaluation has been carried out in a 'controlled' environment (within hospital premises). The purpose of Phase 1 was to facilitate the users of the system to gain some experience on using the services, Having this knowledge in mind, the evaluation has continued with the second phase of the procedure, which included patients beyond the 'controlled' environment (at patients' homes).

These steps are summarized as follows:

- Phase 1 (2 months) – controlled environment
  - five healthcare professionals
  - ten patients with suspected cardiac problems or patients with known cardiac problems
- Phase 2 (extend beyond 'controlled' environment) (4 months)
  - five healthcare professionals
  - ten patients with suspected cardiac problems or patients with known cardiac problems

Informed consent was obtained in writing from all patients or their next of kin if the patient was not ethically competent. Relevant information was given orally and in writing. Patients were assured that their decision to be included in the evaluation did not affect the care provided. The patients' right to stop participation in the process at any time and without giving a reason was an important part of the informed consent. An ethical problem was the intrusion on patients with unknown technology. Therefore, it was considered very important to provide the patients with complete information about the project and the characteristics of the evaluation before their enrolment. In any case, the law of the country on the storage and transmission of personal data has been followed.

Due to the similarities of the monitoring methods in this evaluation to the hospital equipment, no extra discomfort was caused to the patient. The potential risk could have been that technical errors caused wrong or delayed information for the health professional so that the clinical decision to send the patient to hospital could have been delayed.

The evaluation has sought the subjective opinion of the professionals and patients involved in the process regarding the DYMOS's service provision, its usability, user interaction, satisfaction, suitability, usefulness, and acceptance.

3.6 Results

The evaluation of the system yielded some very interesting results. The main outcome was that the system proved to decrease the use of resources when compared to conventional approach. The other important benefits identified were the following:

- Improved communication within healthcare team (nurses and other professionals, both hospital and not hospital based) and between healthcare team and hospital, thus providing capability to consult within a team of experts, without the need to move patient from his/her home to each one of them. This results in the reduction of number of visits to health professionals and reduces burden not only on patient but also on his/her relatives and makes better use of the scarce and expensive medical professionals and scarce hospital beds.
- Provision of continuity of care through the presence of a healthcare team by the patient at any given time, irrespective of locality or movement.
- Improved and secure timely access to patient information, in accordance with their authorization levels, through unified information space centred on the patient. As an added benefit, all the professionals treating the patient have access to the same set of data.
- Improved cost-effectiveness through improved communications and better planning of resources and services.
- Improved health practices (shift towards evidence-based) and reduction of bureaucratic overhead.
- Business potential is great due to a number of reasons: (1) patients' preferences to stay in their homes rather than being institutionalized, as long as they feel secure, (2) decrease in the need for hospital beds and (3) better allocation of the professionals' time.

The economic outcomes of the use of the DYMOS's service are quite promising. It is expected that remote monitoring provided by linked collaborative medical teams should yield cost savings because of the expense of hospital stays together with costs for transportation.

During the evaluation methodology, a questionnaire (Table 3.2) was developed to evaluate the DYMOS's services. The results from 10 healthcare professionals are presented in Table 3.2.

Most of the users had the same opinion and in most of the cases were in favour of the system. The above results are uniform, showing a favourable position on the DYMOS's services like 'freshness' of the information, collection of services, personalized interface, collaboration features and appointment scheduling. Minor drawbacks were

- The limited life of the battery of the mobile devices. The issue of the small battery life though is global for all mobile devices. In the near future, new technologies will come to solve this problem.
- The level of help provided within the system could have been more.

Table 3.2 Evaluation methodology questionnaire

	Strongly Disagree	Disagree	Neither	Agree	Strongly Agree
1. The information provided by the system is up to date.					10
2. The level of user satisfaction arising from the navigation to the system is excellent.					10
3. The system delivers the services that were conformed during the analysis phase.				10	
4. The input methods of the system (keyboard, pen, etc.) are satisfactory.			4	5	1
5. The battery life of the hardware is acceptable.	7	2	1		
30. The Collaboration System meets my expectations.			2	8	
31. The Collaboration System is very easy to use.			1	3	6
32. The Appointment Scheduling System meets my expectations.				1	9
33. The Appointment Scheduling System is very easy to use.				1	9

According to the professionals, the last two drawbacks were not categorized as too serious as they did not stall their work.

3.7 Conclusion

In this chapter we have extensively investigated various applications' collaboration features within the eHealth context. As we have specifically observed during the analysis conducted, there is a common collaboration model used by many eHealth approaches/projects with, however, a given weakness of employing modules that could support multi/cross-organization collaboration. In this regard, we have proposed a set of new features, expanding the current model, in an attempt to more comprehensively approach the particular problem. These elements have been incorporated in the proposed system DYMOS and positively evaluated through the experimentation phase and the use of real-case scenarios.

The main original assumptions made about the DYMOS's services were to improve quality of life and satisfaction of patients by providing them better assistance at any time and place through the use of a shared care model, improve collaboration among professionals and decision-making, improve the professionals' work conditions by reducing work load and enhancing clinical working processes for remote follow-up of patients with cardiac problems by providing better communication ways based on state-of-the art technologies, and improve cost-effectiveness of home care provision of cardiac patients.

Through the running and the evaluation results of the trial, the achievement of the above initial assumptions can be supported. Furthermore, the evaluation has provided knowledge about ways of offering the patient the opportunity to be cared at home for longer uninterrupted periods by making use of new technologies and the building up of a virtual linked and collaborative care team around him/her. Through this setup an efficient and cost-effective collaboration among medical professionals for a 24/7 care provision has been registered. An increased professional satisfaction linked to the service being provided has been registered through the evaluation of the provided questionnaires.

In addition, through the use of a shared medical record and wireless mobile technologies, decision-making among professionals has become more time effective, saving unnecessary telephone calls, explanations about the patients conditions and waiting time of consulting the physicians, which are normally heavy loaded.

Moreover, the quality of patient's life has been improved by having the opportunity of staying in the surrounding of his/her beloved, avoiding long hospitalization periods, feeling confident that he/she receives 24/7 better assistance and care from his/her virtual assigned medical team. Additionally, the quick access and possibility of easy communication with the doctor make the patient feeling psychologically more positive.

Even though no final quantitative impact of the DYMOS's services has been measured, initial cost estimations have shown a high potential of care cost decrease. This can be associated with timely better utilization of resources, avoiding duplication of work, unnecessary communication among professionals and delays in accessing the patient information. Overall, it can be concluded that the system satisfied the initial assumptions made, and a deployment of such services could reveal a high beneficial potential for any system or entity.

References

1. Georgiadis TD. Dynamic creation of collaborating system and database management, using mobile agents, M.Sc. Thesis, Computer Science Department, University of Cyprus, June 2002.

2. Pitsillides A, Samaras G, Pitsillides B, Georgiades D, Andreou P, Christodoulou E. Virtual collaborative healthcare teams for home healthcare. Special issue on Advanced Mobile Technologies for Health Care Applications. J Mobile Multimedia 2006;2(1): 023–036.
3. Pitoura E, Samaras G. Data Management for Mobile Computing. Boston: Kluwer Academic Publishers, ISBN 0-7923-8053-3.
4. C-CARE Project: Continuous Care, IST-1999-10217, Website: http://cordis.europa.eu/fetch?ACTION=D&CALLER=PROJ_IST&RCN=55034.
5. HEALTHMATE Project: Personal intelligent health mobile systems for Telecare and Teleconsultation, IST-2000-26154, Website: http://www.healthmate-project.org.
6. HUMAN Project, IST-2001-33483, Website: http://www.human-project.ws/.
7. COCOON Project: Building knowledge driven and dynamically adaptive networked communities within European healthcare systems, IST FP6- 507126, Website: http://swa.cefriel.it/COCOON.
8. NOESIS Project: Platform for wide scale integration and visual representation of medical intelligence, IST FP6-507960, Website: http://www.noesis-eu.org/.
9. PIPS Project, IST FP6-507019, Website: http://193.178.235.132/.
10. CHS Project: Citizen Health System, IST-1999-13352, Website: http://lomiweb.med.auth.gr/index.php?q=en/node/186.
11. ARTEMIS Project: A semantic Web service-based P2P infrastructure for the interoperability of medical Information systems, IST FP6-002103, Website: http://www.ist-world.org/ProjectDetails.aspx?ProjectId=647fbec760dc48d58f54f933d632b78b&SourceDatabaseId=7cff9226e582440894200b751bab883f.
12. MPOWER Project: Middleware platform for eMPOWERing cognitive disabled and elderly, IST FP6- 034707, Website: http://www.mpower-project.eu.
13. MobiHealth Project, IST-2001-36006, Website: http://www.mobihealth.org.
14. TOPCARE Project: A Telematics Home Care Platform for Cooperative Health Care Provision, IST-2000-25068, Website: http://www.topcare.info/.
15. AUBADE Project, IST-2002-507605, Website: http://www.aubade-group.com.
16. CLINICIP Project, 506965, Website: http://www.clinicip.org.
17. INTREPID Project: A Virtual Reality Intelligent Multi-sensor Wearable System for Phobias' Treatment, IST-2002-507464, Website: http://www.ist-world.org/ProjectDetails.aspx?ProjectId=34901e26065047afb9aebd4e15794570&SourceDatabaseId=7cff9226e582440894200b751bab883f.
18. MyHeart (Fighting Cardio-Vascular Diseases by Preventing Lifestyle & Early Diagnosis), IST FP6-507816, Website: http://www.extra.research.philips.com/euprojects/myheart.
19. HealthService 24 Project, eTEN-517352, Website: http://www.healthservice24.com.
20. Mobi-Dev Project: mobile devices for healthcare applications, IST-2000-26402, Website: http://cordis.europa.eu/fetch?ACTION=D&CALLER=PROJ_IST&RCN=54810.
21. WIDENET Project: Offering World-Wide Services through an International Network on Health Records, IST-1999-14203, Website: http://cordis.europa.eu/fetch?ACTION=D&CALLER=PROJ_IST&RCN=54336.
22. BIOPATTERN Project, IST-2002-508803, Website: http://www.biopattern.org.
23. DICOEMS Project: Emergency risk management e-health platform, IST FP6-507760, Website: http://www.dicoems.com/.
24. SemanticMining Project, IST-2002-507505, Website: http://www.semanticmining.org/.
25. IDEAS Project, Integrated Distributed Environment for Application Services in e-Health, IST-2001-34614, Website: http://www.ideas-ehealth.upv.es/.
26. HEARTFAID Project: A knowledge based platform of services for supporting medical-clinical management of hearth failure within elderly population, FP6-IST-2004-027107, Website: http://www.heartfaid.org.
27. Ioakim G. Dynamic wofkflows in wireless environment, M.Sc. Thesis, Computer Science Department, University of Cyprus, May 2007.

Chapter 4
An Empirical Study of Sections in Classifying Disease Outbreak Reports

Son Doan, Mike Conway, and Nigel Collier

Abstract Identifying articles that relate to infectious diseases is a necessary step for any automatic bio-surveillance system that monitors news articles from the Internet. Unlike scientific articles that are available in a strongly structured form, news articles are usually loosely structured. In this chapter, we investigate the importance of each section and the effect of section weighting on the performance of text classification. The experimental results show that (1) classification models using the headline and leading sentence achieve a high performance in terms of F-score compared to other parts of the article; (2) all section with bag-of-word representation (full text) achieves the highest recall; and (3) section weighting information can help to improve accuracy.

Keywords: Infectious Diseases Surveillance Systems · Disease Outbreak Reports

4.1 Introduction

In infectious disease surveillance systems such as the Global Public Health Intelligence Network (GPHIN) system [1] and ProMed-Mail [2], the detection and tracking of outbreaks using the Internet have been proven to be a key source of information for public health workers, clinicians, and researchers interested in communicable diseases.

For any automatic bio-surveillance system, the identification and classification of articles that relate to infectious diseases is a necessary first step in monitoring news articles from the Internet. This reduces the load on later processing steps that often involve more knowledge-intensive methods.

In practice, though there are a large number of news articles whose main subject is related to diseases but which should not necessarily be notified to users together with a relatively small number of high-priority articles that experts should

S. Doan (✉)
Department of Biomedical Informatics, Vanderbilt University Medical Center, Nashville, TN 37203, USA
e-mail: doan@nii.ac.jp

A. Lazakidou (ed.), *Web-Based Applications in Healthcare and Biomedicine*,
Annals of Information Systems 7, DOI 10.1007/978-1-4419-1274-9_4,
© Springer Science+Business Media, LLC 2010

be actively alerted to. Alerting criteria in our approach broadly follow the World Health Organization (WHO) guidelines and include news related to newly emerging diseases, the spread of diseases across international borders, the deliberate release of a human or engineered pathogen, etc.

The use of conventional approaches in the classification process, i.e., bag-of-word, inevitably fails to resolve many subtle ambiguities, for example semantic class ambiguities in polysemous words like "virus," "fever," "outbreak," and "control," which all exhibit a variety of senses depending on the context. These different senses appear with relatively high frequency in press news reports, especially in headlines where context space is limited and creative use of language is sometimes employed to catch attention. A further challenge is that diseases can be denoted by many variant forms. Therefore, we consider that the use of advanced natural language processing (NLP) techniques like named entity recognition (NER) and anaphora resolution are needed in order to achieve high classification accuracy.

In recent years, there have been many studies on text classification in general [3, 4], or on semi-structured texts [5], and XML classification [6]. Other research has investigated the contribution of linguistic information in the form of synonyms, syntax, etc. in text representation [7–9] or feature selection [10].

In this chapter, we focus on an empirical study of canonical sections in news articles. The sections of news are based on the thematic superstructure approach by van Dijk [11]. In the experiments reported in this chapter, we adopt a simple approach by dividing sections in news reports into four canonical sections, namely Head, Lead, Content, and Comment, and explore the importance of each section. The main contribution of this chapter is firstly to provide empirical evidence about the importance of each section within news articles related to the relevancy criteria of our domain. This study also suggests that the use of all section with bag-of-word representation in practical systems is very important because it achieves very high recall, which is a very important measure in practice.

The rest of this chapter is organized as follows: in Section 4.2, we provide a brief overview of related work on the importance of sections in topic classification. Next, we introduce an approach based on van Dijk in Section 4.3. In Section 4.4, we outline the BioCaster schema for the annotation of terms in biomedical text; Section 4.5 provides details of the method, experimental results and analysis on the gold standard corpus. Finally, we draw some conclusions in Section 4.6.

4.2 Related Work

The first qu estion raised relates to how we can identify sections in a news article. So far, there has been surprisingly little work on identifying sections in this genre. Most previous work we are aware of has dealt with scientific articles with clear document structures. These structures usually are Title, Abstract, Introduction, Materials and Methods, Results, and Discussion. Mizuta and Collier [12] analyzed the structure of articles using zone identification, in which a general schema for identifying zones within biological articles was proposed. This schema consisted of Background, Problem setting, Outline, Textual, Method and Result.

Based on available structures, there are several works on studying the effects of sections within scientific papers. Sinclair and Webber [13] studied the classification of scientific article into GeneOntology codes. They explored several document representations like bag-of-words, bag-of-nouns, bag-of-stemmed nouns on two classifiers (maximum entropy and naïve Bayes) and found that naïve Bayes achieved the best results with bag-of-words document representation. They reported that both Title and Abstract achieved better result than other sections. Additionally, "all section" (that is, full-text) achieved the highest recall measure.

Related to document representation, Yetisgen-Yildiz et al. [14] reported that using a combination representation of bag-of-phrases and bag-of-words can improve the text classification in MEDLINE articles; however, the improvement is small (0.03% F-score).

Shah et al. [15] studied the information distribution within biological articles and showed that Abstracts provided the highest keyword density, but other sections might be better sources for the extraction of biologically relevant data.

Schuemie et al. [16] analyzed further the distribution of information in biomedical full-text articles. They gave two criteria, information density and information coverage, to measure the distribution of information within text. They found that Abstracts contain the highest information density. Moreover, 30% gene symbols in the Abstract were accompanied by their names, compared to 18% in the full text.

A recent study on section weighting by Hakenberg et al. [17] investigated several weight methods for sections and found that by setting putting the greatest weight on Abstract and Introduction sections, the system achieved the best performance in terms of F-score.

In this work, we are working with news articles that have relatively loose structures. Based on the work of van Dijk, we simply divide a news article into four canonical sections: Head, Lead, Content, and Comment. For document representation, we use the methodology described in [13] with a bag-of-words representation. For information density analysis, we used information density as described in [16] for analyzing concepts in Summary related to the main topic. Finally, for section weighting, we used the best results reported in [17] by setting the Summary weight to 3. Additionally, we range the weight to 5, 10 to show the effect of section weighting.

4.3 Simply Thematic Structures in Epidemic News

Identifying structures inside news articles is non-trivial. In a scientific article we can easily recognize separate sections such as Title, Abstract, Introduction, Method and Conclusion by their titles. News is different to scientific article in two respects: length and structure. Length is typically less than 600 words from major news agencies and structure is often flexible depending on the context of the story and the reporter.

We firstly consider a thematic approach to news proposed by van Dijk [11].

In his work, he proposed a thematic schema of news, namely Headline, Lead (together forming the Summary), Main Events, Context, History (together forming the Background), Verbal Reactions, and Comments. The Headline, according to van Dijk, "has a very specific thematic function: it usually expresses the most important topic of the news item." The next section is Lead, which often opens a news article. Headline and Lead both directly express the highest level macro-propositions of the news. Together, then, they function as a summary for the news article, thus they form the Summary section. The next section is the Background, which includes several subcategories, such as Main Events, Context, History, and reflects the content of the news. The following section is Verbal Reactions, which is defined as quotations and reflects opinions of peoples related to the news. Finally, Comment section often contains conclusions, expectations, speculations, and other information about the news. From these descriptions of the various sections that constitute a typical news article, two obvious questions arise: How to identify these sections within news article and how important is each section to the main topical relevance of news articles? As we discussed earlier, the structure of a news article is quite loose, thus it seems very difficult to apply van Dijk's sections directly to news articles. In discussions with experts in public health, we realized that in many (thought not all) cases the main topic and its relevance to infectious disease can be detected when they scanned the headline and the first sentence of a news article rather than the whole text. By incorporating this idea to the van Dijk approach, we assume a simplified news structures with four main sections as follows:

1. Headline: Title of a news article, on the top of a news.
2. Lead: The first sentence in a news article following the Headline. Headline and Lead form the Summary section.
3. Content: Background and Verbal of a news article. It is the section following the Lead.
4. Comment: The last sentence of a news article.

The structure of a news article can be schematically represented as follows:

<HEADLINE> . . . </HEADLINE>
<TIME> . . . </TIME> (optional)
<LOCATION> . . . </LOCATION> (optional)
<SENTENCE 1> . . . </SENTENCE 1>
<SENTENCE 2> . . . </SENTENCE 2>
. . .
<SENTENCE n-1> . . . </SENTENCE n-1>
<SENTENCE n> . . . </SENTENCE n>

For example:

<HEADLINE> Cholera in Angola – update </HEADLINE>
<TIME> 21 June 2006 <TIME>

<SENTENCE 1> As of 19 June 2006, Angola has reported a total of 46,758 cases including 1893 deaths with an overall (case fatality rate, CFR 4.0%).</SENTENCE 1>

...

<SENTENCE 7> WHO is sending Interagency Diarrhoeal Disease Kits to the most affected provinces and continues to support the Ministry of Health in its surveillance, water and sanitation, social mobilization and logistics activities.</SENTENCE 7>.

Here, the Headline is "Cholera in Angola – update," Lead is "21 June 2006." As of 19 June 2006, Angola has reported a total of 46,758 cases including 1893 deaths with an overall (case fatality rate, CFR 4.0%)." We assume that it includes information about time and organization that is of central importance to the news story. Content is the text between <SENTENCE 2> and </SENTENCE 6>. Comment is the text between <SENTENCE 7> and </SENTENCE 7>. The Summary section is the text inside <HEADLINE> and </SENTENCE 1>.

4.4 Data Set

In addition to section headings, we wanted to explore the use of terminology and its classes in our classification models. Below we present a brief summary of the schema and then follow this with a description of the data set used in our experiments.

4.4.1 BioCaster Annotation Schema

The BioCaster annotation schema is a component of the BioCaster text mining project. This schema has been developed for annotating important concepts that reflect information about infectious diseases. These key concepts are classified as Type and Role in which Type is identified using Name Entity Recognition (NER) and Roles are associated as attributes to the Name Entities (NEs). In total, there are 18 NEs denoted by convention in upper case. These include PERSON, LOCATION, ORGANIZATION, TIME, DISEASE, CONDITION, OUTBREAK, VIRUS, ANATOMY, PRODUCT, NONHUMAN, DNA, RNA, PROTEIN, CONTROL, BACTERIA, CHEMICAL and SYMPTOM. Of them, PERSON has the attribute case, NONHUMAN and ANATOMY have the attribute transmission, and CHEMICAL has the attribute therapeutic. They are marked up into text in XML format as follows:

<NAME cl="Named Entity" attribute1="value1" attribute2="value2" ... </NAME>,

where "Named Entity" is one of the names for the 18 BioCaster NEs and attribute1, attribute2, ... are the names of the NE's attributes, "value1", "value2", ... are values corresponding to attributes. Further details of the annotation guidelines are discussed in Ref. [18].

For example,

<NAME cl="DISEASE">Cholera</NAME> in <NAME cl="LOCATION"> Angola </NAME> - update <NAME cl="TIME">21 June 2006 </NAME> As of <NAME cl="TIME"> 19 June 2006</NAME>, <NAME cl="LOCATION">Angola</NAME> has reported a total of <NAME cl="PERSON" case ="true" number="many">46 758 cases</NAME> including <NAME cl="PERSON" case="true" number="many"> 1893 deaths</NAME> with an overall (case fatality rate, CFR 4.0%). ...

<NAME cl = "ORGANIZATION">WHO</NAME> is sending Interagency Diarrhoeal

Disease Kits to the most affected provinces and continues to support the Ministry of Health in its <NAME cl = "CONTROL"> surveillance </NAME>, water and sanitation, social mobilization and logistics activities.

Information about important concepts obtained from annotations can serve as clues for recognizing four sections inside news articles defined in Section 4.3.

4.4.2 BioCaster Gold Standard Corpus

The BioCaster gold standard corpus was collected from Internet news and manually annotated by two doctoral students. The annotation of a news article proceeded as follows. First, NEs are annotated following the BioCaster schema and guidelines. Second, each annotated article is manually assigned into one of four relevancy categories: alert, publish, check, and reject. The assignment is based on guidelines that we made following discussions with epidemiologists and a survey of World Health Organization (WHO) reports [19]. These categories are currently being used operationally by the GPHIN system, which is used by the WHO and other public health agencies. Where there were major differences of opinion in NE annotation or relevancy assignment between the two annotators, we consulted a public health expert in order to decide the most appropriate assignment. Finally, we had a total of 1000 articles that were fully annotated.

We grouped the 1000 articles into two categories: reject and relevant. The reject category corresponds simply to articles with label reject while the relevant category includes articles with labels alert, publish, and check. We conflated the alert, publish, and check categories because we hypothesized that distinguishing between non-reject (relevant) categories would require higher-level semantic knowledge such as pathogen infectivity and previous occurrence history, which is the job of the text mining system and the end user. Finally, we had a total of 650 news articles belonging to the reject category and 350 news articles belonging to the relevant category.

4.5 Experiments

4.5.1 Method

We used the BioCaster gold standard corpus to investigate the effect of canonical sections on the performance of classification. The experimental process was as follows. We randomly divided the data set into 10 parts. Each part has 35 articles belonging to the relevant category and 65 articles belonging to the reject category. Then, we implemented 10-fold cross-validation: nine parts for training and the remaining part for testing. For training sets we extracted canonical sections as features to build a classifier. The remaining part was used for testing. The classifier we used in this chapter is the standard naïve Bayes [20], maximum entropy (baseline maxent), and Support Vector Machine (SVM) classifiers. In the pre-processing we did not use either a stop list or word stemming. The experiments were implemented in Linux OS, using the Bow toolkit [21] for naïve Bayes and maximum entropy; and SVM^{light} [22] for SVM.

In document representation, we used bag-of-words representation for naïve Bayes, which was reported in [13] that it offers the best result compared to other methods like bag-of-nouns, bag-of-stems, bag-of-stemmed nouns. We used term frequency as term weight and linear kernel in SVM because they were reported as the best results compared to other weighting methods [23]. For section weighting we used the same section weighting methods described in [17] in which both Abstract and Introduction were set to 3 while the remaining sections were set to 1. In addition, we set the weights of both Headline and Lead sections to 3, 5, and 10 and the remaining sections to 1.

The features for training data are grouped as follows:

1. The baseline
   - Baseline: Using full-text only as the baseline method.
2. Section features
   - Head: Only the Head section is used as features, i.e., all text, NEs and NE's attributes in the Headline section.
   - Lead: Only the Lead section in headline is used as features, i.e., all text, NEs and NE's attributes in the Lead section.
   - Content: Only the Content section is used as features, i.e., all text, NEs and NE's attributes in the Content section.
   - Comment: Only the Comment section is used as features, i.e., all text, NEs and NE's attributes in the Comment section.
   - All sections: All Sections are used as features, i.e., all text, NEs and NE's attributes in the whole news article. These features are reported by Doan et al. that they achieved the best result in annotated text classification [24].

3. Summary features

   - Summary text: Only full-text in summary section is used as features, i.e., only full-text in the Summary section.
   - Summary NEs: Only NEs in summary section are used as features, i.e., only NEs and their attributes in the Summary section.
   - Summary text + NEs: Both text and NEs are used as features, i.e., all full-text, NEs and their attributes in the Summary section.

4. Features of section weights: Both text and NEs are used as features, i.e., all full-text, NEs, and their attributes in the whole news article. Of them, the Summary section is weighted as follows:

   - Summary text + NEs 3: The Summary section is set to 3, all remainings are set to 1.
   - Summary text + NEs 5: The Summary section is set to 5, all remainings are set to 1.
   - Summary text + NEs 10: The Summary section is set to 10, all remainings are set to 1.

In order to investigate some linguistic properties related to the main topic of news, we use the concept of information density described in [16] in which we define the information density of each NE in Summary as its frequency in the Headline section over the whole corpus. We will describe this in detail in Section 4.5.3.

4.5.2 Performance measures

In our experiments we use two performance measures, standard precision/recall and accuracy. Both are calculated based on the two-way contingency table shown in Table 4.1. There a is the frequency of assigned and correct cases, b is the assigned and incorrect cases, c is the none assigned but incorrect cases, and d counts the none assigned and correct cases [25]. Then,

$$\text{Precision} = a/(a+b), \text{and Recall} = a/(a+c).$$

$$\text{Accuracy and } F\text{-score are defined as accuracy} = (a+d)/(a+b+c+d),$$

$$F\text{-score} = 2 \times \text{Precision} \times \text{Recall}/(\text{Precision} + \text{Recall}).$$

Table 4.1 A Contingency Table

	YES is correct	NO is correct
Assigned YES	a	b
Assigned NO	c	d

4.5.3 Results and Discussions

The results of experiments for each algorithm are shown in Table 4.2.We next discuss the effectiveness of sections based on evaluations of algorithms, sections, NEs, and section weighting. Algorithm evaluation of the three algorithms: naïve Bayes achieved the best *F*-score with 85.60%, while SVM achieved 81.63% and MaxEnt achieved 84.15%, respectively. These confirmed the results in [13] for scientific papers. Hereafter, we will focus on the improvement in naïve Bayes.

4.5.3.1 Sections Evaluation

We now investigate the effectiveness of each section in a news article. Interestingly, we saw the Lead section achieves the best *F*-score with 85.6% using naïve Bayes. It indicates that the first sentence in a news article plays a very important role in deciding whether the news article should be alerted or not. This reflects the public health experts' comment mentioned in Section 4.3 that they can often judge the relevancy of a news article by scanning the first sentence. The contribution of each section to accuracy can be ranked in the following order: Lead > Content > All Section > Headline for naïve Bayes. However, it is not conclusive because we observed they are not consistent in SVM and MaxEnt methods in Table 4.2. We also noticed that in both naïve Bayes and SVM the highest recall achieved is 98.29 when using baseline method, which is all sections with bag-of-word representation. This suggests that the bag-of-word representation method still plays very important role in practice not only due to its simplicity but also due to its performance.

Table 4.2 Experimental Results for Three Algorithms, the Number in Each Column Indicates Accuracy, Precision/Recall and *F*-score Measures, Respectively

Features	Naïve Bayes	SVM	MaxEnt
Baseline	81.60/65.90/98.29 78.90	68.70/53.54/98.29 69.32	81.70/86.15/56.86 68.51
Headline	84.00/82.31/69.14 75.15	84.50/75.47/84.57 79.76	79.70/80.48/55.43 65.65
Lead	88.90/78.38/94.29 85.60	77.20/61.62/98.86 75.92	77.70/86.71/42.86 57.36
Content	87.90/75.28/97.43 84.93	85.80/81.46/78.29 79.84	88.70/83.57/84.29 83.93
Comments	85.60/71.55/97.71 82.61	76.40/60.97/100.0 75.75	85.20/82.58/73.14 77.57
All sections	88.10/80.00/88.10 83.85	86.40/84.36/75.71 79.80	73.10/90.10/26.00 40.35
Summary text only	54.60/43.50/99.43 60.52	40.00/36.85/100.0 53.86	59.10/45.99/96.57 62.31
Summary NEs only	82.70/71.64/83.71 77.21	82.30/67.88/96.57 79.72	81.10/74.47/69.43 72.00
Summary text + Nes	88.40/78.40/92.29 84.78	84.50/71.47/95.14 81.63	84.70/86.35/66.86 75.37
Summary text + NEs 3	88.20/76.01/96.86 85.18	81.20/81.92/60.86 69.84	89.00/84.88/83.43 84.15
Summary text + NEs 5	88.30/76.66/95.71 85.13	75.00/80.66/37.14 50.87	88.00/84.34/80.29 82.27
Summary text + NEs 10	88.50/77.91/93.71 85.08	68.20/75.40/12.29 21.13	87.70/86.03/77.43 81.50

4.5.3.2 NE Evaluation

Now we consider the effect of NEs in the "top sections" (Summary NEs only) on classification accuracy. We can see that using NEs in Summary have comparable *F*-score to Headline for three algorithms (77.21% vs. 75.15% for naïve Bayes, 79.72% vs. 79.76% for SVM, and 72.0% vs. 65.65.% for maximum entropy).

Looking at the distribution of NEs, we recognize the distinctive tendencies between NEs. Ignoring general NEs like PERSON, LOCATION, ORGANIZATION, TIME, we observed that there are big differences in NEs: NEs that tend to be the relevant category (relevant NEs) while their frequency in the relevant category is much higher than the reject category. Also, NEs tend to be the reject category (irrelevant NEs) while their frequency in the relevant category is much lower than the reject category. The list of relevant NEs are DISEASE, CONDITION, OUTBREAK, VIRUS, SYMPTOM and irrelevant NEs are NONHUMAN, CONTROL, ANATOMY, PRODUCT, BACTERIA, CHEMICAL, PROTEIN, DNA, RNA.

Through this analysis we can see some interesting properties related to linguistic properties of the text. First, the relevant category contains articles about the name of infectious diseases (DISEASE, OUTBREAK) or situations of diseases like conditions, symptoms, or virus cases the disease; secondly, the relevant category contains articles about entities that are not directly related to diseases like proteins, DNA, RNA, drug products. Furthermore, the existence of NONHUMAN and BACTERIA in irrelevant category also indicated about the information of "species": documents that are not directly related to people should not belong to the relevant category.

4.5.3.3 Section Weighting Evaluation

Now we consider the effect of section weighting on performance. We can easily see that the top section, i.e., Summary, achieved high performance. The *F*-score of both algorithms naïve Bayes and maximum entropy are higher than the baseline when using section information. In practice, we observed that SVM does not work well in section weighting: when the weights are set to greater values, the recall tends to drop significantly. We also saw that using section weighting achieved more stable and higher results for both naïve Bayes and maximum entropy. The results suggested that Summary section achieved the highest performance when it is weighted to 3.

4.6 Conclusions

This chapter has focused on analyzing the contribution of section information to the automatic classification of news articles related to disease outbreaks. The experimental results indicated that:

1. Top sections within news, i.e., Headline and Lead play an important role in deciding the main topic of the news.

2. All section with bag-of-word representation (full text) achieves the highest recall.
3. Using section weighting can improve the performance of text classification.

In the future we will investigate automatic algorithms for identifying main sections within news articles based on their contributions to the main topic.

References

1. Public Health Agency of Canada. Global Public Heath Intelligence Network (GPHIN), 2004. http://www.gphin.org.
2. International Society for Infectious Diseases. ProMed Mail, 2001. http://www. promed-mail.org.
3. Sebastiani F. Machine learning in automated text categorization. ACM computing survey, 2002:34(1):1–47.
4. Yang Y, Liu X. A re-examination of text categorization methods. In Proc. of 22th SIGIR, ACM International Conference on Research and Development in Information Retrieval, 1999:42–49.
5. Kudo T, Matsumoto Y. A boosting algorithm for classification of semistructured text. In Proceedings of the 2004 Conference on Empirical Methods in NLP, 2004:301–308.
6. Zaki MJ, Aggarwal CC. XRules: an effective structural classifier for XML data. In Proceedings of the ninth ACM SIGKDD International Conference, 2003:316–325.
7. Bloehdorn S, Hotho A. Boosting for text classification with semantic features. In Proceedings of the Workshop on Mining for and from the Semantic Web at the 10th ACM SIGKDD 2004, 2004:70–87.
8. Frürnkranz J, Mitchell T, Riloff E. A case study in using linguistic phrases for text categorization on the WWW. In Working Notes of the AAAI/ICML Workshop on Learning for Text Categorization, 1998:5–13.
9. Hotho A, Staab S, Stumme G. WordNet improves text document clustering. In Proceedings of the SIGIR 2003 Semantic Web Workshop 2003, 2003.
10. Scott S, Matwin S. Feature engineering for text classification. In Proceedings of International Conference on Machine Learning 1999, 1999:379–388.
11. van Dijk TA. Structures of news in the press. In: Discourse and Communication. Berlin: De Gruyter, 1985:69–93.
12. Mizuta Y, Collier N. Zone identification in biology articles as a basis for information extraction. In Proceedings of Natural Language Processing in Biomedicine and Its Applications (JNLPBA) 2004, 2004:29–35.
13. Sinclair G, Webber B. Classification from fulltext: A comparison of canonical sections of scientific papers. In Proceedings of Natural Language Processing in Biomedicine and Its Applications (JNLPBA) 2004, 2004:66–69.
14. Yetisgen-Yildiz M, Pratt W. The effect of feature representation on MEDLINE document classification. In AMIA Annu Symp Proc., 2005:849–853.
15. Shah PK, Perez-Iratxeta C, Bork P, Andrade MA. Information extraction from fulltext scientific articles: where are the keywords? BMC Bioinformatics 2003;4(1):20.
16. Schuemie MJ, Weeber M, Schijvenaars BJA, van Mulligen EM, van der Eijik CC, Jellier R, Mons B, Kors JA. Distribution of information in biomedical abstracts and full text publications. Bioinformatics 2004;20:2597–2604.
17. Hakenberg J, Rutsch J, Leser U. Tuning text classification for hereditary diseases with section weighting. In Proceedings of the First International Symposium on Semantic Mining in Biomedicine (SMBM), 2005:34–37.
18. Kawazoe A, Jin L, Shigematsu M, Barrero R, Taniguchi K, Collier N. The development of a schema for the annotation of terms in the BioCaster disease detection/tracking system. In

Proceedings of the International Workshop on Biomedical Ontology in Action (KR-MED 2006), 2006:77–85.
19. World Health Organization. ICD10, International Statistical Classification of Diseases and Related Health Problems, Tenth Revision, 2004.
20. Mitchell TM. Machine Learning. Mc Graw Hill, 1997.
21. McCallum AK. Bow: A toolkit for statistical language modeling, text retrieval, classification and clustering, 1996. http://www.cs.cmu.edu/_mccallum/bow.
22. Joachims T. Making large-scale SVM Learning Practical. In: Sch¨olkopf B, Burges C, Smola A, eds., Advances in Kernel Methods – Support VectorLearning. Cambridge: MIT Press, 1999.
23. Aronson AR, Bodenreider O, Demner-Fushman D, Fung KW, Lee VK, Mork JG, Neveol A, Peters L, Rogers WJ. From indexing the biomedical literature to coding clinical text: experience with MTI and machine learning approaches. In Proceeding of ACL Workshop on BioNLP 2007: Biological, Translation and clinical language processing, 2007:105–112.
24. Doan S, Kawazoe A, Collier N. The role of roles in classifying annotated biomedical text. In Proceeding of ACL Workshop on BioNLP 2007: Biological, Translation and clinical language processing, Prague, Czech, 2007:17–24.
25. Yang Y. An evaluation of statistical approaches to text categorization. Inf Ret J 1999;1:69–90.

Chapter 5
A Web-Based Application to Exchange Ophthalmologic Health Records Using Open-Source Databases

Isabel de la Torre Díez, Roberto Hornero Sánchez, Miguel López Coronado, María Isabel López Gálvez, and Beatriz Sainz Abajo

Abstract Electronic Health Record (EHR) refers to an individual patient's medical record in digital format. Several models of standardization for EHR exchange have been proposed and multiple organizations formed to help evaluate and implement them. In this chapter, we present a web-based application (TeleOftalWeb) to store and exchange EHR and fundus photographs. We apply Health Level 7/Clinical Document Architecture (HL7/CDA) Release One and Digital Imaging and Communications in Medicine (DICOM) standards. It has been built on Java Servlet and Java Server Pages (JSP) technologies. EHR and fundus photographs are stored in an open-source database, eXist. Its architecture is triple-layered. The application verifies the standards related to privacy and confidentiality. Data transmissions were carried over encrypted Internet connections such as HyperText Transfer Protocol over SSL (HTTPS).

Keywords: Diabetic Retinopathy · Digital Imaging and Communications in Medicine (DICOM) · Electronic Health Record (EHR) · Extensible Markup Language (XML) · Health Level 7/Clinical Document Architecture (HL7/CDA) · Java

Terms and Definitions

HTTPS HyperText Transport Protocol Secure. It is the protocol for accessing a secure web server. Using HTTPS in the URL instead of HTTP directs the message to a secure port number rather than the default web port number of 80.

ISO International Standardization Organization. It is a worldwide federation of national standards bodies. The work of preparing International Standards is normally carried out through ISO technical committees.

I. de la Torre Díez (✉)
Department of Signal Theory and Communications, University of Valladolid, Campus Miguel Delibes, s/n, 47011 – Valladolid, Spain
e-mail: isator@tel.uva.es

A. Lazakidou (ed.), *Web-Based Applications in Healthcare and Biomedicine*,
Annals of Information Systems 7, DOI 10.1007/978-1-4419-1274-9_5,
© Springer Science+Business Media, LLC 2010

Java It is an object-oriented applications programming language developed by Sun Microsystems in the early 1990s. Java applications are typically compiled to bytecode, although compilation to native machine code is also possible. The language itself derives much of its syntax from C and C++ but has a simpler object model and fewer low-level facilities.

JDBC Java Database Connectivity. It is an API for the Java programming language that defines how a client may access a database. It provides methods for querying and updating data in a database.

JPEG Joint Photographic Experts Group. JPEG is a lossy compression technique for colour images. Although it can reduce files sizes to about 5% of their normal size, some detail is lost in the compression.

JSP Java Server Pages: It is a Java technology that allows software developers to dynamically generate HTML, XML or other types of documents in response to a web client request. The JSP syntax adds additional XML-like tags, called JSP actions, to be used to invoke the functionality. It lets you separate the dynamic part of your pages from the static HTML.

PDF Portable Document Format. It is a file format developed by Adobe Systems. PDF captures formatting information from a variety of desktop publishing applications, making it possible to send formatted documents and have them appear on the recipient's monitor or printer as they were intended.

SSL Secure Sockets Layer, a protocol developed by Netscape for transmitting private documents via the Internet. SSL uses a cryptographic system that uses two keys to encrypt data, a public key known to everyone and a private or secret key known only to the recipient of the message.

XML Extensible Markup Language is a general-purpose specification for creating custom markup languages. It is classified as an extensible language, because it allows the user to define the mark-up elements. XML purpose is to aid information systems in sharing structured data, especially via Internet.

XSL-FO Extensible Stylesheet Language Formatting Objects. It is a markup language for XML document formatting, which is most often used to generate PDF. XSL-FO is part of XSL, a set of W3C technologies designed for the transformation and formatting of XML data.

XSLT Extensible Style Language Transformation, the language used in XSL style sheets to transform XML documents into other XML documents. An XSL processor reads the XML document and follows the instructions in the XSL style sheet, then it outputs a new XML document or XML-document fragment.

5.1 Introduction

The information systems are a necessary part of the telemedicine services. They provide storage, retrieval, connection and evaluation of the medical information. Moreover, they administrate all the medical data about a patient [1]. One of these systems is the Electronic Patient Record (EPR). An EPR is a fundamental part of health information technology and its use is growing quickly. It is indicative of the advances in medical informatics and facilitates the doctor–patient relationship. It can be organized either on a document-based backbone or on a structured database system. An EPR transmitted through the Internet is especially important. It contains a private material of medical information for a patient. Electronic records in health fall under the purview of health informatics. It is a combination of computation, computer science and medical record keeping. Recent technological advances have enabled the introduction of a great number of telemedicine applications in healthcare computing [2].

In most European countries, the National Health Service (NHS) is investing large amounts in information technology (IT) [3]. In this context, the idea of Electronic Health Records (EHR) has been around for a decade or more [4]. EHR is a secure, real-time, point-of-care and patient-centric information resource for physicians. EHR must enable the communication of healthcare information to support shared patient care, improved quality of care and effective resource utilisation. EHR may contain data about medical referrals, medical treatments, medications and their application, demographic information and other non-clinical administrative information. Some benefits of the EHR systems are their universal access, coding efficiency and efficacy, easier and quicker navigation through the patient record [5]. In spite of the advantages of EHR, there are several barriers to their adoption such as training, costs, complexity and lack of a national standard for interoperability [6].

Many EHR-related initiatives have been announced in Canada. In May 2006, the government of British Columbia announced spending of $150 million towards the creation of online computerized medical records for doctors [7]. EHR-related initiatives are under way and each addresses a specific part of health care, primary, acute and community care. For example, the Ontario Primary Care Network in Canada is a pilot project involving approximately 40 physicians and 300,000 patients. Individual physicians are implementing office systems for the capture of patient information and support office administration. Community care providers are piloting projects to improve the delivery of services to their customers [8].

Nowadays, telemedicine applications often involve many institutions using different systems and technologies. This complicates the necessary technical standardization [9]. International and national institutions and organizations are concerned with the standardization of EHR systems such as, CEN Technical Committee (CEN/TC) 251, ISO Health Informatics Standards Technical Committee (ISO/TC 215), openEHR, Health Level 7 (HL7), Integrating the Healthcare Enterprise (IHE), Digital Imaging and Communication in Medicine (DICOM) to name but a few [10].

CEN/TC 251 is the body within Europe mandated to develop standards for health informatics. It is a workgroup within the European Union working on standardization in the field of Health ICT. The goal is to achieve compatibility and interoperability between independent systems and to enable modularity in EHR systems.

ISO/TC 215 has defined the EHR and also produced a technical specification ISO 18308 describing the requirements for EHR architectures. It provides standardization in the field of information for health. It ensures compatibility of data for comparative statistical purposes and to reduce duplication of effort and redundancies.

OpenEHR is the next-generation public specifications and implementations for EHR systems and communication, based on a complete separation of software and clinical models. It is dedicated to the development of an open, interoperable health computing platform, where a major component is clinically effective and interoperable EHR. It does this by researching clinical requirements and creating specifications and implementations.

IHE is an initiative to integrate existing standards into a comprehensive best practice solution. It does not create new standards, but rather drives the adoption of standards to address specific clinical needs.

HL7 is a not-for-profit organization involved in development of international healthcare standards. It is used for many different medical environments. HL7 Document is intended to be the basic unit of a document-oriented EPR. The patient medical record is represented as a collection of documents. The HL7 standard defines the message, segment, field, etc. The HL7 Clinical Document Architecture (CDA) is an extensible markup language (XML)-based document markup standard that specifies the structure and semantics of clinical documents for the purpose of exchange.

In order to HL7 standard, there are mobile clinical information systems by using HL7 to integrate the patient data [11], EHR applications in different medicine areas such as oncology [12] and emergency departments [13].

DICOM is a cooperative standard. It was developed from 1990 to 1996, mainly by the American College of Radiology (ACR) National Electrical Manufacturers Association (NEMA) committee in the United States, with contributions from European standardization organizations, the Japanese Industry Radiology Apparatus (JIRA), the IEEE, HL7 and ANSI as well as from European manufacturers and societies. The goal of the DICOM Standard is to achieve compatibility and improve workflow efficiency between imaging systems and other information systems in healthcare environments worldwide. This standard allows the exchange of medical images and related information between systems from different manufacturers. One of the DICOM advantages is that only a part of the defined keys are specified [14].

In ophthalmology, the diabetic retinopathy is one of the major causes of blindness among the people. According to World Health Organization (WHO), diabetic retinopathy is considered to be the result of vascular changes in the retinal circulation. In the early stages, vascular occlusion and dilations occur. It progresses into a proliferative retinopathy with the growth of new blood vessels. Many approaches are proposed by the authors to automate and detect the presence of diabetic retinopathy in fundus images [15]. The evaluation of digital images allows the diabetic retinopathy to diagnose. In this chapter, we present a web-based application, TeleOftalWeb, to store and exchange ophthalmologic EHR and fundus images by using XML and Java technologies. We employ EHR systems specifications as HL7/CDA and ISO/TC 215. Thanks to the use of XML-based technologies and HL7 specifications, this application allows the EHR standardization. It ensures interoperability among different applications and institutions.

We have designed, developed and evaluated a web-based application to store and exchange EHR in ophthalmology, TeleOftalWeb. We apply HL7/CDA Release One and DICOM standards. EHR and fundus photographs are stored in XML native database, eXist. Its architecture is triple-layered. The application server is Tomcat 5.5.9. The application is platform-independent, thanks to using XML and Java technologies. TeleOftalWeb provides a telemedicine service, EHR and fundus images in different formats. It manages a database with information about patients and their eyes' fundus photographs. Moreover, it allows the images visualization and processing. Any specialist may access their records immediately and see medical images. For security, all data transmissions were carried over encrypted Internet connections such as Secure Sockets Layer (SSL) and HyperText Transfer Protocol over SSL (HTTPS). The application verifies the standards related to privacy and confidentiality. It has been tested by ophthalmologists from the University Institute of Applied Ophthalmobiology (IOBA), Spain. *Currently, more than 1000 health records and 2000 fundus photographs have been included.*

5.2 System Overview

5.2.1 Application Architecture

TeleOftalWeb has been built on Java Servlet and Java Server Pages (JSP) technologies. The EHR and medical images are stored in the native XML database, eXist. Its architecture is a typical three-layered with two database servers (relational and native XML), one application server and a thin client. Figure 5.1 shows the application architecture. The client application consists of an interface based on JSP

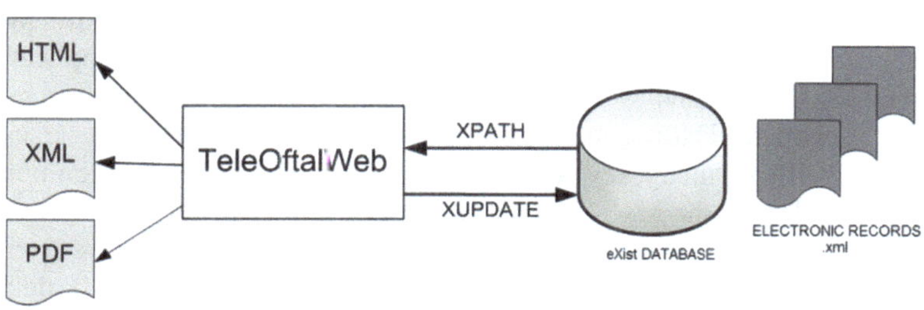

Fig. 5.1 Application architecture

running on the web server. The server application communicates with the databases to retrieve data. *The application is platform-independent, thanks to use XML and Java Technologies.* In communication with the native XML database, we used the languages XPath and XUpdate. XPath is employed to find information in an XML document. It models an XML document as a tree of nodes. There are different types of nodes, including element nodes, attribute nodes and text nodes. The primary purpose of XPath is to address parts of an XML document. XUpdate makes heavy use of XPath for selecting a set of nodes to modify or remove. XUpdate is a simple XML update language. XUpdate is a pure descriptive language that is designed with references to the definition of XSL Transformations (XSLT).

The development environment was NetBeans IDE 4.1 of Sun Microsystems. The IDE runs on many platforms including Windows, Linux, Solaris and the MacOS. Java was the basis application programming language. We included all tools and Application Programming Interface (API) as Javascript, JSP, Java Servlets and Java Database Connectivity (JDBC). Combining Java and XML leads to the attractive dual portability of code and data. Wherever Java programs can run, they can also access XML information. This enables Java and XML information to interoperate efficiently and effectively on different platforms [16].

The users can access and retrieve medical information and images through web browsers such as Mozilla Firefox, Microsoft Internet Explorer and others. EHR can be displayed in the following formats: portable document format (PDF), hypertext markup language (HTML) and XML. The medical records and the images can be viewed in this portable format. The users can view and store Joint Photographic Experts Group (JPEG), DICOM and other type of images in the user module. *For security, all data transmissions were carried over encrypted Internet connections such as Secure Sockets Layer (SSL) and HyperText Transfer Protocol over SSL (HTTPS).*

5.2.2 Data Modelling

We chose free open-source database servers. For the manager module, we used a relational database to store the personal and authentication data. The database manager was MySQL Server 5.0 with the Connector/J-3.1.11. MySQL is a multi-threaded, multi-user and SQL relational database Server (RDBMS). In the MySQL database, we stored all the user data and access information to web application. It has two tables: "users" and "permissions". The table "users" contains personal user data. The user identification, user name, password and user type appear in table "permissions". The primary key is the same in both tables (identification number). The data modelling in the MySQL database is shown in Fig. 5.2.

An XML database is a data persistence software system that allows data to be imported, accessed and exported in the XML format. There are two XML databases classes: XML-enabled and native XML. The first one maps all XML to a traditional database (such as a relational database), accepting XML as input and rendering

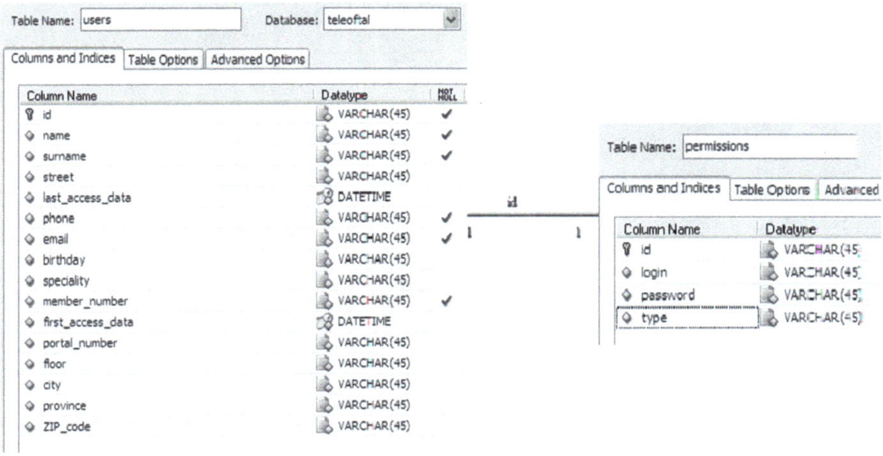

Fig. 5.2 User data modelling in MySQL database

XML as output. The native XML database has an internal model that depends on XML and uses XML documents as the fundamental unit of storage.

We applied a native open-source XML database, eXist 1.1.1, to manage and store the EHR and medical images. The Java servlet inserts the record into the eXist database. It stores and indexes collections of XML documents in both native and mapped forms for highly efficient querying, transformation and retrieval. The EHRs are stored in eXist database (see Fig. 5.5) according to the ANSI/HL7 CDA Release One template. CDA distinguishes three different levels of granularity, where each level iteratively adds more markup to clinical documents although the clinical content remains constant at all levels [17].

The scope of the CDA is the standardization of clinical documents for exchange. A HL7/CDA structure may include texts, sounds, pictures and all kind of multimedia contents. It can refer to external documents, procedures, observations and acts. It includes information about authors, authenticators, custodians, participants, patients and so on [18].

The XML-based architecture described in the CDA Release One standard has been used to define the health information format. Thanks to the use of XML-based technologies and HL7 specifications, our application fulfils the EHR standards. Its development methodology is a continuously evolving process that seeks to carry out specifications that facilitate interoperability between healthcare systems. EHR with fundus photographs are stored in eXist database according to the HL7/CDA Release One template. In Fig. 5.3, CDA Header in an EHR in TeleOftalWeb is showed. The CDA Header identifies and classifies the document and provides information on the document authenticator, the patient, the encounter, the provider and other service actors. Document-related information includes the id, set id, version, type and various timestamps. The id element uniquely identifies the specific clinical document. The type and version elements identify the clinical document template. Encounter

```
<clinical_document_header>
<id EX="9a4e9e2d.xml" RT="TeleOftaWeb3.2"/>
<document_type_cd V="11488-4" S="LOINC" DN="Consultation note"/>
<origination_dttm V="2008-10-27"/>
<originator>
    <originator.type_cd V="AUT"/>
        <participation_tmr V="2008-10-27"/>
        <person>
        <id EX="11" RT="TeleOftaWeb3.2"/>
        </person>
</originator>
<provider>
        <provider.type_cd V="CON"/>
        <person>
        <id EX="11" RT="TeleOftaWeb3.2"/>
        </person>
</provider>
<patient>
        <patient.type_cd V="PATSBJ"/>
        <person>
        <id EX="8" RT="TeleOftaWeb3.2"/>
                <person_name>
          <nm>
            <GIV V="1"/>
                                  <FAM V="1"/>
                        </nm>
                </person_name>
                <addr>
          <STR V="dsaf"/>
                        <HNR V="8"/>
                        <ADL V="8"/>
                        <CTY V="dsfadsf"/>
                <STA V="sdafas"/>
                <ZIP V="8"/>
                <CNT V="EspaÃ±a"/>
                </addr>
                <phon V="888888888"/>
                <local_header descriptor="email">xxx@x.es</local_header>
        </person>
        <birth_dttm V="1988-01-11"/>
        <administrative_gender_cd V="M" S="2.16.840.1.113883.5.1"/>
        <local_header descriptor="numeroSS">8</local_header>
</patient>
<local_header descriptor="compartidos">
        <local_header descriptor="person">
                <local_attr name="V" value="11"/>
                <local_attr name="type" value="owner"/>
        </local_header>
      <local_header descriptor="person">
<local_attr name="V" value="354642123"/>
<local_attr name="type" value="shared"/>
</local_header>
</local_header>
 </clinical_document_header>
```


Fig. 5.3 CDA Header in the application

data include the id, code, timestamps, service location and local header. The id and code elements uniquely identify the relevant encounter and its type in the regional network, while attribute-value pairs in the local header facilitate interoperability with the EHR system.

Moreover, Extensible Stylesheet Language Formatting Objects (XSL-FO) was used to format XML data. XSL-FO is a complete XML vocabulary for laying out text on a page. An XSL-FO document is a well-formed XML document that uses this vocabulary. One of the EHR output formats is a PDF. It is a necessary process to get from a XML document to a PDF printable document. First, the XML must be fed to an XSLT processor with an appropriate stylesheet in order to produce another XML document which uses the XSL-FO namespace. It is intended for an XSL-FO formatter. The second stage is to feed the output of the first stage to the XSL-FO formatter that can produce a printable document styled for visual presentation.

The body of the clinical document consists of section elements. Sections correspond to reusable XML fragments. Each CDA section may contain CDA structures such as paragraph, list and table elements, nested CDA sections, or coded_entry elements. CDA structures contain CDA "entries" such as content, link, coded_entry and local_markup. Sections including only a link are used to refer to external multimedia objects. In Fig. 5.4, we can see the EHR body structure in TeleOftalWeb. CDA

```
<section>
        <caption>FiliaciÃ³n</caption>
            <paragraph>
        <content>
        <local_markup descriptor="patient">
                <local_markup descriptor="person">
                <local_markup descriptor="id">8</local_markup>
                <local_markup descriptor="person_name">
                <local_markup descriptor="nm">
                <local_markup descriptor="GIV">1</local_markup>
                <local_markup descriptor="FAM">1</local_markup>
                </local_markup>
                </local_markup>
                <local_markup descriptor="addr">
                <local_markup descriptor="STR">dsaf</local_markup>
                <local_markup descriptor="HNR">8</local_markup>
                <local_markup descriptor="ADL">8</local_markup>
                <local_markup descriptor="CTY">dsfadsf</local_markup>
                <local_markup descriptor="STA">sdafas</local_markup>
                <local_markup descriptor="ZIP">8</local_markup>
                <local_markup descriptor="CNT">EspaÃ±a</local_markup>
                </local_markup>
                <local_markup descriptor="phon">888888888</local_markup>
                <local_markup descriptor="email">asdfa@yahoo.es</local_markup>
                </local_markup>
                <local_markup descriptor="birth_dttm">1988-01-11</local_markup>
                <local_markup descriptor="administrative_gender_cd">M</local_markup>
                <local_markup descriptor="numeroSS">8</local_markup>
                </local_markup>

        </content>
        </paragraph>
</section>
```

Fig. 5.4 Structure of the body in the EHR

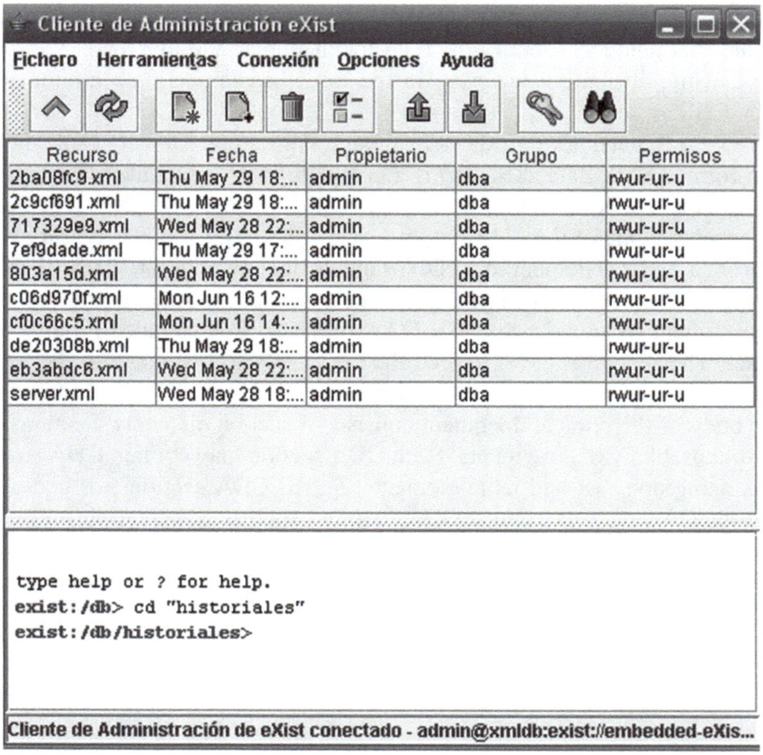

Fig. 5.5 Manager interface in eXist database

<body> occurs in the <levelone> element. A <section> has an optional <caption>, followed by nested <section> elements or structures, followed by optionally repeating <coded_entry> elements.

Fundus photographs in any digital format are introduced in the EHR template. Physicians can view, store and manage them. For example, DICOM images are converted into JPEG images. We developed a software tool to convert DICOM images into JPEG. Then, they are encoded in Base64 to be stored in eXist database according to HL7/CDA Release One standard.

5.3 Results

We present the two application modules: manager and user. Then, we describe the experience of introducing diabetic patient's health records from a screening program of diabetic retinopathy in a rural area of Spain [19].

5.3.1 Application Manager Module

The manager module interface is shown in Fig. 5.6. The manager can access to the web platform. Manager has to introduce the login and password. Figure 5.7 shows

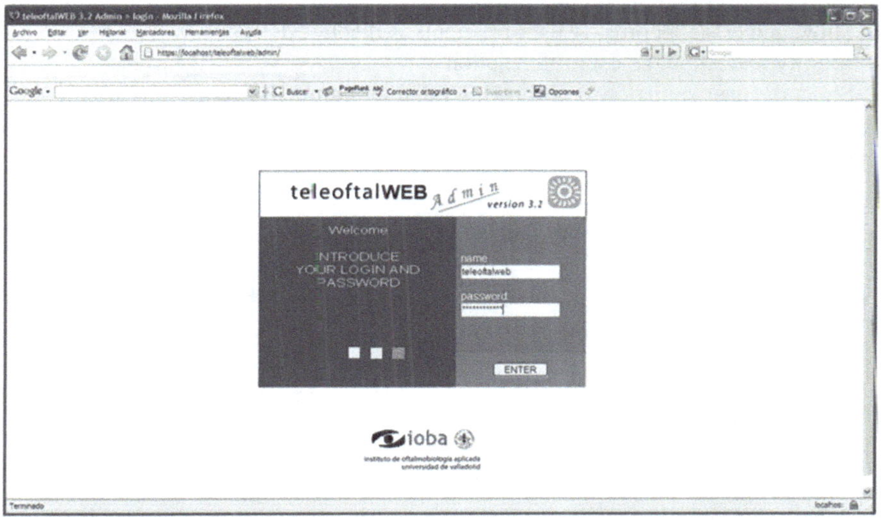

Fig. 5.6 Manager module

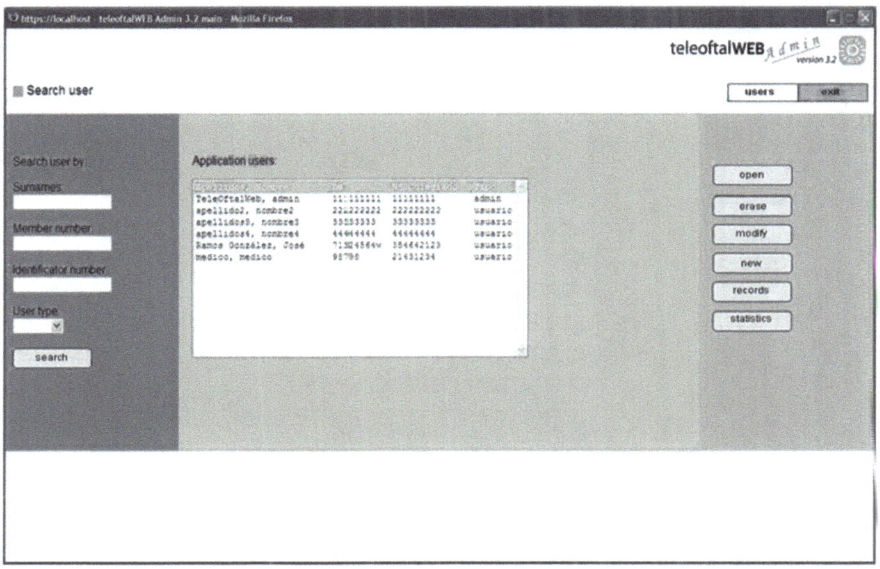

Fig. 5.7 Users in the application

the application users. The two user roles are: manager and user. The application manager can do the following actions:

- Create users. The manager has to introduce the following compulsory information: surname, name, identification number, member number, phone, e-mail, specialty, user type, login and password.
- Show and erase records. A list of patients is displayed.
- Modify and show the user information.
- Show the user statistics. It is showing the total number of records by users.
- Search users by different criteria such as surname, identification number, type of user and member number.

5.3.2 Application User Module

The authorized users can access to this module. They have their login and password. The users can do the following actions:

- Create new records (see Fig. 5.8). They have to introduce the necessary data: patient affiliation information, patient precedents, medical exploration and diagnostic. The affiliation information is always necessary to complete the record.
- Erase records.
- Search revisions.
- Create new revisions in a record.

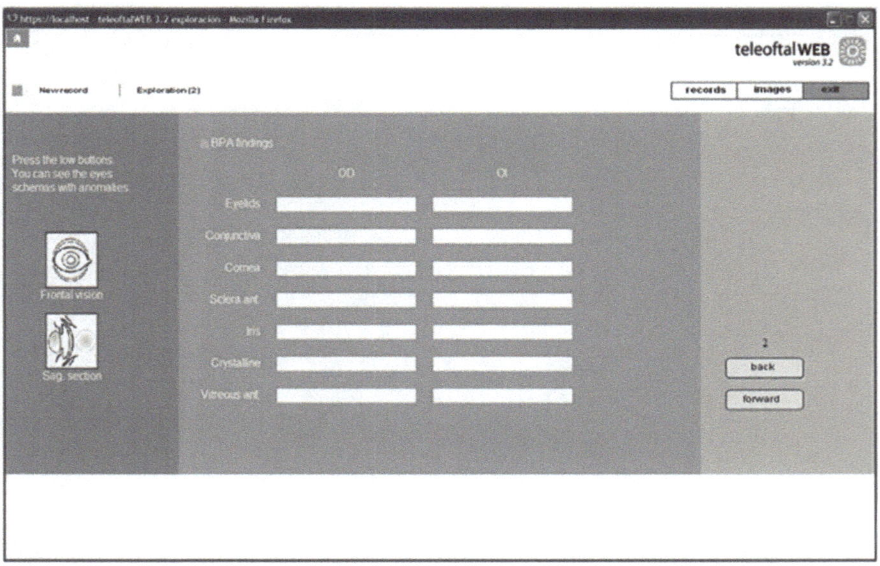

Fig. 5.8 Create a new record

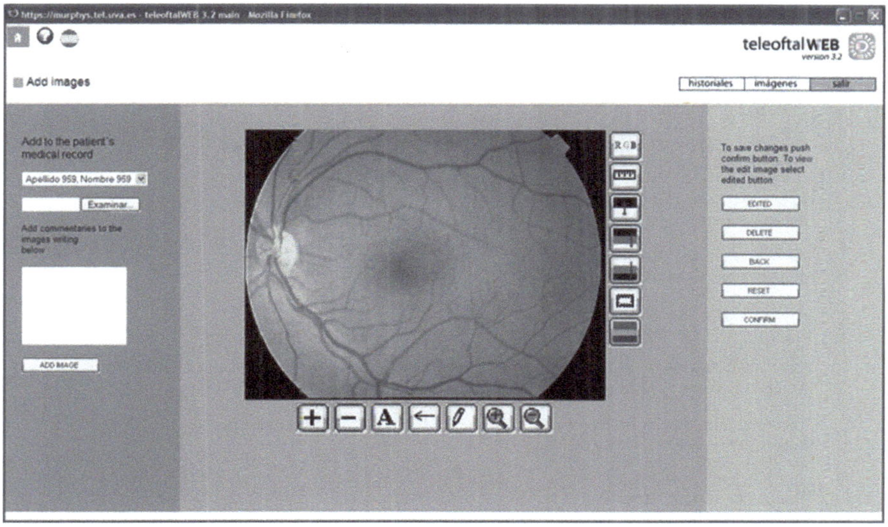

Fig. 5.9 Images editor

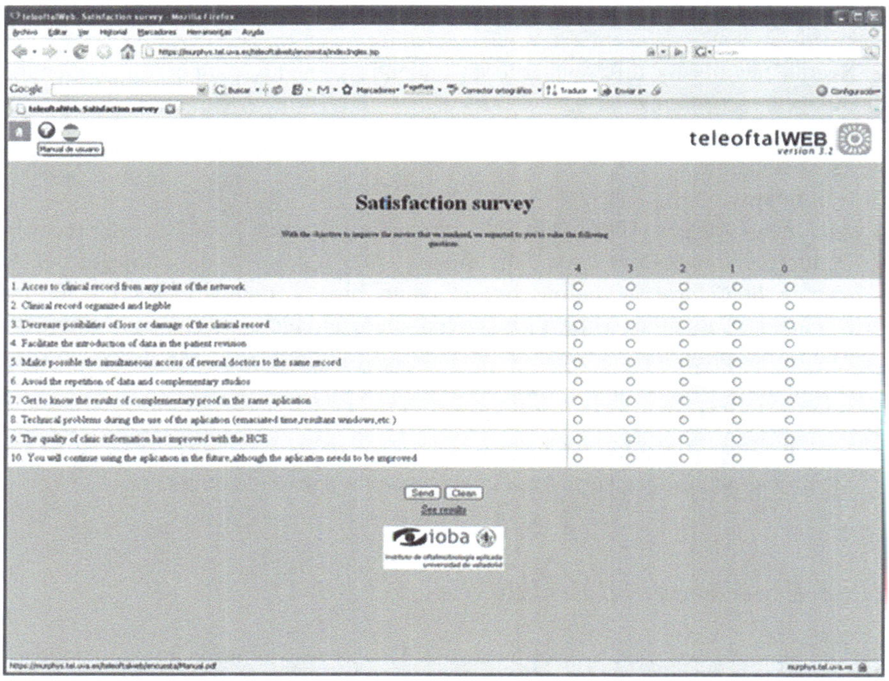

Fig. 5.10 Web usability survey

Questions\Physicians	1	2	3	4	5	6
Access to clinical record from any point of the network	4	4	4	4	4	4
Clinical record organised and legible	3	4	4	3	4	4
Decrease possibilities of loss or damage of the clinical record	3	4	4	4	3	3
Facilitate the introduction of data in the patient revision	3	3	3	4	3	4
Make possible the simultaneous access of several physicians to the same record	4	3	3	3	4	4
Avoid the repetition of data and complementary studies	4	4	4	4	4	4
Get to know the results of complementary proof in the same application	4	4	4	4	4	2
Technical problems during the use of the application (emaciated time, resultant windows, etc.)	2	2	1	2	2	4
The quality of clinic information has improved with the EHR	2	2	2	2	2	2
You will continue using the application in the future, although the application needs to be improved	4	4	3	4	4	4
SUS score	67.5	75	67.5	80	80	75

Fig. 5.11 Survey results

- Search records by different criteria: patient's surname, patient's identification number, record creation date and record origin. The user can share the records with other application users.
- Erase revisions.
- Edit images.
- Add new images (JPEG, DICOM and others formats) in different records. Figure 5.9 shows this action. The images editor allows to show images and to change their shape and colour, to make them bigger or smaller. The images can be changed into other colours (red, green, blue) and the users can add comments. The reset option allows the users to see the original image. The users can keep the modified images in the XML native database.
- Erase images in the records.
- Search images in different formats according to the following criteria: image identification number, surnames, image creation date and comments.

5.3.3 Experience and Evaluation

The application was used by six physicians. The process to introduce each patient's record with two DICOM and JPEG fundus photographs in the system was around 10 min. More than 1000 EHR are introduced in the system.

Our application allows to store and exchange all the records and fundus photographs. Physicians used the application with different web browsers to store and exchange EHR. In each record there are the following parts: anamnesis, exploration, diagnosis and treatment. The EHR is associated with the fundus photographs in all type of digital formats.

A web survey with ten questions about the application usability was done (see Fig. 5.10). We used System Usability Scale (SUS) to make the questionnaires. It is a Likert scale. SUS has proved to be a valuable evaluation tool, being robust and reliable. It correlates well with other subjective measures of usability [20]. The SUS score is more than 50 for all the physicians. Its average value is 74. The questions such as clinical records are organized and legible, access to EHR from any place, information quality in the application were strongly agreed. The results can be viewed in Fig. 5.11. According to these results, our web-based application is useful for the physicians because SUS score is always more than 50. All physicians who used the application can access to EHR from any point of the network.

5.4 Discussions and Conclusion

A web-based application has been developed and evaluated to store and exchange EHR and fundus photographs in ophthalmology using HL7/CDA and XML technologies. The EHR system facilitates new interfaces between care and research environments, leading to great improvements in the scope and efficiency of research. The EHR in our application contains information about patient affiliation information, patient precedents, medical exploration and diagnostic.

We apply XML and Java technologies to interoperate efficiently and effectively on different web platforms. The extensive use of HL7/CDA standard is desirable, not only in cardiology environment but also for all fields present in medicine [21]. We apply it in an ophthalmologic application. There are several EHR applications in different medicine areas such as oncology and emergency departments. In the telematic system for oncology [12], they use a data warehouse as EPR server. The authors do not present a standardization process for the EHR. In our application, we applied EHR standards. The information system designed for emergency department [13] has been implemented by prototyping a web-based. It is a multi-platform and multi-user system, using the Java programming language. There are few standards for modern-day electronic records systems as a whole; there are many standards relating to specific aspects of EHR. The standards differ in the progress achieved in the standardization process; each of the content formats seems to be suitable for implementing EHR.

There are important barriers in the EHR adoption such as the lack of national information standards and code sets. Moreover, the lack of available funding and interoperability can be presented. We treat to solve some of these problems to the EHR adoption in ophthalmology.

The main advantages of this application are adaptation to the standard HL7/CDA, facilitating the interoperability between institutions and applications. Moreover, the transactions are secure. The web-based application allows to improve data access for patient data management. The physicians can analyze the patient records from everywhere. They only need a computer with Internet. Physicians can detect one of the most important eye diseases between diabetic people, the diabetic retinopathy. It is the most common diabetic eye disease and a leading cause of blindness in adults. It is caused by changes in the blood vessels of the retina.

According to our review, we analysed several studies about EHR systems. These systems have been presented using XML-based clinical document architecture to exchange discharge summaries [22]. There are EHR applications in different specialties such as pediatric [23], ophthalmology [24], emergency departments and oncology [12]. In the telematic system for oncology, they use a data warehouse as EPR server. The authors do not present an EHR standardization process. Information system for emergency department has been implemented by prototyping a web-based application. It makes uses the XML-based openEHR standard. Moreover, DICOM is also used in other image-related medical fields, such as pathology, endoscopy, dentistry, ophthalmology and dermatology. Its wide availability is central for implementing the EHR [25]. The DICOM Structured Report (SR) is the diagnostic report that encodes the interpretation and the impressions of the physician. The information contained in a SR is grouped into nine information modules. Those modules contain all the information needed to identify the patient, the study and the series in which the document is contained.

In summary, we have designed, developed and evaluated a web-based application to store and share EHR in ophthalmology by using HL7/CDA and DICOM standards. The records and the fundus photographs in all type of formats are continuously updated and are available concurrently for use everywhere. We verified that the application was useful for the physicians.

References

1. Horsch A, Balbach T. Telemedical information systems. IEEE Trans Inf Technol Biomed 1999;3(3):166–175.
2. Hung K, Zhang Y. Implementation of a WAP-based telemedicine system for patient monitoring. IEEE Trans Inf Technol Biomed 2003;7(2):101–107.
3. Mocanu ML, Dorobantu M, Mocanu C, Burdescu D. A distributed database system for glaucoma monitoring. Eur J Biomed Inform 2004;50–58.
4. Ferreira A, Correia R, Antunes L, Palhares E, Marques P, Costa P, da Costa Pereira A. Integrity for electronic patient record reports. Proceedings of the 17th IEEE Symposium on Computer-Based Medical Systems (CBMS′04), 2004:4–9.
5. Smith D, Newell LM. A physician's perspective: deploying the EMR. J Healthcare Inf Manag 2002;16(2):71–79.
6. Gans D, Kralewski J, Hammons T, Dowd B. Medical groups' adoption of electronic health records and information systems. Health Aff (Project Hope) 2006;24(5):1323–1333.
7. Canadian Institute for Health Information. Understanding family physician usage of electronic health records in Canada: results from the 2004 National Physician Survey, 2006:1–11.
8. Office of Health and the Information. Toward Electronic Health Records. Canada: Highway Health Canada, 2001.
9. Holle R, Zahlmann G. Evaluation of telemedical services. IEEE Trans Inf Technol Biomed 1999;3(2):84–91.

10. Bott OJ. Electronic Health Record: Standardization and Implementation, 2nd OpenECG Workshop, Berlin, Germany, 2004:57–60.
11. Choi J, Yoo S, Park H, Chun J. MobileMed: a PDA-based mobile clinical information system. IEEE Trans Inf Technol Biomed 2006;10(3):627–635.
12. James A, Wilcox Y, Naguib RNG. A telematic system for oncology based on electronic health and patient records. IEEE Trans Inf Technol Biomed 2001;5(1):16–17.
13. Amouh T, Gemo M, Macq B, Vanderdonckt J, Wahed A, Reynaert MS, Stamatakis L, Thys F. Versatile clinical information system design for emergency departments. IEEE Trans Inf Technol Biomed 2005;9(2):174–183.
14. Neri E, Thiran J, Caramella D, Petri C, Bartolozzi C, Piscaglia B, Macq B, Duprez T, Cosnard G, Maldague B, De Pauw J. Interactive DICOM image transmission and telediagnosis over the European ATM network. IEEE Trans Inf Technol Biomed 1998;2(1):35–38.
15. Satyarthi D, Raju BAN, Dandapat S. Detection of diabetic retinopathy in fundus images using vector quantization technique. Annual India Conference, 2006:1–4.
16. Fan R, Ceded L, Toser O. Java plus XML: a powerful new combination for SCADA systems. Comput Control Eng J 2005;16(5):27–30.
17. Eichelberg M, Aden T, Riesmeier J, Dogac A, Laleci G. Electronic health record standards – a brief overview. 4th International Conference on Information and Communications Technology (ICICT 2006), Cairo, Egypt, 2006.
18. Treins M, Curé O, Salzano G. On the interest of using HL7 CDA release 2 for the exchange of annotated medical documents. Proceedings of the 19th IEEE Symposium on Computer-Based Medical Systems (CBMS'06), 2006:524–532.
19. Hornero R, López MI, Acebes M, Calonge T. Teleophthalmology for diabetic retinopathy screening in a rural area of Spain. In Eighth Annual Meeting of the American Telemedicine Association (ATA'2003), 2003:111.
20. Brooke J. SUS: a "quick and dirty" usability scale. In: Jordan PW, Thomas B, Weerdmeester BA, McClelland AL (eds.) Usability Evaluation in Industry. London. 1996.
21. Marcheschi P, Mazzarisi A, Dalmiani S, Benassi A. HL7 clinical document architecture to share cardiological images and structured data in next generation. Comput Cardiol 2004; 617–620.
22. Paterson GI, Shepherd M, Wang X, Watters C, Zitner D. Using the XML-based clinical document architecture for exchange of structured discharge summaries. In Proceedings of the 35th Hawaii International Conference on System Sciences, 2002:119–128.
23. Ginsburg M. Pediatric electronic health record interface design: the PedOne system. In Proceedings of the 40th Hawaii International Conference on System Sciences, 2007:1–10.
24. Chew SJ, Cheng HM, Lam DSC, Cheng ACK, Leung ATS, Chua JKH, Yu CP, Balakrishnan V, Chan WK. OphthWeb-cost-effective telemedicine for ophthalmology. Hong Kong Med J 1998;4(3):300–304.
25. Noumeir R. DICOM structured report document type definition. IEEE Trans Inf Technol Biomed 2003;7(4):318–328.

Chapter 6
An Image-Centric, Web-Based, Telehealth Information System for Multidisciplinary Clinical Collaboration

Patricia Goede, Lori Frasier, and Iona Thraen

Abstract Web-based technologies are changing the face of traditional telehealth applications by providing cost-effective clinical data capture and sharing solutions. Access to medical images in coordination with clinical workflow and face-to-face technologies can integrate clinical service delivery, diagnosis, and treatment across geographic, disciplinary, and organizational boundaries. For example, medical images are used for a variety of purposes and range in their complexity from a simple digital photograph of a physical mass taken by a primary care provider to a magnetic resonance image (MRI) reviewed by a radiologist that might describe the details of the mass; to a histopathology slide that a pathologist might use to diagnose the malignancy of the mass. Each of these images is managed by separate domain-specific information systems which are often located in technology silos and are constrained by disciplinary, organizational, and geographic barriers.

TeleCAM is a telehealth information system that provides a standards-based technological infrastructure for the collection, storage, and display of digital images via the web. Aggregating images across domains, workflow, time, and geographies can greatly enhance clinical collaboration, diagnostic efficiencies, continuity of care, and ultimately patient care outcomes. This chapter will provide a short review of the history of telemedicine and describe in detail the technological specifications, features, and management strategies of a web-based solution. Several clinical applications will also be described in order to visualize the full capacity of this web-based solution.

Keywords: Image-Centric · Web-Based · Telehealth Information System · Clinical Applications

---

P. Goede (✉)
VisualShare, Salt Lake City, USA
e-mail: patricia.goede@hsc.utah.edu

A. Lazakidou (ed.), *Web-Based Applications in Healthcare and Biomedicine*,
Annals of Information Systems 7, DOI 10.1007/978-1-4419-1274-9_6,
© Springer Science+Business Media, LLC 2010

6.1 Traditional Telemedicine

Telemedicine, more commonly referred to today as telehealth, dates back to as early as 1906 depending on who you read and how you define the concept. For purposes of this discussion, telemedicine/telehealth is defined as the transfer of medical/health information of multiple formats across distances using telecommunication technologies. The distance traveled and the quality of the information transmitted are limited by the technologies of the time. Einthoven, the father of electrocardiography, is credited with having investigated the transmission of ECG signals over the telephone lines in 1906 and having written about it an article published by the "*Archives Internationales Physiologie*" [1]. Further evidence of its historical roots is in the use of radios to connect physicians with offshore ships with medical emergencies in the 1920s. Norway established a service for ship support by radio links during this same time period [2]. *The Radio News* magazine of 1924 envisioned a physician contacting and examining his patient over the radio. This visual representation of the possibilities preceded the actual invention of the TV in 1929.

It was not until 1945 that France used telemedicine for consultation services and in the early 1950s that demonstrations and ongoing development efforts started to take off. In 1951, the New York World's Faire demonstrated a cross-state application of telemedicine followed in the late 1950s with teleradiology in Montreal and the use of tele-education and telepsychiatry in Nebraska [3]. In the early 1960s, the National Aeronautics and Space Administration was contributing to the developments of telemedicine through monitoring physiological measures in space suits. Funding and technology was provided by NASA for early demonstrations [4].

By the mid-1970s, 15 telemedicine projects in the United States were identified [5]. Moving forward to the 1980s–1990s, international use of telemedicine applications expanded to France, Norway, Portugal, Spain, and Greece. As technology grew and changed, new geographies and applications developed. What started out as simple radio communication progressed to include phone lines, ISDN, to full and fractional T-1 lines, ATM, Internet, intranets, satellites, and more recently the use of cells and mobile devices. Clinical applications include but were not limited to "dermatology, oncology, radiology, surgery, cardiology, psychiatry, and home health care" [4].

Developments and applications of telehealth technologies are only limited by imagination and local resources. New 21st century developments and applications include home-based measuring devices (blood pressure, glucose, heart rates, etc.), social service applications (corrections, child maltreatment, geriatric care), and multi-site, multi-participant research such as the Genome project. Web-based technologies (web video conferencing, Internet 2.0, VPNs) are challenging the traditional store and forward and videoconferencing technologies by bringing more cost-effective solutions to the desktop and remote devices for real-time interactions, image and content transfer, and mobile device data capture and display. Other factors such as increased memory effecting storage capacities, improved transmission and data compression protocols, GRID computing and annotation strategies are impacting the ability to transmit data in multiple formats and in synchronous and asynchronous time interactions.

6.1.1 Strengths and Limitations of Traditional Telehealth Infrastructures

Traditional telehealth infrastructures support synchronous interactions between patients and providers usually employing video-conferencing equipment. Real-time consultation, patient examinations, and collection of patient measures using peripheral devices can transport the patient across great distances into the provider's office. This face-to-face interaction allows the remote provider to explore patient concerns in-depth, extends specialty consultations beyond tertiary environments and urban concentrations, and puts a face to the voice in the clinical experience. Opportunities to field questions from the patient, to clarify any misunderstandings, and to "touch" the patient greatly enhances the experience. Limitations of this technology also exist. Costs associated with the traditional telehealth equipment, the need for enhanced bandwidth for transmission quality, scheduling and staffing costs, and the format of video can limit the ongoing adoption of this technology.

6.1.2 Description of Gaps and Needs

Web technology is creating a wide variety of information solutions that improve remote telehealth interactions but additionally disrupt the status quo. Current and past systems are cumbersome by comparison to an agile and client server "lite" remote access solution. Real-time interactions with traditional telemedicine supports practitioner hands-on interactions through video but remains limited in the exchange of data, the ability to bank and analyze the raw materials for research and quality improvement while consuming massive amounts of digital bandwidth. Additionally, asynchronous viewing, critiquing, or consultation by other members in the healthcare continuum are also limited. One could argue that this may be due to the nature of the documentation, i.e., video. But as digital recordings improve as well as compression and transmission capabilities, it is not unlikely that patient interactions will be captured in digital snippets. Also web technologies such as web cams may replace current video equipment intensive systems.

Variation in data types (image, structured data, text, video) presents another gap or need. More commonly, data types are variable, stored in differing data structures and on differing databases. The historical version of telehealth has remained relatively isolated from the rest of the healthcare system infrastructure. As electronic medical records, cross-continuum interactions, health and human services interfaces, and patient-centered healthcare evolve, the ability to remotely negotiate these multiple chasms is challenging. Emerging web-based technologies such as data service layer data grids [6] and annotation software [7] will create the necessary bridges on behalf of the patient.

The current telehealth infrastructure, while meeting the needs of the patient, is limited in its ability to aggregate cases and over time. Aggregation and long-term repositories provide the necessary infrastructure for program evaluation, quality assurance and improvement, and research. Recent web-based data access technologies support the ability to maintain the integrity of the home data and data systems while providing for manipulation and analysis. Additionally, the layering of XML (eXstensible Markup Language) output files and SVG (Scalable Vector Graphics) supports annotation use and reuse of images without corrupting the original digital file. Integration of these technologies can create a virtual research laboratory while maintaining and supporting individual patient care at the home remote site.

6.1.3 Costs

The costs of web-based telehealth are like any other technology-related costs. They go down over time. As the web becomes more and more ubiquitous, security protocols strengthen around virtual private networks, memory increases with decreasing costs, and devices become smaller and smaller, costs for telehealth will change. Application service providers will grow over time and provide more cost-effective solutions to telehealth usage. Clinical care will remain clinical, but the capture, storage, use and reuse across remote sites of that clinical data are changing rapidly under the influence of web-based technologies. Current dinosaurian-like telehealth infrastructures will be disrupted by the more agile and mobile web-based technologies.

6.2 Twenty-First Century Telehealth

The use of imaging technology to obtain expert consultation of medical exams is not new. Prior to digital technologies, both videotapes and 35 mm photos were routinely collected by less experienced medical providers and sent to their colleagues with more expertise. The advent of electronic mail and digital images has allowed for more rapid consultation, and the need to protect these images and patient information resulted in the development of proprietary commercial software applications. The value of software applications that meet the remote communication and collaboration needs of healthcare providers and their patients is considerable. However, existing applications contain adoption barriers, because they do not meet the specific workflow and interface needs of their own customers nor do they permit single-copy-centralized image sharing and image collaboration. These barriers indicate that a solution serving the geographically distant healthcare providers must place interface usability, user workflow and image centric remote communication as top priorities in order to be successfully adopted.

The existing process of clinical case consultation can be improved by providing clinicians and practitioners with secure case communication and collaboration tools. These tools must fulfill the need to create and submit child abuse cases for expert consultation, integrate clinical coding standards (e.g., ICD-9/10, CPT), manipulate images form multiple sources (e.g., clinical photos, radiographs, histology), preserve archive quality images while allowing multi-user, non-destructive visual identifiers and protect all information from unauthorized access.

Physicians and healthcare providers require a solution that fulfills their teleconsultation needs regardless of location. Telehealth solutions typically are designed to link clinics that are geographically distant from each other. Small hospitals and clinics typically do not have the means to link up to a traditional or dedicated telemedicine infrastructure used for clinical case review. Healthcare providers require the ability to track the incremental accumulation of case material from initial creation at a remote clinic through to the final evaluation by a consulting physician at a clinic in a different location or tertiary care center.

Web-based telehealth applications are, if architected and deployed properly, a viable solution for health care providers that are geographically distant from each other. Telehealth solutions can be used for diagnosing patients when paired with video conferencing and alone when one provider needs a consult from a colleague but has no ability to access a telemedicine framework. Web-based telehealth solutions must meet the workflow needs of health care providers and provide a means to evaluate clinical notes and textual data with imaging in an environment that supports decision-making. For consistency we will use the terms of producer and consumer and recognize that the producer–consumer model is an iterative cycle in the workflow. Telehealth solutions must be developed with a consistent user interface for clearly defined fields for adding clinical notes, seamless image import or upload, support for visual annotation of features on an image, and linking the annotated set of features on images to textual descriptions (i.e., lexicons, clinical note, pathology report, or diagnosis).

6.3 TeleCAM/VisualStrata as an Example of Web-Based Telehealth Application

6.3.1 Increasingly Collaborative Nature of Biomedical Imaging in Clinical and Basic Science Research

Providing clinicians, medical educators, and basic scientists with solutions for sharing and collaboration will improve the process of clinical and scientific discoveries. The biomedical-imaging environment, like many others, has both clinical and scientific image-based components. Images are generated from multiple imaging modalities that include clinical photos, radiographs, histology, and microscopy. At each stage of the clinical management of a clinical or research study, multiple images are acquired from multiple imaging modalities. Furthermore, each image is interpreted by one or more experts and, generally, must be shared by one or more experts. Investigators must have the ability to add visual annotations and notations that identify regions of interest on images. Moreover, investigators that fill a collaborative role must have the ability to incrementally add annotations to the same image without destroying or corrupting the image and the previous set of annotations. Relationships between images, expert knowledge, and the context from which images are generated and collected are necessary so that investigators can compare experimental results for validation, exploratory analysis, and hypothesis testing. Consequently, there is a critical need to capture the growing and evolving base of expert knowledge so that downstream experts can easily utilize previous results.

Existing solutions do not facilitate the incremental and collaborative collection of expert knowledge that readily makes the collection information available to other experts. Instead, clinicians, medical educators, and basic scientists generate multiple copies of image data with unlinked textual results that reside in multiple data repositories and are unavailable for collaboration. Linking images beyond one-time data extraction has potential value to collaborators and sets up cross-disciplinary communication. Repetition of work by image re-interpretation and duplication is reduced.

A client–server solution that adheres to a defined methodology of structured output reuse of data, integrates lexicons or standard vocabularies, and provides the ability to incrementally add information to the image base without destroying the image would improve collaboration across heterogeneous image repositories. The image and associated textual information are coupled and linked in a structure that facilitates access and retrieval and reduces replication of reference images that complicate access and retrieval.

Examples of the process and output are illustrated in Fig. 6.1 (pathologist–clinician–scientist). Briefly, an investigator, in this example a basic scientist, identifies abnormal morphology in a tissue sample. The annotated image is accessed by a clinical specialist who in turn adds an interpretation (expert knowledge) incrementally to the pathologist's findings, without destroying the pathologist's annotations. The basic scientist could reuse the clinical findings to determine a region of interest that will be the central focus of a molecular pathways experiment and incrementally add experimental results as annotations with linked textual results. This process of successive addition of expert knowledge to the same image is iterative. More digital images, each with annotations, may be added to form an integrated case file. Basic research results may also be added to the file. At any step in the process, the consultation and collaborating team may use the annotated content.

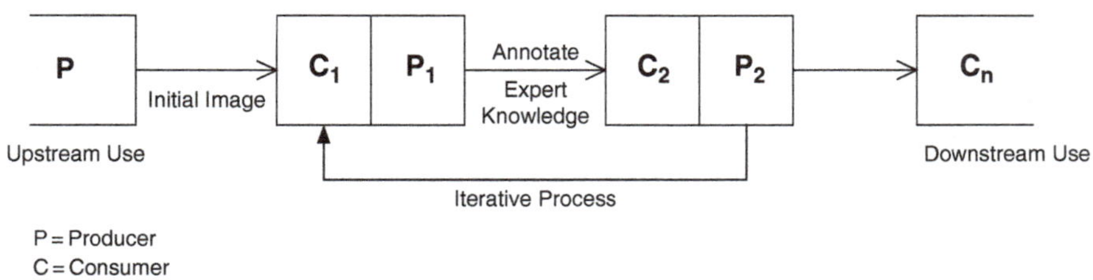

Fig. 6.1 Generic model for producers and consumers

6.3.2 Lack of Image Data Integration Across Scales/Instruments

An increasing number of specialty-specific, biomedical imaging devices used in clinical and research facilities generate large volumes of raw image data. For example, light microscopy generates images from immuno-histochemistry stained tissue whereas electron microscopy is used to examine tissue at the cellular level. The same methodology applies to the staining and mapping of neurotransmitters in different layers of the retina that allows an investigator to determine cell–cell interactions. Biomedical imaging devices commonly found in clinical practices often generate image-based results that are visible light and are exported as standard image formats such as TIFF or JPEG. Each of the resulting images is used by one or more experts within different specialties and in different contexts throughout a clinical or research investigation. The typical process is for each expert to interpret images independently from other experts without the ability to easily share their results. Additionally, existing systems generate images and associated information in a proprietary manner, reducing the ability to share and collaborate beyond the system with other specialists.

6.3.3 Integration of Standard Vocabularies and Lexicons

The biomedical imaging and expanding the clinical and research knowledge base in above is a significant issue. Most of the existing clinical and research imaging systems have limited collaboration capabilities that lack a consistent, methodical, and structured process. There are very few solutions that are available that allow for consistent, context appropriate communication and collaboration (results sharing), integration of third-party lexicons and encoding standards (FCAT, SNOMED, UMLS, ICD9, TNM), and standardization of output into a structured format that supports collaboration. If each expert is allowed to add knowledge in an unstructured and inconsistent manner, the end result will be isolated islands of information that are difficult for individuals, as well as collaborating experts, to extract meaning and value.

6.3.4 Limited Ability for Reuse and Management of Structured Visual Information

As the volume of image data expands, so does the challenge of managing and tracking the image data as well as the visual knowledge associated with each image or image set. Current individual and workgroup processes are creating, one image at a time, large "piles" or volumes of disparate, uncataloged image data and added visual information on various file systems. Moreover, image files are often copied multiple times for a variety of similar purposes such as presentations, collaboration, web presentation, and publication.

Clinicians, medical educators, and basic scientists lack software tools and solutions to author, manage, link, and reuse image content to communicate results, compose presentations (e.g., case presentations, research presentations, and teaching presentations) or publications (e.g., peer reviewed journals, textbooks). Each image collection has one specific use within a single context, which necessitates multiple duplications of the same annotated image, as opposed to annotating a single image that can be reused with some, all, or none of the annotations for multiple purposes in multiple contexts. An obvious drawback to multiplication of images compounds the problem of reuse and management.

6.3.5 Maintaining Data Integrity – Structured Information Supported by Metadata Formats and Curation Standards

In biomedical imaging environments, it is becoming more and more common that clinicians and basic scientists share results of clinical or basic science research studies that contain an imaging component. As a result, there is demand for multispecialty client authoring tools that capture the incremental stream of visual expert knowledge generated while preserving previous work and the original image in an unaltered state. The visual expert knowledge must remain linked to the original image and investigator, be available to other investigators, and remain in a uniform state that allows timely access to the data. This can only be achieved by structuring maintaining revision control over the collections of data. Establishing a common methodology for the purposes of consistent, context-appropriate communication and collaboration, integration of third-party lexicons or vocabularies (FCAT, SNOMED, UMLS, ICD9, TNM), standardization and interoperability of authoring tools, and interactive presentation mechanisms is critical to visualization and data sharing.

6.4 Model for Image Sharing and Collaboration – The process of Collaboration

Producers and consumers rely on the images and the expert clinical and research information associated with the image for collaboration, treatment, and potentially to determine clinical outcomes. A generic model outlining producers and consumers and how information flows is shown in Fig. 6.1. This model illustrates how consumers can become producers by generating additional information for subsequent consumers, and how producers may be involved in iterative activities depending on the clinical and research process and the information conveyed.

"Upstream Use" and "Downstream Use" define the basic flow of images and information in the model. An individual that is downstream initially takes the role of a consumer of upstream information. A consumer transitions into the role of a producer when the information is used as the basis of an analytic procedure. As a producer, an individual may generate images, author new textual information, or

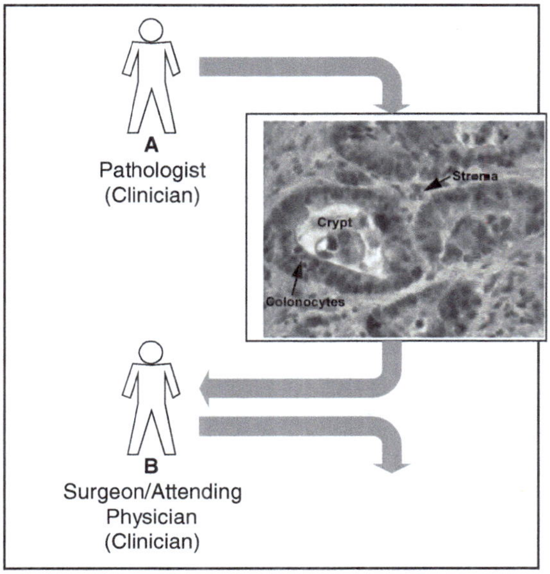

Fig. 6.2 Producer and consumer

create incremental value-added annotations and comments as part of a procedure. Our experience indicates that this initial model captures the fundamental mechanism of information flow for multi-specialty communication and collaboration.

An example of a pathologist (A) and surgeon (B) in a producer–consumer scenario interacting with a single image is shown in Fig. 6.2. In this use-case, the pathologist (A) is the producer (producing images from the tissue sample) for review by the surgeon (B) acting as consumer. This example illustrates the producer–consumer use-case visual annotation on one image. The pathologist (A) annotates a region of interest (ROI) indicating the stained colonocytes, the crypt, and the stroma on the histopathology. The surgeon reviews the pathologist's findings to determine if the polyp was completely removed.

The needs assessment and subsequent requirements analysis will determine the roles of the individuals – pathologist, surgeon, cancer specialist, clinical scientist, and basic scientist – and image acquisition equipment – microscopes, cameras, and scanners – within the colon cancer research program at the Huntsman Cancer Institute. These individuals and equipment will be grouped into two categories: producers and consumers. Producers generate image data (e.g., endoscopic, microscopic, and surgical) and related information including graphs, diagrams, pedigrees, notes, and reports.

The information sharing using annotations shown in Fig. 6.2 are extended in Fig. 6.3 to include additional expert knowledge in the form of clinical notes, pathology report information, or notations added to a single image. In this scenario, the pathologist (A) acting as a producer identifies and annotates a region of interest

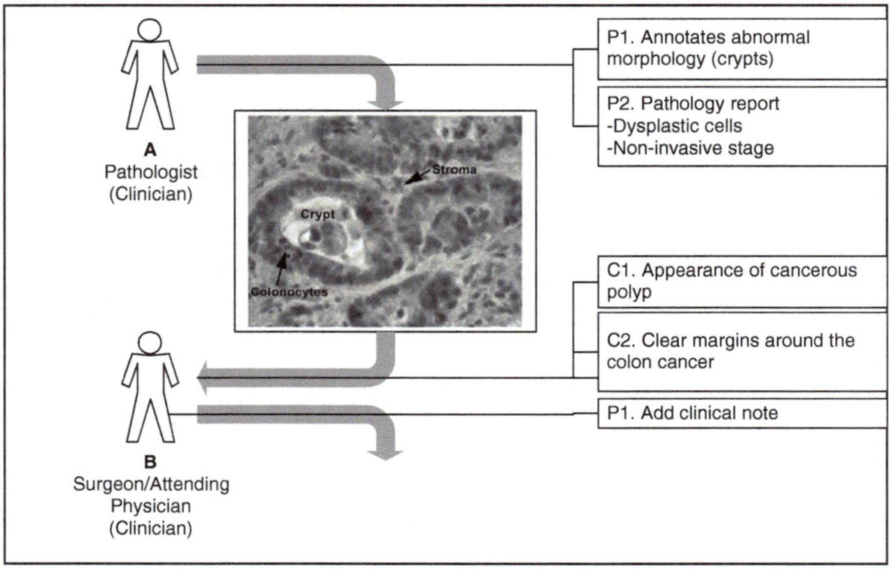

Fig. 6.3 Producer (pathologist) and consumer (surgeon) interaction with one image

(ROI) and adds a textual description of the findings that are linked to the image contained in the pathology report. The surgeon (B), acting as consumer, further reviews the pathologist's annotations and switches roles to become a producer by contributing additional expert knowledge in the form of annotations and clinical notes that remain linked to the image.

Another example involves the cancer specialist and surgeon as producer and consumer, respectively. The cancer specialist produces images, with expert annotations from a colonoscopy study. The surgeon receives the annotated images as a visual reference to develop a surgical plan. These images might also be used by a primary care clinician to illustrate the surgical procedure to a patient. In each of the simple examples above, multiple people interact with the same image for complementary but different purposes.

For a given patient study, many images are generated from different imaging modalities. For instance, at many molecular imaging centers, a given study can yield many images from a combination of imaging modalities including, but not limited to, colonoscopy, pathology, microscopy, and molecular imaging. The collection of imaging studies and information as expert knowledge may evolve to fill a much larger role by allowing imaging experts to query the data to resolve questions on how multi-spectral imaging is coupled to morphological features to determine protein localization or physiological responses or maintain relationships between the data that allow the collection to be consumed by a much larger laboratory information system or asset management system. In addition, for each image the number of consumers and producers may grow as new clinical and research

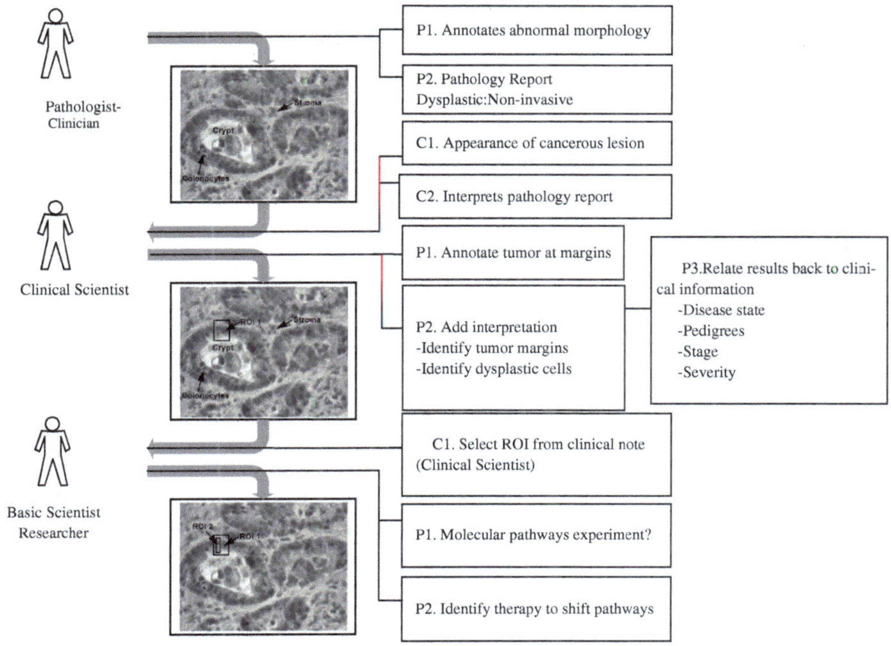

Fig. 6.4 Producer (pathologist) and consumers (clinician and basic scientist) incremental addition and selection of annotations and expert knowledge for one image

questions are asked, which will require a system that quantifies and catalogs experimental conditions and maps them to image collections for sharing and collaboration (Fig. 6.4).

6.4.1 Federated Data Repositories (e.g., BIRN) That Allow for Multiple and Immediate Access to Data Collections

The solution for creating cohesive information systems in a global information enterprise, or fully integrating information systems at the semantic, syntactic, and logic levels, has been described as a federated information system based on the "canonical data model" [8]. Nearly every organization has available and uses commercial-off-the-shelf (COTS) software applications; yet these applications rarely allow or promote collaboration. Moreover, such applications are commonly used to create and present material for collaboration and are general enough to handle most tasks, but do not support the conceptual framework or workflow of clinicians and scientists. The inability to share results from clinical and scientific experiments that contain an imaging component adds a level of complexity to an already difficult problem of sharing heterogeneous data. When disparate applications do not operate as a single system, the result is duplication and inconsistent data, reducing information accuracy and data integrity.

Information system integration has been a problem for as long as such systems have existed. Moreover, integrating the clinical and basic science knowledge base into federated data repositories has proved to be a difficult process. The continued proliferation of physically distributed, autonomous, and heterogeneous systems continues to raise the demand for better integration capabilities. In light of the given criteria for heterogeneity, it is clear why many past and present integration efforts fall short of their promises. For example, it is a common mistake to assume that integration woes can be solved solely through a sufficiently high-level syntactic communication medium such as CORBA, DCOM, or more recently XML web services.

6.4.2 Advantages of Federated Data Repositories

A federated database repository provides the functionality of a database system as a means to integrate other information systems. The FDBS approach provides the classical external and conceptual levels of the database system [9] while allowing the internal level (or storage) to be adapted to other information systems. This approach unifies the semantic, syntactic, and data model disparities of the underlying systems.

When based on a fully general data model and appropriate design, a FDBS approach has the potential to provide all of the following capabilities:

- Fully addresses all types of heterogeneity (including imaging results).
- Minimizes loss of autonomy – the unique facets of each system can be utilized.
- Full location, schema, and language transparency.
- Manageable data access restrictions.
- Read and write access.
- Tight federation – schema appears unified.
- Centralized or distributed architecture.
- Top-down or bottom-up approach – integration achieves some specific purpose, or is to meet a more general need.
- Virtual or materialized data.

The completeness of the underlying data model of a federated data repository is especially important when interfacing with other data models. For a single system to act as a general integration solution, it must be based on a fully complete data model (schema) where the concepts of the data model are the simplest and complete for which the values and operations of all other systems can be represented.

6.4.3 Extending the Federated Data Repository

Part of the answer to image management problems is an enterprise server-side solution that facilitates integration of image-text collections, revision and access control of image-text collections, and collaboration. Image data and added visual expert knowledge must be collected in a way that allows clinicians and basic scientists to maintain their existing workflow processes and reuse images for multiple purposes while not closing the door on server-side cataloging. Thus, another focus is the social issues surrounding data sharing that promote individual and workgroup practices that encourage the reuse of images to reduce the rate of "pile-up". Advantages of this approach include

- Ease of integration
- Flexible, open, portable architecture
- Support of disparate languages and systems
- Streamlines image management
- Secure architecture
- WWW/Internet access
- Metadata support
- Preserves original image data
- Lexicon integration
- Cost savings through reuse

6.5 Web-Based Technological Architecture, Standards, and Protocols

Web-based telehealth applications in large part must support or facilitate image-based communication, collaboration, and review process and promote data interchange by discouraging data duplication and data isolation (e.g., data islands).

6.5.1 Image-Based Communication and Collaboration

Image-based communication and collaboration is the core of any telehealth system for clinical diagnosis and peer review. Telehealth solutions must link images with clinical data and are the foundation of the dialog between two or more people. At the same time, text records that provide a context for the image review remain vital. For example, little can be gleaned from an image of a bruise in a child's groin without knowing the age and history of the child. This injury in a 5-year-old that came home from the park with his mother might suggest a fall on the monkey bars. On the other hand, this injury in a 2 ½-year-old might suggest something entirely different. Therefore, *images plus supporting records* are the recipe for efficient, accurate, and complete image communication and review, thus establishing the need for customizable, flexible text records associated with images.

6.5.2 Customization of Text Records

Customization of text records is an important feature for web-based telehealth applications. The options for text records can be grouped into four categories: (1) upload of a report as a file (e.g., text, MS Word, or PDF), (2) entry of a report via copy-paste of text from another system into a large text field, (3) customization wizards for creating data entry screens (e.g., history, physical exam) and data fields (e.g., chief complaint, abuse history, medical allergies), and (4) real-time data interchange from another system (e.g., patient record system). Below we discuss each option and solution with an emphasis on data customization and data interchange.

6.5.3 File Upload

Uploading a file and associating it with a specific image consultation event is a simple and effective means to provide text information as a context for reviewing images. File upload and association is a feature already included in current web-based telehealth application for images as well as lab reports. There is typically no need to further edit the information in uploaded files because the purpose of this information is to support the image consultation and case review process. There are advantages and disadvantages to storing and presenting information as a file. The advantages are that it is a simple and effective means to include necessary information. The obvious disadvantages are that the information is not easily modified unless a new file is uploaded in place of the original, and searching the file for key-words is problematic. The effort required to expand the ability to optionally replace screens with file uploads is minimal and will be discussed further in the following section on data customization wizards.

6.5.4 Copy-Paste

The copying-pasting of bulk text information (text blobs) from another system into a large text field within web-based telehealth systems is also a simple way to bring existing information from an outside system. The advantages and disadvantages of using the Copy-Paste of text blobs are the same as that for File Uploads. In each of the two options – File Upload and Copy-Paste – it is important that customers understand that the information is a copy of the reference record located elsewhere and may not necessarily represent the current state of the information. However, in most situations the case consultation and review will take place right away where the state (e.g., time sensitivity of the information) of the text record is not an issue. If the state of information is important, then either manual updating will be necessary to integrate into the case management workflow or electronic data interchange from an outside system to/from another system (See section on data interchange below) will be necessary.

6.5.5 Data Customization

Allowing organizations to create their own data entry screens, data entry fields and link them together into a step-wise workflow is a desirable feature for a large enterprise. The authors have developed a system that uses the Mode-View-Controller approach and architectural pattern.

The MVC is very flexible such that each screen has three associated files: a Model file, a View file and a Controller file. Currently, each of the three files is manually created once, with the expectation that there will be little to no change. Based on what we now know from our prototype customers, it is clear that there could be a great deal of change for any given customer. Fortunately, the MVC architecture supports the concept of allowing a customer to create a custom set of Model, View, and Controller files. In any given situation, the customer would choose to create a new screen or edit an existing screen (TeleCAM currently has Demographic, History, Vitals, General Physical Exam, Genital Exam Female (or Genital Exam Male), Genital Exam Anus, Examiner Diagnosis, Consultant Review, Conclusion in addition to the image management and communication screens). Figure 6.5 illustrates how the MVC facilitates the process of creating or modifying an input screen. From there the customer would make a variety of decisions including: type of data entry field or pre-set combinations of fields; provide descriptive labels; provide help tips; select whether or not a field is optional or required; and choose from different types of validation (e.g., "validate as a name" or "validate as an email address" or "validate as an integer not greater than 300 and not less than 45"). Once the data entry fields on a given screen are provided and the specific screen is ordered with respect to other screens, the back-end programming would generate Model, View, and Controller files based on the customer's preferences as well as make any necessary database model changes.

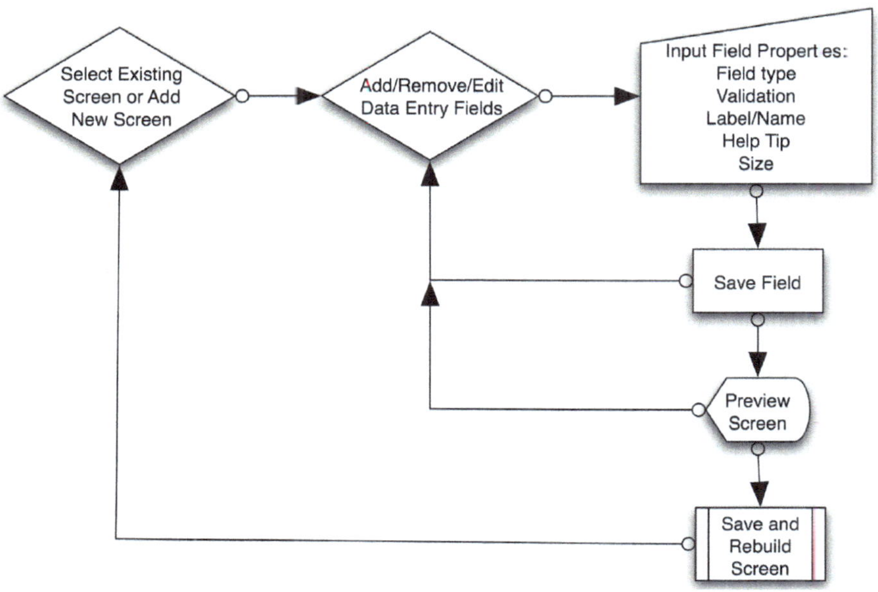

Fig. 6.5 A diagram illustrating how to create or modify existing data input screens

6.5.6 Data Interchange

Data interchange is in many ways the holy grail of the technical world. Data interchange implies that data entered into a software system once is then shared ubiquitously (e.g., securely to the right systems) between authorized systems. In reality, the process is much more difficult but not necessarily because of the technical difficulty. Instead data interchange is difficult because of the necessary agreement on the how's, why's, and where's between the people representing the two software systems sharing the information. Imagine being able to change your contact phone number at your bank and know it will be updated at all other bank accounts, insurance companies and so on. Crossing barriers between multiple organizations with personal data is a sensitive issue. On the other hand, it is easy for a single organization like Amazon [10] or Google [11] to create an electronic data interchange process for their affiliate resellers, because there is only one governing organization defining the process.

It is also important to note that many healthcare providers intentionally do not want clinical data (images with text) linked, in real-time, with the broader patient record despite the obvious benefits of efficiency and data accuracy.

One of the modern solutions for data interchange is web services [12]. Web services provide the common dialect for the execution of functions producing data on remote servers over the Internet for consumption by a remote client, regardless of differing operating systems and programming environments. In other words, my computer using type A operating system and type X programming language could request information (e.g., a list of popular best selling books) via a web service from a computer using type B operating system and type Y programming language. The choice of computer operating system and programming language by either party in the electronic exchange is not a factor. All communication is possible because there is an established, standard means (or dialect) of communicating the request whereby system A knows how to make the request and system B knows how to respond to the request. This marvelous request–response interaction can take place regardless of what technical choices are made on system A and B. The two most common web service implementations are Simple Object Access Protocol (SOAP) [13] and XML-Remote Procedure Call (XML-RPC) [14]. Both of these implementations are based on Extensible Markup Language (XML) [15]. XML is a popular way to represent structured data whether it is the title and author of a book, an address book record, or patient intake information. In fact, much of TeleCAM uses XML for storing data as a file or representing graphical elements such as a line or circle.

Our effort at providing data interchange begins by developing a web service method that allows a system to generically produce data for an outside software system or consume data from an external software system. These methods will be kept simple, yet effective by making the "contract" or agreement between a web-based system and an outside system "Read-Only" and "One-Way". Below we discuss in detail the "Read-Only; One-Way" agreement, the two methods, and the technical development plan for data interchange.

6.5.7 Read-Only; One-Way

Initially, we are interested in two methods: that of "consuming" data *from* an external system (see Fig. 6.6a) and "producing" data *for* an external system. In each situation the data will be "read-only" such that the data consumed from an external system will not be modified by a user. Likewise, the data produced for an external system will not be modified by a user of the external software system. This agreement or contract is simple and strict.

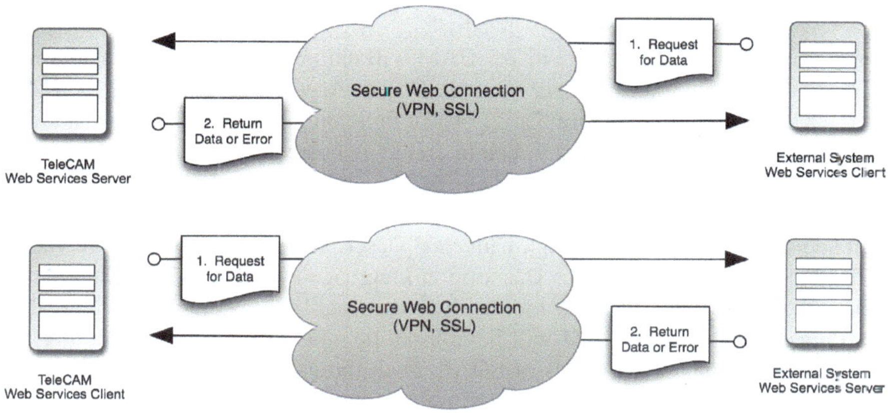

Fig. 6.6 (**a**) Method for *consuming* data from an external system – read only. (**b**) Method for *producing* data from an external system – read only

The process will, at this time, always be one-way or unidirectional such that the state of the data and data synchronization are not a technical challenge. The "consumer" in each of the methods illustrated in Fig. 6.6a,b agree to not modify the data and always rely upon, or depend on, the "producer" as the definitive source. The information may be requested by a consumer and returned by a producer at any time, so the consuming system is never without a current copy to display.

The information format for production and subsequent display of the information by the producing and consuming systems must also be established. In order to keep the data interchange process simple and straightforward, the format of the information will be a simple XML structure that allows the producer to either "blob" all the information into a single container or to subdivide the information into a "tree" of data.

The arbitrary tree structure can be "read" and broken apart by the consuming system and formatted accordingly, whereas a blob cannot be broken apart in any consistent way due to its lack of structure. Despite the limitations of lumping the data into one blob, this option may be sufficient depending on the specific use scenario.

The simplicity and strictness of the "read-only" and "one-way" agreement allows us to provide this service early in our commercialization and software lifecycle process while meeting our objective of establishing data linking mechanisms to third-party software systems. Moreover, we are able to provide the simple methods without the complicated negotiation process between third-party vendors or the technology departments of our customers. Adoption of the solution described herein does not restrict or exclude, in any way, an extension of our data interchange solutions to a two-way or read–write process in the future.

6.5.8 Technical Implementation of Data Interchange

Implementing data interchange in TeleCAM will require using one of two common web service technologies: SOAP (Simple Object Access Protocol) [13] or XML-RPC (XML Remote Procedure Call) [14]. Both SOAP and XML-RPC are industry standards that are used for many data interchange business applications. The most public are those offered by companies like Amazon [10] and Google [11]. Both of these public services use SOAP. SOAP is a specification that depends on several additional specifications (e.g., Universal Description Discovery and Integration (UDDI) [16] and Web Services Description Language (WSDL) [17] for automated discovery of services that are most valuable in publicly available services. The web services inside TeleCAM will be non-public and therefore do not require the additional automation protocols of SOAP. Therefore, the use of XML-RPC as the simplest approach is probably the best implementation choice. Examples of XML-RPC use include RedHat Inc. [18] and the Jabber/XMPP protocol [19]. RedHat uses XML-RPC to remotely manage live, real-time updates to remotely installed RedHat Linux Operating systems. Jabber/XMPP uses XML-RPC to send commands to a remote XMPP-based instant messaging server. In both the XML-RPC examples above, the remote exchange is predefined with both the consumer (client) and the producer (server) in mind. There are no outside, anonymous parties requiring access. This means that the automated discovery of the web service is not necessary. This "inside" relationship between consumer and producer is the same for TeleCAM. In other words, any consumer (or producer) of data from TeleCAM will be a known party that has been authorized and committed development effort to accommodate the specifics of the exchange. XML-RPC is a good match for this pre-defined data exchange process between two "inside" parties.

6.6 Features

6.6.1 Interface Features That Support the Clinical Workflow

Based upon the volume of cases, difficulty of reviewing remote cases and shortcomings of existing commercial solutions, the authors developed and deployed a telehealth solution to support the needs of primary care providers to improve child abuse detection and prevention case evaluations. The telehealth system, TeleCAM^{TM}, allows the practitioner at a remote clinic – using a standard web browser with SSL or VPN support – to easily and securely create a case by entering initial case information (e.g., medical assessment, images, and laboratory reports) and assign the case to a consulting physician for review.

At each stage in the lifecycle of a clinical case, text fields are modified, report files may be added (e.g., word processing documents, PDF) and images are acquired and visually annotated by two or more providers in an iterative collaboration. Figures 6.3 and 6.4 depict the workflow of two practitioners collaborating over a single image. The practitioners are engaged in a real-time "visual dialog" that does not destroy or alter the original image because TeleCAM already supports same time/different place dialog [8, 9]. This same-time/different place dialog is composed of region-of-interest annotations, textual labeling, and real-time text messaging. While Figure 6.1 shows only two participants, it is common for more specialists to be involved in more complex cases.

All information entered and modified in TeleCAM^{TM} is revision tracked (including the visual dialog) and logged per user. When the consulting physician has reached a conclusion (positive child abuse confirmed, negative child abuse confirmed or inconclusive) the case is closed, and the case enters the final lifecycle stage where it may be moved to a secure, static archive for reference. Table 1 summarizes the list of features.

Table 6.1

Feature name	Description
Custom user roles	Provide ability for the customer to create different user roles and access control for each role
Grand rounds capability	Provide ability to associate a case as a teaching/training case for the purpose of conducting grand rounds group (case) review
Notifiers	Send email notifiers to the relevant team members when a patient case reaches a certain workflow milestone
Multiple image upload and management	1. The ability to drag-and-drop multiple images for upload 2. Improve the speed of image loading/viewing during the review process 3. Extend the image operations to work with multiple selected images
Image downloading	Provide ability to download one or more (see Multiple Image Uploading and Management feature) at a time
Dashboard	The presentation of cases at different workflow milestones to facilitate and expedite case management
Custom text record definition	The ability for the customer to modify or add new data input screens
Data interchange	The ability to consume (or produce information for) information from an outside software system (i.e., Electronic Patient Record System)
Ad Hoc reporting	The ability to create custom, ad hoc case statistical reports that span multiple sites (e.g., clinics)

These features were identified as value-add features necessary to aid in the clinical workflow and support the complete case collection and multi-person information sharing and communication

6.7 Architecture and Use of Communication Protocols

6.7.1 Multi-user Visual Annotation and Reuse of Annotated Images for Training, Education, and Decision Support

Annotating digital images with symbols and text is a fundamental task that clinicians and healthcare providers must perform when preparing material for clinical and academic use [8, 9, 20, 21]. Image annotation, in the broad sense, includes any means that allows an author to label, point to, or otherwise indicate some feature of the image that is to be the focus of attention [22–25]. Each image may contain several annotations or groups of annotations that are necessary to convey a certain point. Providers should be able to perform image annotation quickly and easily to optimize workflow and time management. However, image annotation is made difficult by the lack of tools for annotation of digital media for use in a context-appropriate (i.e., colleagues, trainees, patients) that also promotes reuse of the annotated material [22, 26–29].

Commercial-off-the shelf (COTS) software is customarily used to create and present material. Such software is general enough to handle most presentation tasks. However, COTS software does not support the author's conceptual framework or workflow [9, 30]. Difficulties and limitations arise for several reasons, including (1) lack of optimal file format that supports reuse, (2) lack of a methodology for annotating digital material in a hierarchical fashion that does not embed the annotations within the raster-based image, and (3) lack of support for multi-specialty or multi-modality imaging in electronic medical record systems and mechanisms to index and catalog annotated material for reuse.

Three unanswered questions that clinicians and basic scientists have are (1) how to annotate digital material in a widely accepted manner, using a clearly defined set of rules (a methodology) that supports re-use of the annotated images, (2) how to create material for context-appropriate reuse for case conferences, lectures, and publications, without having to maintain several different file formats for each use, and (3) how to share annotated images and expert knowledge that promotes communication and collaboration. Furthermore, investigators who use imaging methods are amassing large volumes of digital images, which contain a clinical or basic science research component or both. Locating images based on keyword searches are absent, leaving most investigators to the hunt-and-peck approach to locate their images. More importantly, the images are isolated from intellectual content, such as expert knowledge or database information that prevents the data from being shared [22, 24, 29].

Flattened image annotations result in undesirable side effects. Examples of side effects are repetition of work, increased authoring effort, increased organizational requirements, increased complexity, difficulties to automate image cataloging, and limited instructional capability. These side effects, coupled with the problems of flattened, raster-based images, can be minimized or eliminated by not flattening the annotations to the image, which is one of the goals of our grant proposal.

The solution is to develop a software solution that promotes communication and collaboration around breast cancer imaging, starting with an annotation methodology that is the foundation for software that facilitates visual annotation of digital image data generated in the clinic and laboratory and tracks the inherent structure and identifies relationships or intellectual groupings of the annotations [18, 19, 24]. This methodology will keep annotations accessible as vector data, not embedded in the image. A second phase of this development effort is to develop the foundation that supports storage of annotations in a standard format as vector files, linked to the original image, and more importantly, linked to the bioinformatics content in databases (e.g., pedigrees). Such a solution is the basis of our proposal, which will be developed in the context of breast cancer because the breast cancer program at our institution affords a multi-specialty paradigm (internists, radiologists, oncologists, geneticists, epidemiologists, statisticians, informaticists, and basic scientists) in which to implement our innovative and novel solution for image collaboration and communication.

6.8 Clinical Applications

The diagnostic process in clinical medicine has historically been based upon the medical history and physical examination of the patient. Integration of increasingly technological information into the process has evolved with medical science. In early modern medicine, the gram stain or microscopic cellular analysis of blood or urine was all that might be available to the clinician. Advancement in the fields such radiology, microbiology, pathology, genetics, and many other areas has changed the basic need of the clinician to incorporate “hands on” medicine with modern technology. The ability to link clinical information for storage, consultation, research, and analysis has also advanced rapidly in digital imaging technologies, broadband, fiberoptic, and internet applications.

Telemedicine and telehealth applications in patient care began evolving in the 1990s and were rapidly adopted in many parts of the world to link urban medical centers with rural providers and patients [31]. The potential applications seemed endless. Ideally, the clinician and patient would be linked by cameras and monitors streaming a real-time interaction at any distance. Small networks in specific locations such as states and provinces, countries developed. As the Internet became ubiquitous, the ease of teleconsulting using established Internet capabilities and less costly digital technologies became available. Image-centric specialties where visualization of a clinical finding is central to the diagnostic process are especially well suited to Internet-based technologies. Historical information accompanied by high-quality image transmission transmitted as a single record provides additional opportunities. When databases are associated with transmissions, research, quality improvement, and patient tracking are easily accomplished.

The diagnosis of child maltreatment has traditionally utilized images as an important diagnostic modality. A child presents with an apparent lesion, bruise, burn, abrasion, laceration, or other visible injury, which leads to the initial abuse concerns.

As clinicians developed expertise in analyzing histories that caregivers provided to account for these lesions, transmission of images and consultation with those experts becomes a key feature in the diagnosis. Child sexual abuse became a visually based specialty in the 1980s when pediatricians adapted the instrument of gynecologists, the colposcope, to obtain externally magnified genital images. Initially 35-mm photography and analog video capture was used to study normal genital anatomy as well as the sequelae of abuse. Digital imaging technology support the storage and transmission of colposcopic. Peer review networks evolved with the purpose of clinical discussions regarding the significance genital findings.

Most child abuse specialists are located in tertiary medical centers and large specialty hospitals, yet many children with allegations of abuse present for care in communities who may have few resources to deal with such issues. Legal implications are tremendous in child maltreatment cases. Failure to recognize abuse places a child at risk for further trauma. Overinterpretation of findings can result in false allegations, families disrupted, and inappropriate prosecution with possible incarceration of innocent people.

Child maltreatment is only one example of an image-centric specialty that has benefitted from the use of web-based telehealth. Ophthalmologists are increasingly using digital images to track diabetic retinopathy, retinopathy of prematurity, and progression of macular degeneration. Pediatric ophthalmologists especially are sparsely distributed and whereas many hospitals and centers have the capability to treat premature infants in local Neonatal ICUs. RetCAM™ images can easily be transmitted to a referral center for tracking and consultation.

Radiology is a classic example of digital imaging. CT scans have always been obtained in digital format, but prior to digital imaging systems were printed on standard X-ray films. Digital imaging technologies are rapidly replacing film acquisition. Storage and transmission of such images have been perhaps at the leading edge of development of propriety technologies. Most systems in radiology are not cross compatible and require specialized readers transmitted with the images. Outsourcing radiology services has become commonplace, where highly trained radiologists in very distant locations read images and transmit results.

Cardiology, like radiology, uses specialized images that are often obtained in digital format. Cardiologists are increasingly utilizing technicians to obtain echocardiograms and transmitting them using web-based technologies. Moving images can be interpreted at a distance by a cardiologists far removed from the patient. The primary care physician receives the diagnostic information and provides treatment under the guidance of the specialist.

Pathology is a similar image-centric specialty, with gross, microscopic, and specialized immunologic tests that lend themselves well to digital acquisition and review. Extremely high-resolution images can be stored and archived. Data sets associated with images can be an enormous resource for researchers in cancer, genetics, and other disease states.

Image-centric web-based applications are becoming common in clinical medicine. Clinical information and biological databases linked with the ease of access and ubiquity of secure web-based applications will be a tremendous asset in future clinical applications as well as biomedical research.

References

1. Einthoven. Archives Internationales Physiologie. Wikepedia: Telehealth, 1906;4:132. Accessed on 2/18/2009. http:users.forthnet.gr/ath/giovas/telemed.
2. Pederden S. History of Telemedicine, Chapter 1. http://www.uninet.edu/conganat/ICVHAP/conferencias/017/history.htm. Accessed on 2/18/2009.
3. Wootton R. History of Telemedicine, Chapter 1. http://www.uninet.edu/conganat/ICVHAP/conferencias/017/history.htm. Accessed on 2/18/2009.
4. Brown N. A Brief History of Telemedicine, Telemedicine InformatinExchange, 1995. http://tie.telemed.org/articles, Accessed on 2/18/2009.
5. Bashshur RL, Armstrong PA, Youssef ZI. Telemedince: results of the intial experience. Aviation Space Environ Med 1977;48(1):65–70.
6. Hurwitz and Associates. Reducing complexity of data integration and application development through a data service layer. November 13, 2003.
7. Goede PA, Lauman JR, Lauman BS, Cochella C, Katzman GL, Morton DA, Albertine KH. A methodology and implementation for annotating digital images for context-appropriate use in an academic health care environment. JAMIA 2004;11(1):Jan/Feb.
8. Marshall C. Annotation: from paper books to the digital library. Proceedings of the 1997 ACM International Conference on Digital Libraries (DL97), 1997.
9. Caruso R, Postel G. Image editing with Adobe Photoshop 6.0. Radiographics 2002;22: 993–1002.
10. http://www.linux.org.
11. http://www.W3C.org/XML.
12. http://www.W3C.org/SVG.
13. Adobe Systems, San Jose, CA.
14. http://www.xmlrpc.com/.
15. http://www.w3.org/XML/.
16. http://www.oasis-open.org/committees/uddi-spec/doc/spec/v3/uddi-v3.0.2-20041019.htm.
17. http://www.w3.org/TR/wsdl.
18. Lieberman H, Rosenweig E, Push S. Aria: an agent for annotating and retrieving images. IEEE Computer 2001;34(7):57–62.
19. Chronaki C, Zabulis X, Orphanoudakis S. I^2Cnet medical image annotation service. Med Inform Special Issue 1997;22(4):337–347.
20. Caruso R, Postel G, McDonald C, Aronson B, Christensen J. Software-annotated, digitally photographed, and printed MR images: suitability for publication. Acad Radiol 2002;9: 346–351.
21. Davidson H, Lauman J, Goede P, Harnsberger HR. CAT: a methodology for annotating digital teaching file images. Scientific Program Proceedings in Radiology (RSNA). InfoRAD exhibit 2000:698.
22. Goede P. CAT: an annotation methodology for the medical image annotation tool MIAT). Seattle, WA: National Center for Research Resources (NCRR) Sponsored BioInformatics Approaches to Neuroimaging in Clinical Research, 2002:January 25–27.
23. Wagner F, Wolff A. Map labeling heuristics: provably good and practically useful. association for computing machinery. Annual Symposium on Computational Geometry, 1995, 2001:109–118.
24. Goede P, Lauman J, Cochella C, Katzman G, Morton D, Albertine K. A methodology and implementation for annotating digital images for context-appropriate use in an academic healthcare environment. JAMIA (submitted).

25. Wagner F, Tycho S, Wolff A, Kapoor V. Three rules suffice for good label placement. Algorithmica 2001;30(2):334–349.
26. Albertine KH. Use and re-use of content from an imager's perspective. National Center for Research Resources (NCRR).
27. Heaps N, Davidson H, Lauman J, Harnsberger H. Arrow Magick: Labeling Digital Radiological Images on the Web. Telemed J 1999;5:95.
28. Lober B, Brinkley J. A portable image annotation tool for web-based anatomy atlases. Proceedings of the American Medical Informatics Association, 1999.
29. Lauman J. Image annotation and re-use issues in medical academia. Proceedings of American Society for Experimental Biology, 2001.
30. Chronaki C, Zabulis X, Orphanoudakis SC. Maintaining medical image annotations in I^2Cnet. Proceedings of EuroPACS'96, Heraklion, Crete, Greece, 1996:141–145. http://www.ics.forth.gr/ICS/acti/cmi_hta/publications/papers/1996/eup96ann/eup96ann.html. Accessed July.
31. Brauer GW. Telehealth: the delayed revolution in health care. Med Prog Technol 1992;18(3):151–163.

Chapter 7
SOAP/WAD-Based Web Services for Biomedicine

Thomas Meinel and Ralf Her Wig

Abstract Information on biomedical data has increased exponentially in the recent years. In consequence, publicly available data of various types are dispersed across a large number of web-based repositories that are dedicated to specific research issues. Additionally, increasing access to this biomedical information has given rise to numerous developments of advanced methods and tools in the field of computational biology. Web service technology has been developed in order to allow a direct and automated access to those distributed data resources and tools. Web services are software systems that support the communication and interoperability between machines independent of computer platforms or computer languages; the transfer of biological data using SOAP (Simple Object Access Protocol) in combination with the Web Service Description Language (WSDL) is one of the major standards in the bioinformatics community. The combination of distributed web services is used to generate even complex workflows that are able to address the increasingly complex questions of biomedical research. The purpose of this review is to introduce to SOAP/WSDL-based web services and to demonstrate their usage, from both the provider's and the user's perspectives. We introduce the basic standards and technology, describe the combination of web services into workflows, present use cases of web services and workflows related to health care and describe the utility of web services for biomedicine.

Keywords: SOAP/WSDL · Simple Object Access Protocol · Web Service Description Language · Web Service Technology

7.1 Introduction

Biomedicine requires more and more the comprehensive gathering of complex data to support specific scientific analyses. Data repositories are dispersed worldwide. Biomedicine faces therefore the need for sophisticated, automatic procedures of data

---

T. Meinel (✉)
Max Planck Institute for Molecular Genetics, Vertebrate Genomics Department, Bioinformatics Group, Ihnestrasse 63-73, D-14195 Berlin, Germany
e-mail: meinel@molgen.mpg.de

A. Lazakidou (ed.), *Web-Based Applications in Healthcare and Biomedicine*, Annals of Information Systems 7, DOI 10.1007/978-1-4419-1274-9_7,

© Springer Science+Business Media, LLC 2010

retrieval, exchange and distributed computing. Web service technology in general has been developed as a framework for such data exchange. In the life sciences, in particular in bioinformatics, standards for web services [1] have been introduced and successfully implemented by data providers, often as a complement to single user-oriented web interfaces. An existing body of publications introduces to evolution, current status and perspectives of web services [2–5].

Web services that are established specifically for biomedicine are rather rare. Respective literature is focused on knowledge domains like gene annotation, data mining, meta-analyses [6] or literature parsing [7]. Generally, single-standing techniques are proposed [8] as well as definitions and approaches for web service orchestration and workflow configuration systems [9]. Life science fields related to biomedicine like bioinformatics or systems biology have generated a large number of repositories that are already accessible by web services (Table 7.1). Here, standardization is the key to achieve interoperability between computers as well as individual web services. This is a relevant issue also for specific web services in biomedicine.

Table 7.1 Web Service WSDL Accessions, According to Fig. 7.2

Web service	Ref.WSDL file or description URL
OMIM	[24] http://www.ncbi.nlm.nih.gov/entrez/query/static/esoap_help.html
iHOP	[25] http://ubio.bioinfo.cnio.es/biotools/iHOP/wsdl/iHOP-SOAP-document-literal.wsdl
GenomeMatrix	[26] http://genomematrix.molgen.mpg.de/cgi-bin/ws/esoaposti/wsdl
ConsensusPathDB	[27] http://cpdb.molgen.mpg.de/ws/CPDB.wsdl
KEGG	[28] http://www.genome.jp/kegg/soap/doc/keggapi_manual.html
Reactome	[29] http://www.reactome.org:8080/caBIOWebApp/docs/services.html
SABIO-RK	[30] http://sabio.villa-bosch.de/webservice.jsp
PyBioS	[31] registration required at: http://pybios.molgen.mpg.de
DICOM	[32] registration required at: http://iris.med.duth.gr
DIOS	[33] registration required at: http://dios.registry.cz

A fundamental feature for the development and integration of complex information systems is the utilization of the (Web) *Service Oriented Architecture* SOA, which addresses the following issues adequately: Web services are autarkic components; they can be improved independently of the accessing applications, and input parameters can be adjusted at run-time to find optimized results. Interoperability, maintainability, accessibility, and application level interaction are advantages of web services that can be combined into integrated applications as workflows.

Data transactions by web services require standardizations that are described in this review. We focus on the SOAP/WSDL-based technology that is a common standard in bioinformatics. We highlight the composition of web services in complex workflows. Moreover, several information domains of biomedicine that are covered by particular web service providers and comprised in web service registries are presented, for example, repositories for diseases, metabolic and signalling pathways, enzyme databases, annotation resources of biochemical entities including genes, biomedical data mining and literature, as well as experimental data resources. Furthermore, we address the important aspect of identifying existing web service functionality for a specific research question that can be solved by exploiting semantics or by searching appropriate registries of web services.

7.2 Web Service Technology

7.2.1 Standardization Initiatives for Web Services

The *World Wide Web Consortium* W3C originally proposed a web service as a software system that is designed to support interoperability of machine-to-machine interaction over a network. The goal of the W3C web services activities is to develop a set of technologies in order to lead web services to their full potential, but they also act as a central information resource. The W3C proposes standardizations that enable web services to act as programmatic interfaces between web service applications of different technical aspects. Web services fit into two frameworks, the message-oriented technique and a biologically oriented set of methods. Machine-readable formats are required for both to allow interactions between multiple web services. SOAP (originally an acronym for *Simple Object Access Protocol*) is utilized for the transmission and the processing of messages between computers. The message is an XML standard and performs the serialization of the data in conjunction with other web-related standards using HTTP as standard protocol. The *Web Service Description Language* WSDL, another W3C standard consequently also on the basis of XML, is established to organize the data structure within a SOAP message including data hierarchies and semantics of parameter terms and data values. A WSDL file comprises definitions for the interface, the endpoint URL and the single web service methods, i.e. the functional operation units of a web service. This assures the communication and the interoperability between computers.

The *Web Services Interoperability Organization* WS-I [10] has been established to specify web services interoperability, for selected groups of web services standards, across platforms, operating systems and programming languages. In this context, some extensions for the W3C standards are defined that represent a "gold standard", a guide that is intended to support the development of web services. Along these rules, SOAP and WSDL specifications should be limited to the necessary minimum for allowing a better operability. Annotation standards are given in the WS-I Basic Profile 1.2 for SOAP and WSDL.

The *EMBRACE Grid Project* was funded [11] to strengthen existing web service activities in computational biology with the goal to collect web services in compliance to the existing body of W3C and WS-I terminologies, descriptions and rules.

7.2.2 SOAP Messaging

Within all necessary standardization of web service messages, SOAP plays the message-specific part. According to the environment, the web has been standardized on addressing resources (by URLs), generic resource interfaces (HTTP), resource representations (HTML, XML, etc.) and media (MIME) types (text/html, text/plain, etc.). XML is a widespread, clearly developed and standardized markup language standard. It is therefore extremely suitable for transferring the content of serialized messages. The XML standard schema is readable for any computer language and can therefore be satisfactorily used for implementations of client–server dependencies. The message is formatted in XML; it is thereby human-readable and easily traceable.

Each SOAP-based web service messaging includes the two transactions *request* and *response*. The main task of SOAP is to serialize the message contents; the core interaction is the data transfer between a requesting computer and the server-side endpoint of the provider's data resource. SOAP normally utilizes HTTP or HTTPS as transfer protocols. SOAP messages are structured in the core message, i.e. the SOAP body includes the encoding style of the message, a facultative header and the message envelope.

The body of a message must comprise the entire information for a successful retrieval of contents of a web service repository. It integrates the requested method as well as parameters and values. General data types, as string, integer or floating point numbers, are used in bioinformatics applications and are defined in the SOAP/1.1 encoding document. Because SOAP is based on XML, it is platform-independent, simple and extensible. The latter feature enables the outsourcing of web service-specific characteristics that depend on the aim and specific functions of a web service and the underlying data resource.

7.2.3 WSDL Documents as Descriptions for Web Services

A WSDL document is generated by the web service provider; it describes the predefined functionality of a particular web service according to the existing database backend and makes a web service transparent for users within a single document. WSDL is introduced as a standard language also to enable the (automatic; see below) building of a client library. WSDL contributes information about specific web service characteristics to the message generation and work, thereby as an extension of the SOAP definitions for the envelope and encoding style rules. A WSDL document declares specifically each method of a web service. A method is a predefined data access operation that stands semantically in a direct connection to the database query between the endpoint of the web service and the data resource's backend. The WSDL file comprises request and response parameters of each method with respective data types.

A WSDL file is structured in different sections. The W3C proposes rules to generate WSDL protocols embedded in an XML hierarchy. It defines data types, service-individual computer access ports, the binding to standard WSDL elements and the binding to the SOAP standard, in conjunction with the binding to the standard SOAP envelope. A WSDL file comprises necessary bindings to the

SOAP envelope through respective declarations. The components *Types*, *Messages*, *PortType*, *Binding* and *Service* of a WSDL file are explicitly described in respective W3C documentations. The *Binding* section defines the HTTP transport protocol and, through the *Service* section, the endpoint URL for the operation. The *PortType* section defines the message specifications for the operation. Both *Binding* and *PortType* are connected to build the interface between technical and content information. Each operation is split into *request* and *response*, a feature that pervades the entire WSDL file. XML namespaces connect single sections and elements of the WSDL document. They play also an important role in a SOAP message because they are intended to avoid name collisions if each of the elements in a message is clearly identified by a namespace – a feature that makes SOAP to a flexible and extensible protocol.

There exist several styles of WSDL files that have an influence on a SOAP message. SOAP supports four modes of messaging (*rpc/literal*, *document/literal*, *rpc/encoded*, and *document/encoded*). A messaging mode is defined by its messaging style (*rpc* or *document*) and its encoding style. Two common types of encoding are used in SOAP messaging, SOAP *encoding* and *literal encoding*. *Literal* means that the XML document fragment can be validated against its XML schema. SOAP *literal encoding* (*encoded*) is not supported by WS-I-conformant web services because it causes significant interoperability problems. A best practice approach, according to the EMBRACE recommendations [11], is the usage of the *document/literal* style that declares the data in a SOAP message explicitly. It is an agreement among WSDL developers in computational biology to follow EMBRACE registry conventions. This *literal* style allows humans to understand the actions of *document/literal* calls. The *Types* section of a WSDL document allows a highly disclosed data hierarchy of the data if the *document/literal* style is used. Finally, all local message elements must be namespace-qualified according to SOAP/1.1 conventions, which is the W3C standard for the interaction with *document/literal* styled WSDL.

An alternative to SOAP/WSDL is the *REpresentation State Transfer* protocol REST, originally an architectural style to guide a redesign of the *Hypertext Transfer Protocol*. It utilizes HTTP methods instead of request messages and XML-formatted response messages, but can also frequently operate in conjunction with a WSDL analogue, the WADL standard (*Web Application Description Language*).

The SOAP/WSDL technique offers a high potential by structured data hierarchies in transfers of serialized data as well as the already established standardization for such web services in bioinformatics and biomedicine. Therefore, developers of biomedical web services are urged to assimilate the standards from bioinformatics. The access to SOAP/WSDL-based web services is limited by the lack of effective login techniques. In biomedicine, however, it is very frequent to operate with personalized, sensitive or confidential data. Thus, data transactions can be generally performed for anonymous or globally valid data, which depends on the data and web service provider; sensible data must be secured by accessory mechanisms.

7.3 Generation of SOAP/WSDL Web Service Components

7.3.1 WSDL Files

Within a WSDL source code, it is commonly agreed to set up WSDL documents in "good style" and to support the single sections with documentation. Tools that facilitate the generation of WSDL files are products of business or non-profit organizations such as the *Eclipse Web Tools Platform*, which support the creation of WSDL files by graphical visualizations of the particular sections in the WSDL document and by consistency inspection of the code. Moreover, validation tools like *soapUI* are provided to test the syntax, perform a message tracing and run performance tests. The WS-I organization offers special validation tools to maintain the compliance of SOAP and WSDL documents.

In addition to the documentation within a WSDL document, most web service providers supply information about the WSDL web service methods, data access via WSDL, database content and example clients in helper web pages. This enhances the transparency of web service methods.

7.3.2 Programming Languages for Servers and Clients

Servers and clients are interoperating computer programs that translate the user's request into an XML message, send (client) and receive (server) the request message, and perform the translation into a database access at the provider's side; the response message is sent back in the same way. The stub program snippet in a server or a client is responsible for the generation and interpretation of an XML-formatted message, using specific modules of a programming language.

Several programming languages provide more or less complex modules for stubs that perform the task to interpret the WSDL file and, accordingly, construct the message by inserting valuable information for requests and responses. Those modules comprise server as well as client functions because the data organization for the serialization is the same as for the de-serialization to regard method parameters, data complexity and concrete values. Older modules (*Perl*: *SOAP:Lite*; *Python*: *SOAPpy*) cannot disclose complex data hierarchies (*complexTypes*), which have to be kept in mind by web services and client developers. Modern modules organize data hierarchies virtually (object-oriented Perl module *XML:Compile:WSDL11*, with dependencies) or as stored class files (using the *Python ZSI toolkit*). The latter files can be generated directly by importing the WSDL file into a helper tool, e.g., *wsdl2py* for *Python* clients.

The server is the endpoint of a SOAP/WSDL messaging. It is accessible by a URI, which is defined in the WSDL file. The server in its function as the database backend access unit is semantically the complement to each of the single WSDL methods. The server is therefore the mediator between web service query message and the query against the database.

```
#!/usr/bin/perl

use SOAP::Lite ;

# connect WSDL file of the GenomeMatrix web service
$service = SOAP::Lite -> service("http://genomematrix.molgen.mpg.de/cgi-
bin/ws/esoaposti/wsdl") ;

# call first GenomeMatrix web service method:
# retrieve all Ensembl genes of human chromosome 21
$result = $service -> GetEnsIdsByRegion("Homo sapiens", 21 , 0, 100) ;
$EnsIDs = ( join( " ", @{ $result->{EnsemblID} }) ) ;

# call second GenomeMatrix web service method: all expression datasets ...
$result = $service -> GetExpressionDatasets("Homo sapiens") ;
# ... and ignore all except leukemia-related datasets
foreach $set ( @{ $result->{microarrayDataset} } ) {
    push @CancerSets, $set  if ( $set =~ m/leukemia/i ) ; }
$cancerSets = join (" ", @CancerSets ) ;

# call third GenomeMatrix web service method:
# filter Ensembl IDs of given Ensembl IDs and given datasets for all genes
# that are significantly down-regulated (log2ratio between -5 and -1)
$result = $service -> GetEnsIdsByExpression("Homo sapiens", -5, -1,
$cancerSets, $EnsIDs ) ;
@result = @{ $result->{EnsemblIDs} } ;

# make unique and display
foreach $EnsID ( @result ){ $filtered{$EnsID} = "" ; }
foreach $EnsID ( sort keys %filtered ) { push @Filtered, $EnsID ; }
print  "" . ( join ( " ", @Filtered ) ) . "\n" ;
```

Fig. 7.1 Generic example client for subsequent accesses by three web service methods combined in a workflow. The biological goal is to retrieve differentially expressed (down-regulated) human genes encoded on chromosome 21 from the *GenomeMatrix* repository [26], which are significant in at least one of all implied *leukaemia*-related data sets. This example is written in *Perl* using the WSDL support of the *SOAP:Lite* module, which must be pre-installed in the operating environment

The client is a program that constructs and sends the SOAP request message to the server and receives the response message. It translates thereby complex data hierarchies into the serialized XML messages forward (request) and backward (response) according to the data complexity given in the WSDL document. Web service providers supply example clients for programmers of web service access routines. Such routines can be seamless integrated into programmed workflows or meta-analyses. Figure 7.1 demonstrates an example client that consists of three subsequent web service methods. Most WSDL programming language modules possess switches that allow for optional message tracing and performance tests.

Users without any experiences in programming can invoke single web service methods and retrieve results with *TAVERNA*, a graphical user interface (see later). This widely used workflow management system has to be configured through the integration of a WSDL file and the web service method of choice by a few mouse clicks. In contrast to a standard web interface, methods can be successively combined by workflow systems such as *TAVERNA* due to the user's definition.

7.4 Workflows and Workflow Management Systems

Computational data pipelines, in silico experiments or meta-analyses in general manage the combination of information derived from several resources. Programmers compile the syntactic structure of such workflows by accessing own repositories, programming the combination of data and including selection criteria like significance parameter. The combination of single data retrievals using web services are the core aspect of building workflows.

7.4.1 Web Service Methods Combined in Workflows

In this review, we are focusing on workflows composed of SOAP/WSDL-based web services. Such client-side workflows can be hard-coded programs that combine web service methods by processing information from one or several WSDL files. Between the single methods, a programmer has influence through operations like filtering or specific decisions. The enactment is either a command-line call in the simplest case or the running of advanced program scripts. A generic example for a workflow in form of a *Perl* program script is given in Fig. 7.1 with the aid of the *GenomeMatrix* web service. *GenomeMatrix* [26] is a knowledge system for the integration and visualization of heterogeneous information on genes and their function. It allows parallel genome analysis and connects multi-species functional information with a collection of manually curated experimental data. The system is capable of displaying multi-species data sets for single genes, pathways or entire chromosomal regions inside an interactive matrix display. The web service is aimed to collect biological experiments from different resources currently with a major portion of microarray studies from GEO or ArrayExpress. The data set includes cancer biopsies as well as drug treatment investigations for which differential expressions and significance tests have been calculated against control experiments.

Web service accesses are frequently batch queries or batch responses that can directly be linked to subsequent web service accesses, which on their own can accept batch requests. The batch feature is an advantage of web services; however, web service accesses can produce a high I/O load due to the serialization and deserialization steps, which can raise problems with some servers like *Apache*.

7.4.2 Workflow Management Systems

The initiation of workflow management systems was aimed at the intuitive managing of workflows by researchers without any knowledge of programming languages. The need to circumvent the creation of own repositories or tools in conjunction with the support from syntactically clear and standardized structure of web services led to the integration of web services into workflows. Such considerations were crucial initial points to generate platform-independent workflow management systems like *TAVERNA* [12], *Biowep* [13], *Kepler* [14] or *Triana* [15].

A lot of literature on workflows and workflow management systems has been published concerning the impact of workflows [16], general architectures [17], specific analyses of in silico experiments [18, 19], or the integration of methods from one particular or multiple resources in bioinformatics. There exists an overwhelming body of information about *TAVERNA* for complex use cases, technical extensions and project-oriented workflow repositories.

TAVERNA is a platform-independent, Java-based toolkit with a graphical user interface for the composition and enactment of workflows. *TAVERNA* possesses not only ab initio plug-ins for web services of several repositories, but also a scavenger for the de novo integration of public repositories accessible through WSDL. This allows for the technology-independent and integrated access to various repositories and tools. Simple drag-and-drop operations combine the single methods; complex data types can be resolved by the XML-splitter function. The *Simple Conceptual Unified Flow Language* SCUFL enables the storage of created workflows as well as the loading of existing workflows. Repositories for collections of workflows exist for a row of applications in bioinformatics [20]. Other prominent architectures or standards are Application Programming Interfaces (APIs) like the Distributed Annotation System *DAS* or *BioMOBY*, which is a project that aims for the discovery of decentralized repositories for native lightweight objects. *TAVERNA* exploits the modularity that exists within those systems.

7.5 Web Services for Biomedicine

7.5.1 Resources from Biomedicine-Related Domains

Web services for biomedicine cover several life science domains: computational biology, bioinformatics, clinical genomics or systems biology. This includes heterogeneous data categories like *disease*, *patient*, *experiment*, *pathway*, *interaction*, *classification*, *annotation* and *literature data mining*. Figure 7.2 gives a schematic picture; example web services are denoted and respective SOAP/WSDL web service accesses are presented in Table 7.1.

The bioinformatics domain offers web services that are mainly created for access of sequence-based repositories on gene transcripts, proteins, transcription factors, protein families, and protein domains or for sequence comparison tools like *BLAST*. The systems biology domain offers accesses to pathway annotations or pathway enrichment analyses [21] as well as to interaction data and to experimental results (collections of microarray analyses; next-generation sequencing (NGS); proteomics). In silico modelling systems [22] for specific disease domains like cancer will challenge appropriate solutions in the near future.

7.5.2 Specific Solutions for Biomedicine

Web services in biomedicine are intended to access internal data like clinical patient records, stem data, images or genealogies, which are afflicted with security, privacy

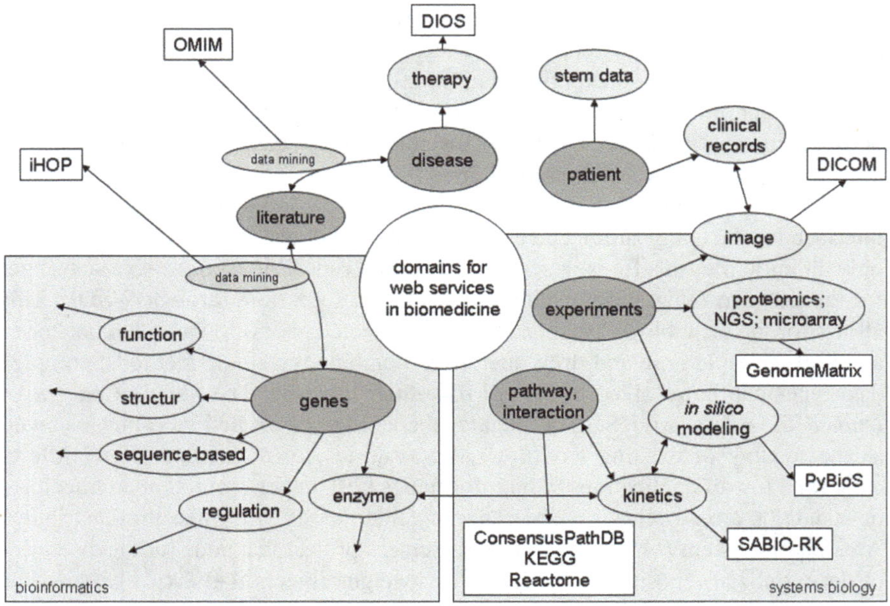

Fig. 7.2 Resource domains of web services for biomedicine (selection) that concern related scientific fields like bioinformatics, systems biology or literature mining. Rectangular boxes denote exemplarily web service providers (compare Table 7.1). Arrows in the bioinformatics box indicate manifold web services in this domain; confer the registries in Table 7.2

and confidentiality. The integration of such data can only be achieved by web services that provide data within an advanced security area, for example, in intranets of collaboration groups. It is a required issue to maintain anonymity if external users have access to the data. It makes sense to configure web services for such internal sources if the complete application is intended to integrate further public resources and a uniform technique shall be employed. Figure 7.2 exemplarily contains the two biomedicine-specific web services (DICOM, DIOS).

The *Digital Imaging and Communications in Medicine* protocol DICOM (Table 7.1) is a current standard for image and related data distribution within healthcare research and education enterprises. It utilizes SOAP-based XML messages for the transfer of ultra-sonographical modalities, radiotherapeutic procedures, and images from several radiology applications. The *DICOM Image Management* DIM web service allows the integration at application level through standardized technologies. The functionality of the service concerns the finding of patients, studies, study details or objects as well as the storage or retrieval of singular results. DICOM consists of an integrated workflow of single web service methods.

The Internet-based system for anti-tumour chemotherapy evaluation DIOS (Table 7.1) addresses the integration of several resources by standardized protocols. Chemotherapeutic regimes that are building the core repository are stored as a library of XML documents according to the XML Schema Definition XSD.

The DIOS web portal enables the web-based access utilizing the SOAP/WSDL technology also for third-party systems.

The two examples make clear that single web service methods very often interact in conjunction with other methods, within internal pipelines or workflows. Documents in standard XSD data formats like XML and *Markup Languages for Microarray and Gene Expression* MAGE-ML or *Bioinformatic Sequence* BSML are standardization components as well as the data exchange format SOAP. In clinical genomics, a field that operates with the use of genetic data in clinical practice, such standards are required if more and more patient data are involved in documentations, and the vision of a personalized medicine becomes reality. The increasing information complexity in IT-driven workflows leads to higher-level infrastructure layers for applications. The IBM *Seventh Layer of Clinical Genomics* CG7L [23] is such a workflow middleware that consists of modular components and classes. It utilizes modular web services for enrichments from electronic clinical records or public resources and encapsulations of patient-individual raw genomic data to connect the interactions with information from ontologies, published studies, or reference databases. Individual clinical history, genotype comparisons, and finding similar family histories are sourced for a case-based reasoning in this commercial decision support system.

7.6 Discovery of Web Services: Semantics and Registries

One crucial issue is the detection of a suitable web service because for a user it is often unclear which service and which method fulfils the intended task. There exist two main strategies: the usage of semantics for the automatic finding of the required method or the generation of registries that collect a large number of web services for a life science domain.

7.6.1 Semantics

The strategy to utilize semantics for web service discovery implies standardizations in (XML-based) data formats and data structures, which can clearly describe semantic relationships of data. For example in WSDL files, semantic data hierarchies are obeyed by the syntax of complex data types. The discovery of web services, moreover, affects web service descriptions. The syntax in semantic web services can be extended by achieving special languages like SAWSDL [34], which can be regarded as a *Semantic Annotation* extension of the *Web Service Description Language* WSDL.

The *Semantic Web* is intended to enable machines to comprehend semantic documents [35]; data integration by the semantic web is conceptualized using a *Resource Description Framework* RDF and ontologies (for further explanations, see [36, 37]) like the *Web Ontology Language* OWL [38]. For bioinformatics, Wolstencroft et al. [39] describe the link between web service discovery and a related ontology. Ceresa and Masseroli [40] review the need for ontologies and present several essential ontologies for E-Health as the *Open Biomedical Ontology* OBO, the *Foundational Model of Anatomy* FMA, the *Unified Medical Language System* UMLS, and further resources. Semantics are employed to address connections between biology, clinical issues, pharmacogenomics or clinical genomics and computer science.

Several authors propose matchmaking algorithms [41, 42] that are using semantics to circumvent the lack of flexibility and expressiveness in web service descriptions. Term look-up [43, 44] or syntactic concept recognition by ontologies [45] is the core function of related tools.

The introduction of semantic *e-Science* into biomedicine is emphasized in a special issue of *BMC Bioinform* 2007 [46] to feature approaches and experiences in a variety of biomedical domains. The two forms of semantics – the user-centric *Web 2.0*, confer here Zhang et al. [47] for the introduction in bioinformatics, and the semantically aware *Web 3.0* – are far extensions of the client-server web service design of the *Web 1.0* [48] that also includes workflows. However, semantics can also be used to build conceptual scientific workflows over web services.

7.6.2 Web Service Collections

Web services collections are intended to comprise the amount of web services that are located at a single institution. Categories organize the variability of tools in the repository; they are accompanied by descriptions of the web services to inform about the granularity of single web services, which expresses the number of web service methods and the data complexity. To convey a detailed educational advertising, extended manuals describe explicitly each single web service method and are often accompanied by example clients. National or international institutions like the *EBI*, the *NCBI* or *DDBJ* initiated platforms to integrate various web services or bioinformatics tools in collections (Table 7.2). *Soaplab* is a special tool collection at the *EBI* according to *EMBOSS* applications. The *KEGG* database offers a large

Table 7.2 Web Services Collections and Registries (Selection)

Institution	URL
Web service collections	
EBI	http://www.ebi.ac.uk/Tools/webservices/
NCBI	http://www.ncbi.nlm.nih.gov/entrez/query/static/esoap_help.html
DDBJ	http://www.xml.nig.ac.jp
Soaplab	http://www.ebi.ac.uk/Tools/webservices/soaplab/overview
KEGG	http://www.genome.jp/kegg/soap/
Web service registries	
EMBRACE GRID	http://www.embracegrid.info/page.php?page=webservices
EMBRACE Registry	http://www.embraceregistry.net
BioCatalogue	http://www.biocatalogue.org/

list of SOAP/WSDL web service methods for several accesses to pathway information. Here, methods and tools are described in detail on Internet pages. Web service collections are valuable resources for biomedicine.

7.6.3 Web Service Registries

Although collections include web services of few large institutions, web service registries unify web services of several institutions that are often providing single applications or specialized repositories. The *EMBRACE Grid* (Table 7.2) opened a web service section that collects life science web services and provides links to respective WSDL files. It was initiated to integrate the major data resources and analysis software tools that provide web services. It is now prelude to the new internationally supported registry called *BioCatalogue*, which integrates web services also from *ENFIN* and *BioSapiens*. The *EMBRACE Registry* invites bioinformatics/computational biology institutions to contribute their services to the collection, shows up single methods in a uniform display, makes selections available by searchable keyword categories, demand obligate test clients, and provide information on access actuality by a permanent repeated testing. Developers of web services in biomedicine are encouraged to distribute and publish their products in registries. The *EMBRACE Registry* [49] as a web service resource for life sciences is an appropriate destination also for web services specialized in biomedicine.

7.7 Concluding Remarks

Recently, Stein [50] reported progress and visions in the retrieval of information for life sciences by cyber-infrastructures. He supposed web services and workflows as central tools that are connected strongly to the data. The combination of resources by semantics will be a straightforward approach. The *Web 3.0* will integrate the usage of objects and relationships additionally to the semantics in a web service. The integration of multiple sciences into one platform or portal is intended to strengthen multiple scientific issues around diseases like the Alzheimer's disease into a translational research [51] across disciplines. Universal accessibility and independence of platforms are required for a modular assembly of multiple operations in workflow management systems (like *TAVERNA*) and further sophisticated features are enabled to be milestones towards those visions.

Of course, disadvantages occur for SOAP/WSDL-based web services. They suffer from lack of the transfer of binary data that is sometimes required; several technical resources like browsers have a larger CPU demand for the I/O of XML-based SOAP messages; changes in databases or database accesses must be manually transferred to WSDL files, which are mirroring database accesses. Confidential and security aspects are not a problem in intranets; current systems require registration formalities. However, the advantages are that inputs of complex data hierarchies or multiple parameters can be used to invoke a web service; time-consuming processes on server-side can be well performed; nested data structures can be applied for complex data types. Standardization of web services is furthermore a required issue, for data types as well as for output data format and data complexity, to enhance the interoperability of web services in workflows.

Web services vary extremely in complexity and hierarchies of the single methods. Some providers tend to offer more methods with fewer hierarchy levels in the single method, which enhances the fine granularity of the whole web service. Such reduction to single, simpler methods allows for an enhanced modularity for internal combinations of single WSDL web service methods, exploiting the hierarchy options given by XML schema definitions. Such pragmatic endeavours are accompanied by the introduction of registries for the discovery of web services and sought methods. It is pragmatic to adopt an existing registry for bioinformatics and life sciences web services also for services in biomedicine; in a registry, special keyword categories facilitate the browsing for biomedicine web services if the catalogue becomes overwhelming. This shall not undermine the advantages and profits of semantics for the discovery of web services.

Workflows become effective with internal or in conjunction with external public data. To support diagnosis and treatment, web services can contribute to decision support applications. The combination of internal and external resources, the usage of semantic metadata and ontologies can lead to a broad acceptance of SOAP/WSDL-based web services in biomedicine and health care.

Acknowledgments This work was supported by the European Union under its 6th Framework Programme with the grant EMBRACE (LSHG-CT-2004-512092).

References

1. World Wide Web Consortium W3C. http://www.w3.org. Accessed on 24 February 2009.
2. Stein LD. Integrating biological databases. Nat Rev Genet 2003; doi:10.1038/nrg1065.
3. Neerincx PB, Leunissen JA. Evolution of web services in bioinformatics. Brief Bioinform 2005;6:178–188.
4. Stockinger H, Attwood T, Chohan SN et al. Experience using web services for biological sequence analysis. Brief Bioinform 2008; doi:10.1093/bib/bbn029.
6. Burgun A, Bodenreider O. Accessing and integrating data and knowledge for biomedical research. Yearb Med Inform 2008;3:91–101.
7. Kim JJ, Rebholz-Schuhmann D. Categorization of services for seeking information in biomedical literature: a typology for improvement of practice. Brief Bioinform 2008; doi:10.1093/bib/bbn032.
8. Vittorini P, Michetti M, di Orio F. A SOA statistical engine for biomedical data. Comput Methods Programs Biomed 2008; doi:10.1016/j.cmpb.2008.06.006.
9. Gonzalez G, Balasooriya J. Web service orchestration for bioinformatics systems: challenges and current workflow definition approaches. IEEE Int Conf Web Services (ICWS) 2007; doi:10.1109/ICWS.2007.202.
10. Web Services Interoperability Organization WS-I. http://www.ws-i.org. Accessed on 24 February 2009.

11. Rice PM, Bleasby AJ, Haider SA et al. EMBRACE: Bioinformatics data and analysis tool services for e-Science. IEEE Int Conf e-Sci Grid Comput 2006; doi:10.1109/E-SCIENCE.2006.57.
12. Hull D, Wolstencroft K, Stevens R et al. Taverna: a tool for building and running workflows of services. Nucleic Acids Res 2006; doi:10.1093/nar/gkl320.
13. Romano P, Bartocci E, Bertolini G et al. Biowep: a workflow enactment portal for bioinformatics applications. BMC Bioinform 2007; doi:10.1186/1471-2105-8-S1-S19.
14. Altintas I, Berkley C, Jaeger E et al. Kepler: an extensible system for design and execution of scientific workflows. International Conference on Scientific and Statistical Database Management 2004; doi:10.1109/SSDM.2004.1311241.
15. Churches D, Gombas G, Harrison A et al. Programming scientific and distributed workflow with Triana services. Concurrency Comput Pract Exper 2006; doi:10.1002/cpe.992.
16. Romano P. Automation of in-silico data analysis processes through workflow management systems. Brief Bioinform 2008; doi:10.1093/bib/bbm056.
17. Romano P, Marra D, Milanesi L. Web services and workflow management for biological resources. BMC Bioinform 2005; doi:10.1186/1471-2105-6-S4-S24.
18. de Knikker R, Guo Y, Li JL et al. A web services choreography scenario for interoperating bioinformatics applications. BMC Bioinform 2004; doi:10.1186/1471-2105-5-25.
19. Cheung KH, de Knikker R, Guo Y et al. Biosphere: the interoperation of web services in microarray cluster analysis. Appl Bioinform 2004;3:253–256.
20. myExperiment Workflow Repository. http://www.myexperiment.org. Accessed on 24 February 2009.
21. Bader GD, Cary MP, Sander C. Pathguide: a pathway resource list. Nucleic Acids Res 2006; doi:10.1093/nar/gkj126.
22. Lee DY, Saha R, Yusufi FN et al. Web-based applications for building, managing and analysing kinetic models of biological systems. Brief Bioinform 2009; doi:10.1093/bib/bbn039.
23. Shabo A, Dotan D. The seventh layer of the clinical-genomics information infrastructure. IBM Syst J 2007; doi:10.1147/sj.461.0057.
24. Amberger J, Bocchini CA, Scott AF et al. McKusick's online Mendelian inheritance in man (OMIM). Nucleic Acids Res 2009; doi:10.1093/nar/gkn665.
25. Fernandez JM, Hoffmann R, Valencia A. iHOP web services. Nucleic Acids Res 2007; doi:10.1093/nar/gkm298.
26. MPI for Molecular Genetics GenomeMatrix. http://genomematrix.molgen.mpg.de. Accessed on 24 February 2009.
27. Kamburov A, Wierling C, Lehrach H et al. ConsensusPathDB – a database for integrating human functional interaction networks. Nucleic Acids Res 2009; doi:10.1093/nar/gkn698.
28. Kanehisa M, Goto S, Hattori M et al. From genomics to chemical genomics: new developments in KEGG. Nucleic Acids Res 2006; doi:10.1093/nar/gkj102.
29. Matthews L, Gopinath G, Gillespie M et al. Reactome knowledgebase of human biological pathways and processes. Nucleic Acids Res 2009; doi:10.1093/nar/gkn863.
30. Rojas I, Golebiewski M, Kania R et al. Storing and annotating of kinetic data. In Silico Biol 2007;7:37–44.
31. Wierling C, Herwig R, Lehrach H. Resources, standards and tools for systems biology. Brief Funct Genomic Proteomic 2007; doi:10.1093/bfgp/elm027.
32. Kaldoudi E, Karaiskakis D. A service based approach for medical image distribution in healthcare Intranets. Comput Methods Programs Biomed 2006; doi:10.1016/j.cmpb.2005.09.007.
33. Klimes D, Kubasek M, Smid R et al. Internet-based system for anti-tumor chemotherapy evaluation. Comput Methods Programs Biomed 2009; doi:10.1016/j.cmpb.2008.10.013.
34. Kopecky J, Vitvar T, Bournez C et al. SAWSDL: Semantic annotations for WSDL and XML schema. IEEE Internet Comput 2007; doi:10.1109/MIC.2007.134.

35. Berners-Lee T, Hendler J, Lassila O. The semantic web. Scientific American Magazine 2001; http://www.sciam.com/article.cfm?id=the-semantic-web. Accessed on 24 February 2009.
36. Shadbolt N, Hall W, Berners-Lee T. The semantic web revisited. IEEE Intell Syst 2006; doi:10.1109/MIS.2006.62.
37. Rubin DL, Lewis SE, Mungall CJ et al. National Center for Biomedical Ontology: advancing biomedicine through structured organization of scientific knowledge. Omics 2006; doi:10.1089/omi.2006.10.185.
38. W3C OWL Reference. http://www.w3.org/TR/owl-ref/. Accessed on 24 February 2009.
39. Wolstencroft K, Alper P, Hull D et al. The myGrid ontology: bioinformatics service discovery. Int J Bioinform Res Appl 2007;3:303–325.
40. Ceresa M, Masseroli M. Clinical and biomolecular ontologies for E-Health. In: Lazakidou AA, Siassiakos KM (eds.), Handbook of Research on Distributed Medical Informatics and E-Health. Hershey: IGI Publishing, 2008.
41. Paolucci M, Kawamura T, Payne TR et al. Semantic matching of web services capabilities. In: The Semantic Web – ISWC 2002. Berlin/Heidelberg: Springer, 2002.
42. Li W, Guo W. Semantic-based web service matchmaking algorithm in biomedicine. International Conference on BioMedical Engineering and Informatics 2008; doi:10.1109/BMEI.2008.278.
43. Harkema H, Roberts I, Gaizauskas R et al. A web service for biomedical term look-up. Comp Funct Genomics 2005; doi:10.1002/cfg.459.
44. Knublauch H, Dameron O, Musen MA. Weaving the biomedical semantic web with the Protege OWL plugin. In: Hahn U (ed.), International Workshop on Formal Biomedical Knowledge Representation 2004. http://sunsite.informatik.rwth-aachen.de/Publications/CEUR-WS/Vol-102/knublauch.pdf. Accessed on 24 February 2009.
45. Jonquet C, Musen MA, Shah NH. Help will be provided for this task: Ontology-based annotator web service. Technical Report 2008. http://www.bioontology.org/publications.html. Accessed on 24 February 2009.
46. Chen H, Wang Y, Wu Z. Introduction to semantic e-Science in biomedicine. BMC Bioinform 2007; doi:10.1186/1471-2105-8-S3-S1.
47. Zhang Z, Cheung KH, Townsend JP. Bringing Web 2.0 to bioinformatics. Brief Bioinform 2009; doi:10.1093/bib/bbn041.
48. Deus HF, Stanislaus R, Veiga DF et al. A semantic web management model for integrative biomedical informatics. PLoS ONE 2008; doi:10.1371/journal.pone.0002946.
49. Pettifer S, Thorne D, McDermott P et al. The embrace registry. EMBnet.news 2008;14:58–62.
50. Stein LD. Towards a cyberinfrastructure for the biological sciences: progress, visions and challenges. Nat Rev Genet 2008; doi:10.1038/nrg2414.
51. Ruttenberg A, Clark T, Bug W et al. Advancing translational research with the Semantic Web. BMC Bioinform 2007; 8:Suppl 3. doi:10.1186/1471-2105-8-S3-S250.

Chapter 8
Web Resources for Gene List Analysis in Biomedicine

Marco Masseroli and Marco Tagliasacchi

Abstract This chapter mainly focuses on the technological and information resources presently available through the web to functionally evaluate lists of genes. It first presents the current biotechnologynanotechnology and molecular biology scenario of the massive production of promising heterogeneous experimental data that need to be evaluated to light new insights on the cellular biomolecular processes and contribute to advances in health care and biomedicine. Then, it describes the technologies to manage, share and computationally use the valuable information and knowledge available in the biomedical and biomolecular domain, and presents the main bio-terminologies and bio-ontologies used to annotate genes and gene products in order to describe their known structural, functional and phenotypic features. Then, it illustrates the main computational analysis techniques that can be used to extract relevant information out of gene and protein annotation profiles, focusing on annotation enrichment analysis and functional similarity metrics. Finally, the chapter presents the resources available online to access existing biomolecular controlled annotations and extract new biomedical knowledge through their analysis, focusing on two representative and well-known web tools. The concise perspective of the field and the selected resources presented help interested readers in quickly understanding the main principles of knowledge representation and analysis in biomedicine and their high relevance for modern biomedical research and e-health.

Keywords: Web Resources · Gene List Analysis · knowledge representation

8.1 Introduction

New biotechnologynanotechnology approaches in molecular biology, particularly high-throughput microarray technologies, allow quickly and simultaneously studying thousands of genes and gene products and their expression levels. Such

M. Masseroli (✉)
Dipartimento di Elettronica e Informazione, Politecnico di Milano, Milan, Italy
e-mail: masseroli@elet.polimi.it

A. Lazakidou (ed.), *Web-Based Applications in Healthcare and Biomedicine*, Annals of Information Systems 7, DOI 10.1007/978-1-4419-1274-9_8,
© Springer Science+Business Media, LLC 2010

technologies are providing unprecedented amount of valuable data that foster the increasing relevance of molecular medicine in health care research and practice. At the same time, advancements in information technologies and biomedical informatics are providing tools and techniques to manage the amount of biomedical data produced, as well as many methods for their analysis. In addition, biomedical domain experts are increasingly annotating biomolecular entities, mainly genes and their protein products, with controlled terminologies and ontologies describing their structural, functional and phenotypic biological features. Availability and analysis of such information is of great value in supporting the biomedical interpretation of biomolecular test results and their use in health care. All these data and information are typically stored in publicly available databanks freely accessible on the web in different formats. Furthermore, over the past decade, several bioinformatics tools have been developed to assist biomedical domain users to explore, analyse and mine such data and information. Most of these tools are web-based applications, which provide ubiquitous access to data and algorithmic resources through the conventional web interface.

Among the biomedical information available on the web, controlled biomolecular annotations have particular relevance, since their analysis and mining can unveil significant biomedical knowledge. Currently, several controlled vocabularies are routinely used to annotate genes and proteins. Some of them have a flat structure, i.e. no explicit relationships between the terms composing the vocabulary exist. Others form ontologies, where semantic relationships are defined between pairs of terms. Controlled annotations enable the analysis of annotation profiles of groups of genes or gene products by means of data mining and knowledge discovery algorithms, which have been implemented and made available as web-based tools. For example, several web tools can be used to perform the enrichment analysis of controlled annotations, which allows isolating the annotation terms most significantly enriched in a group of genes compared to a reference gene group. As each annotation term describes a biomedical feature of the annotated gene, the enrichment analysis can highlight the most relevant biomedical features of a group of genes, thus supporting the interpretation of the common selection of the genes, e.g. selected as candidate associated with a specific pathology through a high-throughput microarray experiment. Furthermore, based on gene annotation profiles, functional similarity metrics between pairs or groups of genes can be computed. This is valuable information since it complements structural similarity metrics, which can be derived from comparison of gene nucleotide sequences, and gene expression level similarities, which can be calculated from microarray experimental data. Such functional similarity metrics enable also the use of clustering techniques to search for groups of genes sharing similar functionalities, and allow the graphical visualization of genes in a "functionality" space.

Since the above described the relevance of web-accessible data and tools in the modern biomedicine and in the health care of the very near future, this chapter focuses on available controlled terminologies and ontologies, computational techniques for their analysis, and currently most relevant web tools that enable accessing available controlled annotations and extracting biomedical knowledge through their analysis.

8.2 Bio-terminologies and Bio-ontologies

Biologists and clinicians mainly collect information and knowledge about facts, and these are difficulty handled by computer systems. As discussed in by Stevens et al. [1], if machines are to compute with factual knowledge, the semantic has to be precisely defined and standardized. The instruments used to reach this goal of defining a precise and standardized semantic are *terminologies* and *ontologies*. Though the first ones are simple collections of the names of the entities involved in a domain, they can be tremendously useful as they define a common vocabulary that can be shared among the applications of that domain. Such vocabularies are *controlled* since they are defined and maintained updated by *curators*, i.e. groups of experts in the domain referred by each vocabulary. Notably, in molecular biology the number, coverage and, most important, usage of such vocabularies are increasing.

Ontologies are the most powerful technology for knowledge representation. They describe a piece of reality: a collection of classes of entities and the relationships among them. Ontologies contain a controlled vocabulary or terminology, plus a *semantic network* that encodes the relationships between each term of the vocabulary. Semantic networks are logical structures used to represent knowledge, in a specific domain, through a graph structure composed of a set of elements, the graph nodes, representing the domain concepts, and relations among them, the graph arches, representing the knowledge of the domain. They are also a reasoning tool, since relations can be found between concepts not directly related. Furthermore, they can be implemented in software and automatically processed.

Ontologies are often used to represent and share knowledge about a domain, by modelling classes of entities pertaining to the domain and the relationships among them. For their peculiar features, ontologies are very useful for automatic classification methods and information analyses that require universal terminologies [2, 3]. Furthermore, in a scenario of increasing automation of knowledge sharing processes and of the inference of functional dependencies among biological and biomolecular agents, the use of ontologies is paramount. In fact, ontologies enable to formalize the knowledge required to execute effective and efficient computational processes. However, in order to be really useful, a bio-ontology, i.e. an ontology suitable for the biomolecular or biomedical domain, must be able to communicate the definition of its terms independently from the reader and the context. This is particularly important in the functional genomics domain, where, for example, it is required to describe the multiplicity of gene functions. Furthermore, a bio-ontology must represent only the terms and relationships absolutely essential to describe the knowledge of the considered domain, in order to remain the most simple possible and increase the spectrum of its usage. In addition, there is also the need of both *organism-specific* ontologies, since genes do not have always the same function in different species, and *cross-organism* ontologies, which regard more species simultaneously, since several genes have the same or analogue functions in different organisms.

In the past few years, several terminologies and ontologies in the biomedical and biomolecular domains have been built, although only few of them are widely used

[4]. The terminologies and ontologies most important and both used to annotate genes and gene products, in order to describe their known functional features, and available to be analysed within the most relevant web tools are described below.

8.2.1 Main Bio-terminologies

Currently, in molecular biology several controller vocabularies are available to describe specific functional features of genes and gene products, and their subcellular and tissue localization. The main examples of such vocabularies are those regarding *biochemical pathways*, provided by the Kyoto Encyclopedia of Genes and Genomes (KEGG) databank (http://www.genome.jp/kegg/) [5], *protein families and domains*, provided by the Pfam databank (http://pfam.sanger.ac.uk/) [6], *inherited disorders*, provided by the Online Mendelian Inheritance in Man (OMIM) databank (http://www.ncbi.nlm.nih.gov/sites/entrez?db=omim) [7, 8], *gene expression* in human anatomical systems, cellular types, developmental stages and pathologies, provided by the eVOC ontologies (http://www.evocontology.org/) [9], and those included in the *Gene Ontology* (http://www.geneontology.org/) [10], following described, which are currently the controlled vocabularies most complete and developed in the biomolecular domain. All such and other controlled vocabularies describing specific gene or gene product characteristics can be used to annotate lists of genes with biological information and semantically analyse them automatically.

8.2.2 The Open Biomedical Ontologies

The Open Biomedical Ontologies (OBO) Foundry (http://obofoundry.org/) [11] is a collaborative experiment to produce a set of orthogonal, well-structured and fully interoperable reference ontologies for shared use across different biological and biomedical domains. It introduces a new paradigm for biomedical ontology development by the establishment of a common design philosophy and implementation, sharing of unique identifier space, inclusion of definitions and provision of gold standard reference ontologies for individual domains of inquiry.

The OBO ontologies tackle several different biological aspects, including organism taxonomies, anatomies, cell types, genotypes, sequence attributes, temporal attributes, phenotypes, diseases, etc. In order to be part of OBO, an ontology must be

- *Open*, i.e. accessible to everyone without any constrain; its origin must be recognized, and subsequent modifications must be distributed under different names and identifiers.
- *Expressed in a common and shared syntax* (OBO syntax, its extension or in OWL), in order to ease use of the same tools and shared implementation of software applications.
- *Clearly specified*, well documented and with a well-defined content.
- Each ontology must be *orthogonal* and *not overlapping* to other OBO ontologies; partial overlapping can be allowed in order to enable combination of ontology terms to form new terms.

- Able to *include textual definitions* of all terms; since several biomedical terms can be ambiguous, the concepts they represent must be precisely defined with their meaning within the specific ontology domain.

8.2.2.1 The Gene Ontology

Among the OBO ontologies, the Gene Ontology (GO) (http://www.geneontology.org/) [10] is the bio-ontology with the broadest coverage and the most wide usage for annotating biomolecular entities. It is a very important effort, started in November 1998, addressing the need for an integrated resource that provides consistent descriptions of gene products in different biomolecular genomic resource. The main aim of GO is promoting consistent annotation of gene and gene products in any organism with the following three orthogonal ontologies:

- Biological processes
- Cellular components
- Molecular functions

The first describes biological processes such as metabolism or signal transduction. The second one helps specifying where a biological process takes place. The last one describes the biochemical activity independently from a precise cellular localization or a precise biological process. They globally hold more than 25,000 controlled functional term categories and subcategories.

The semantic structure of GO is a direct acyclic graph (DAG), i.e. a graph composed of nodes and edges (Figs. 8.1 and 8.2). Each node represents a single

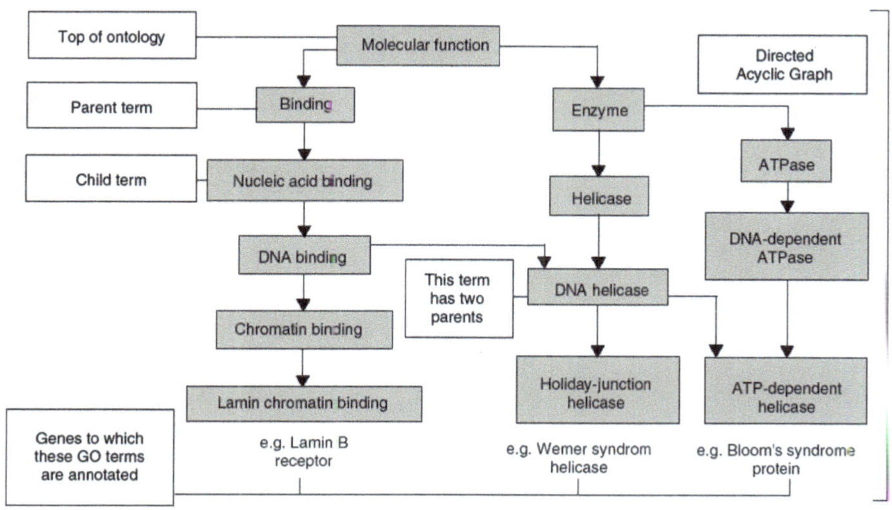

Fig. 8.1 Example of Gene Ontology direct acyclic graph and meaning of its elements

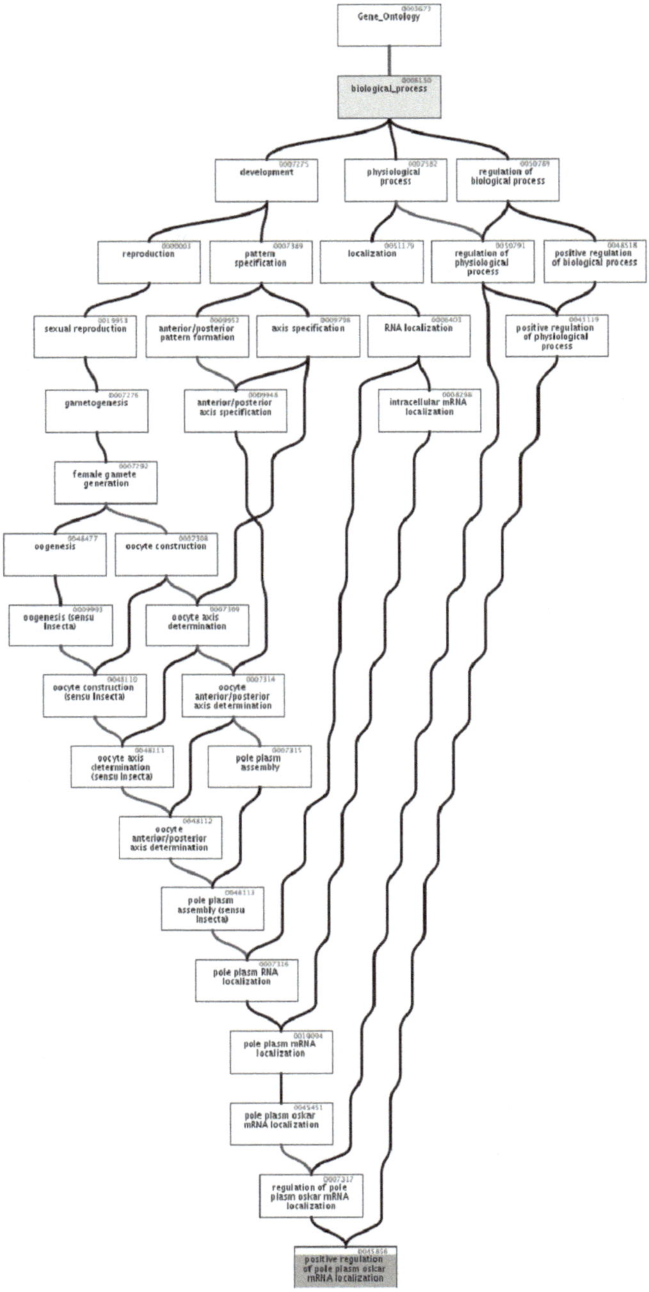

Fig. 8.2 A complex Gene Ontology DAG structure

concept, a GO category, described by a term of the controlled vocabulary. Edges, which link together two nodes, represent relationships between the concepts, and hence between the vocabulary terms. At present, the main types of relations present in the Gene Ontology are *specification* (i.e. the "*IS_A*" relation) and *membership* (i.e. the "*PART_OF*" relation). Through them, either very general terms or very precise terms can be represented. A DAG is very similar to a hierarchical tree structure because no cycles exist between nodes, and edges have a one-way meaning. Nevertheless, a DAG differs from a hierarchy in that a "child" (i.e. a more specialized concept or term) can have many "parents" (i.e. more generic concepts or terms) and may have different types of relations with its different parents.

Despite its broad definition and wide use in the biomolecular domain, GO present some issues mainly due to its still short life, its uneven growing complexity and the fast increasing knowledge of the domain it represents. Nevertheless, the GO remains a very useful instrument both to annotate and describe gene and gene product functions across species and to connect at best several functional annotations concerning individual biological concepts but related to different species, or simply sparsely stored in heterogeneous databases. Therefore, it allows automatically performing controlled searches, functional enrichment analyses and semantic clustering of diverse gene annotations, which is very useful in many genomic analyses (e.g. high-throughput gene expression) to group genes and gene products to some biological high-level concept/term. Besides helping in better interpreting results of such experimental analyses, this ability is fundamental also in the characterization of less known genes. In fact, if in the same cellular component an uncharacterized gene is co-expressed with well-characterized genes annotated to some GO biological process, one can infer that the "unknown" gene's product is likely to act in the same process.

8.3 Analysis of Controlled Annotations

Structural, functional and phenotypic annotations of gene and gene products represent valuable resources that can be analysed for extracting new relevant biological knowledge. In this section we focus on the analysis of annotations of biomolecular entities of an individual organism. We consider the case of annotated genomes, whereby the biomolecular entities are the genes of a given organism, although most of the considerations can be equally applied to annotated proteomes. More specifically, we consider the following analysis techniques, which require as input an annotated genome:

- Annotation enrichment in gene lists
- Functional similarity between genes

Considered annotations are based on a controlled vocabulary such as the ones introduced in Section 8.2 of this chapter. In some cases, semantic relationships between terms of a controlled vocabulary are explicitly defined by means of an ontology, e.g. the Gene Ontology (GO).

Before describing in detail the aforementioned techniques, we introduce the notation that we adopt in the remainder of this section. Consider a controlled vocabulary of n terms and an organism for which m genes have been annotated with at least one term. Let $\mathbf{A}_d \in \{0, 1\}^{m \times n}$ define the matrix representing direct annotations of a specific controlled vocabulary. The m rows of A_d correspond to genes, while the n columns correspond to annotation terms. We assign to each gene and each term a unique numerical identifier in the range, respectively, [1, m] and [1, n], which might differ from the original identifier (typically alphanumerical). The entries of A_d assume values from a binary alphabet according to the following rule:

$$\mathbf{A}_d(i, j) = \begin{cases} 0 \text{ if gene } i \text{ is annotated to term } j \\ 1 \qquad\qquad \text{otherwise} \end{cases}$$

The ith row of the matrix $\mathbf{A}_d$ contains a number of ones equal to the number of available annotations for gene g_i. Conversely, the jth column contains a number of ones equal to the number of times term t_j is used to annotate the genes in the considered genome.

If the specific controlled vocabulary used is part of an ontology, e.g. the Gene Ontology, then annotation curators are asked to always use the most specific ontology term to describe a given feature (e.g. a GO functional category) of the annotated gene. As such, when a gene is annotated to a term, it is implicitly assumed to be annotated also to the more generic terms associated with that feature in the ontology, e.g. all the term ancestors in the GO DAG. This process is sometimes defined as annotation unfolding. Let A_{ij} denote a modified gene-to-term matrix, where the assignment of its entries is given by

$$\mathbf{A}_u(i,j) = \begin{cases} 1 \text{ if gene } i \text{ is annotated to term } j \text{ or to any descendant of } j \\ 0 \qquad\qquad\qquad \text{otherwise} \end{cases}$$

The ith row of the matrix A_{ij} contains all the direct and indirect annotations of gene i, i.e. represents the annotation profile of gene g_i.

8.3.1 Annotation Enrichment Analysis

A relevant problem that arises in functional genomics is to detect significant enrichment and/or depletion of terms used to functionally annotate genes of a set of interest. Given a (possibly large) set of genes together with their functional annotations, hereby denoted *target set*, one might be interested in providing a functional characterization of this set, e.g. by determining which annotation terms are significantly overrepresented (enriched) or underrepresented (depleted) in the available annotation profiles, with respect to a larger gene population, hereby denoted *master set*. For example, in the analysis of data produced by means of a gene expression microarray experiment, the target set consists of those genes that exhibit significant differential expression, whereas the master set contains all genes represented in the microarray. The answer to this problem is provided by *annotation enrichment analysis* techniques. In their common formulation, all annotation terms are considered to be independent from each other. Later in this section we briefly illustrate alternative techniques that are more suitable when this hypothesis does not hold, e.g. for the case of ontological annotation terms.

Enrichment analysis proceeds on a term-by-term basis computing, for each term, a numerical score by means of adequate test statistics, which can be used in two ways:

- Terms can be ranked according to the assigned score in such a way that significantly enriched/depleted terms appear in the top entries of a ranked list. This enables the biologist to focus her/his attention only on few relevant terms.
- By applying a threshold to the score, it is possible to produce a binary decision about the fact that each term is significantly enriched/depleted or not. The choice of the threshold is governed by the target false-positive rate, i.e. the probability of declaring a term significantly enriched/depleted when it is not.

In the following we present the statistical tests that are commonly used to answer to the aforementioned problems.

The input data for annotation enrichment analysis consist of a master set A of genes and a target set B of genes, with $B \subset A$, together with their annotation profiles. Given a term t_j we need to determine whether there is a significant difference in the use of term t_j in the set A with respect to the set B. The problem is cast in the framework of hypothesis testing, whereby a null hypothesis is formulated and the available data are used to either confirm or reject the null hypothesis. Let H_0 denote the null hypothesis, i.e. the fact that a gene belongs to the target set B is independent from the fact that the same gene is annotated to term t_j. Equivalently, the null hypothesis can be formulated by saying that the genes in the set B are picked at random.

Consider the sets depicted in Fig. 8.3, where n_A and n_B denote the cardinalities of sets A and B. Let T_j be the set of genes annotated to term t_j. Adopting the notation

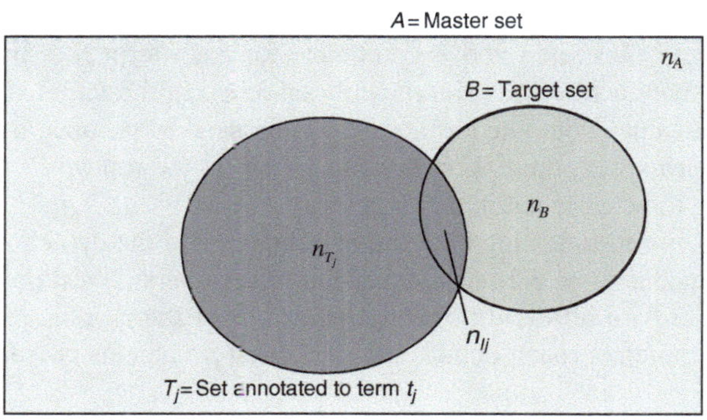

Fig. 8.3 Graphical representation of the A, B and T_j sets used in enrichment analysis

introduced in the previous section, the cardinality of the set T_j, i.e. n_{Tj}, is equal to the sum of the elements in the jth column of the matrix $A_{i,j}$. Consider the set $I_j = B \cap T_j$ of genes belonging to the target set and, at the same time, annotated to term t_j.

If the null hypothesis holds, the cardinality of the set I_j can be represented as a random variable, whose probability mass function is described by the hypergeometric distribution.

$$\Pr(|I_j| = k) = \frac{\binom{n_B}{k}\binom{n_A - n_{T_j}}{n_B - k}}{\binom{n_A}{n_B}}$$

To determine whether term t_j is significantly enriched/depleted, we need to verify if the null hypothesis can be rejected. Generally, when performing the test of a null hypothesis H_0 against some alternative hypothesis, one disposes of a realization x of a random variable X with known distribution under the null hypothesis. In this setting, x is the observed cardinality of the set I_j, n_{Ij}, and the random variable has a probability mass function that obeys the hypergeometric distribution. The statistical test (Fisher's exact test or hyper-geometric test) used to determine the enrichment of term t_j proceeds as follows:

1. Choose a priori the desired significance level α that should not be exceeded. The selected significance level α is equal to the false-positive rate, i.e. the probability of rejecting H_0 when it is true.
2. Compute the p-value p_j, i.e. the probability of finding at least n_{Ij} genes annotated to t_j in the target set under the null hypothesis H_0

$$p_j = \sum_{k \geq n_{I_j}} \Pr(|I_j| = k).$$

3. Compare the obtained p-value with the significance level α. If $p_j \leq \alpha$, then reject the null hypothesis. Equivalently, this means that the fact of belonging to the target gene set is dependent from being annotated to term t_j. Hence term t_j is significantly enriched (at a significance level α) in the target set of genes.

The procedure illustrated above computes, for each term t_j, a binary decision about the fact that each term is significantly enriched in the target set of genes. In addition, the p-values computed at step 2 can be used to produce a ranked list of terms, where terms with the lowest p-value appear at the top of the list since they are more likely to be enriched in the target set.

If one is interested in testing both the enrichment and the depletion of term t_j, a two-sided test needs to be carried out, instead of the one-side test described above. In this case, there are different possible definitions of the p-value proposed in the literature. A simple approach defines the two-sided p-value as twice the one-sided p-value

$$p_j^{\text{two-sided}} = 2 \min\left[\Pr(|I_j| \geq n_{I_j}), \Pr(|I_j \leq n_{I_j}|)\right].$$

Other possible definitions and a discussion on the appropriate choice of the test (one-sided vs. two-sided) are given in Rivals et al. [12].

The significance level α governs the target false-positive rate only if the test is performed on a single term. In practice, one is interested in testing multiple terms for enrichment/depletion at the same time. If all terms are considered to be independent, it can be shown that the false-positive rate is equal to $1-(1-\alpha)^n$, where n denotes the number of terms for which the enrichment is tested. This value tends to 1 when the number of terms is large, as typically occurs in practice for commonly used controlled vocabularies. Therefore, when a statistical test is repeated multiple times, multiple test correction [13] needs to be applied in order to re-calculate the p-values in such a way to avoid a large number of false positives. There are several ways of performing multiple test correction. The simplest method is the *Bonferroni correction*, which can be applied when the tests are independent. The correction computes an adjusted p-value equal to $p_j^{\text{adj}} = n \times p_j$. This method is the most conservative, in the sense that, at a given significance level α, it considerably reduces the number of false positives by favouring an increase in the number of false negatives, i.e. some terms might not be declared as significantly enriched in a set of genes when, indeed, they are enriched. Other multiple correction methods, from the most to the least conservative, are *Bonferroni-Holm* [14], *Westfall–Young* [15] and *Benjamini–Hochberg* [16].

The enrichment analysis method discussed so far assumes that terms are independent from each other. If semantic relationships between the terms of a controlled vocabulary exist, as when they are described by means of an ontology, the independence hypothesis ceases to hold. Recently, some works have addressed this issue proposing methods that take into account term dependencies. In Grossman et al. [17], it is observed that in the case of genes annotated to GO terms, children of enriched terms tend to be also enriched. In order to avoid this inheritance problem, they proposed to take into account also the number n_{T_p} of genes annotated to the parents of the term t_j, and the number n_{I_p} of genes annotated to parents of t_j that also belong to the target set B (Fig. 8.4). Accordingly, they

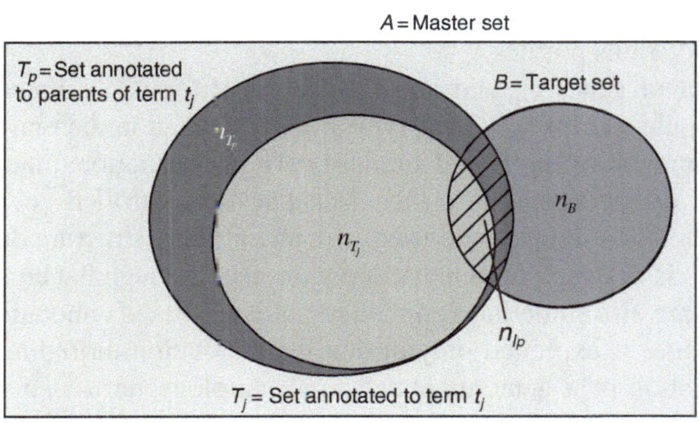

Fig. 8.4 Graphical representation of the A, B, T_j, T_P and I_P sets used in enrichment analysis when an ontology defines dependencies between terms

proposed to modify the probability mass function under the null hypothesis as follows:

$$P\left(|I_j| = k \,\big|\, |B \cap T_p| = n_{I_p}\right) = \frac{\binom{n_B}{k}\binom{n_{T_p} - n_{T_j}}{n_{I_p} - k}}{\binom{n_{T_p}}{n_{I_p}}}.$$

Alexa et al. [18] analysed GO terms in a bottom-up order from the most specific to the more general terms. In their *Elim* method, for each level of the GO hierarchy, if a term t_j is found to be significantly enriched, those genes annotated to t_j are removed from both the master and the target set. Their *Weight* method is more conservative, in the sense that it avoids removing genes from the sets, but rather it introduces a more sophisticated weighting scheme.

Annotation enrichment analysis can be applied also when the target set B of genes is not a subset of the master set A. However, in these cases the enrichment analysis tests need to be modified accordingly, as described by Günther et al. [19].

8.3.2 Functional Similarity Analysis

Computing the similarity between genes or gene products is of paramount importance in many application scenarios, ranging from gene clustering, visualization, search, etc. There are several methods proposed in the literature that compute a similarity score between gene pairs. Traditional strategies are based on the study of the homology of nucleotide sequences, or the knowledge of functional categories (e.g. protein domain families), or the analysis of correlations that arise in microarray gene expression experiments. An issue related to these strategies is that the majority of co-functioning genes are neither sequence related nor synthesize proteins in the same protein family, such as genes in the same pathway. Therefore, an alternative approach to computing functional similarity consists of exploiting the available functional annotations profiles.

Given a pair of genes g_{i_1} and g_{i_2}, and the set of terms annotated to them, the goal is to compute a score $S(g_{i_1}, g_{i_2})$, typically normalized in the range [0,1], which measures the amount of functional similarity. The computational methods that can be used might differ depending on the fact that the controlled vocabulary of the considered annotation terms is endowed with an ontology structure or not. First, we consider methods designed for annotations expressed through flat controlled vocabularies, which are also sometimes applied to ontology-based annotations, where the ontology structure is exploited only during the annotation unfolding step (i.e. the explicit association of a gene annotated to an ontology term also with the more generic ancestor terms in the ontology of the term). Later we discuss more sophisticated methods that explicitly consider the semantic relationships defined by the ontology when assessing the functional similarity.

The simplest methods rely on vector space model techniques commonly used in the field of information retrieval. Let $a_{i_1}^{\mathrm{T}}$ and $a_{i_2}^{\mathrm{T}}$ denote the i_1-th and i_2-th rows of the matrix A (where $A = A_d$ or $A = A_{ij}$ depending on whether unfolding is applied). Hence, each gene is represented by a vector in an n-dimensional space. The similarity between two genes can be computed as the cosine of the angle between the two vectors, i.e.

$$S(i_1,i_2) = \frac{\mathbf{a}_{i_1}^{\mathrm{T}} \mathbf{a}_{i_2}}{||\mathbf{a}_{i_1}|| \, ||\mathbf{a}_{i_2}||}.$$

If two genes share the same annotation profile, $S(i_1,i_2) = 1$, whereas if they do not have any term in common, $S(g_{i_1},g_{i_2}) = 0$. As in conventional information retrieval systems, various weighting schemes can be introduced to account for the fact that terms are not equally likely to occur.

An alternative approach makes use of the *kappa* statistics to define a similarity score between $a_{i_1}^{\mathrm{T}}$ and $a_{i_2}^{\mathrm{T}}$. The kappa statistics can be thought of as the chance-corrected agreement between the annotations of gene g_{i_1} and g_{i_2}, and it is computed as follows. Let $C_{1,1}(i_1,i_2)$ denote the number of times when $a_{i_1}^{\mathrm{T}}(j) = a_{i_2}^{\mathrm{T}}(j) = 1$, for some term j, i.e. the number of terms in common in the annotation profiles of the two genes. Similarly, $C_{0,0}(i_1,i_2)$ is the number of times when $a_{i_1}^{\mathrm{T}}(j) = a_{i_2}^{\mathrm{T}}(j) = 0$. Finally, let $C_1(i_1)$ the number of terms annotated to gene g_{i1}, consequently, $C_0(i_1) = n - C_1(i_1)$. The score computed by means of the kappa statistics is given by

$$S(g_{i_1} g_{i_2}) = \frac{O(i_1,i_2) - A(i_1,i_2)}{1 - A(i_1,i_2)},$$

where $O(i_1,i_2)$ denote the fraction of terms for which the two annotation profiles are in agreement, i.e.

$$O(i_1,i_2) = \frac{C_{1,1}(i_1,i_2) - C_{0,0}(i_1,i_2)}{n}$$

and

$$A(i_1,i_2) = \frac{C_1(i_1)C_1(i_2) - C_0(i_1)C_0(i_1)}{n^2}.$$

When terms of a controlled vocabulary are not independent from each other, such as when they are part of an ontology, the computation of the functional similarity between genes should take this fact into account. In this case, first, the similarity between pairs of terms, $S(t_{j_1},t_{j_2})$, is computed. Second, the functional similarity between pairs of genes $S(g_{i_1},g_{i_2})$ is determined. To address the first task, there are several methods that have been proposed. In the following we summarize the most relevant ones, which have been applied, for example, to assess the similarity between GO terms. *Edge counting methods* measure the similarity between two terms based on distance, expressed as the number of ontology edges, between the ontology nodes associated with the two terms. The shorter this distance, the higher the similarity [20]. Variations may define weights for the edges according to their position in the ontology [21]. Compared to edge counting methods, *information-theoretic methods* [22] have been shown to be significantly less sensitive to edge density variability, which is generally present among different branches of a bio-ontology. They consist of determining the amount of information that two terms share in common. For each term t_j, $p(t_j)$ is the probability of finding t_j or a descendant of t_j in the available annotations of the considered m genes,

$$p(t_j) = \frac{1}{m}\sum_{i=1}^{m} \mathbf{A}(i,j).$$

Hence, the *information content* of a term is equal to $\mathrm{IC}(t_j) = -\log p(t_j)$. These types of methods exploit the assumption that the more information two terms share in common, the more similar they are. Let $\mathrm{LCA}(t_{j_1},t_{j_2})$ be the *least common ancestor* between term t_{j_1} and t_{j_2}, i.e. the term with the least probability among all the ancestors that are in common to both terms. Based on this concept, several metrics have been proposed. *Resnik's metrics* [20] defines the similarity between two terms as

$$s(t_{j_1},t_{j_2}) = \mathrm{IC}[\mathrm{LCA}(t_{j_1},t_{j_2})].$$

Intuitively, the similarity score is large when the probability of the least common ancestor is small. This occurs when the least common ancestor is a specific term in the ontology close to the two terms t_{j_1} and t_{j_2}. An issue of the Resnik's metrics is that it is not bounded in the interval [0,1]. This is fixed by the *Lin's metrics* [23],

$$s(t_{j_1},t_{j_2}) = \frac{2\,\mathrm{IC}[\mathrm{LCA}(t_{j_1},t_{j_2})]}{\mathrm{IC}(t_{j_1}) + \mathrm{IC}(t_{j_1})}.$$

Another similarity metrics proposed by Jiang and Conrath [24] is

$$s(t_{j_1},t_{j_2}) = \frac{1}{\mathrm{IC}(t_{j_1}) + \mathrm{IC}(t_{j_2}) - 2\,\mathrm{IC}[\mathrm{LCA}(t_{j_1},t_{j_2})] + 1}.$$

Computing the functional similarity between two genes is equivalent to determining the similarity between two sets of terms, i.e. those used to annotate the genes. There is no clear consensus about what is the best strategy of combining the term-to-term similarity scores $S(t_{j_1},t_{j_2})$ to compute the gene-to-gene similarity $S(g_{i_1},g_{i_2})$. Below we report some of the most widely adopted options. Let $\sum$ denote a $n_{i_1} \times n_{i_2}$ matrix where each row represents one of the terms used to annotate gene g_{i1} and each column one of the terms used to annotate gene g_{i2}. In Lord et al. [25], the similarity between two genes is set equal to the maximum similarity among all possible term pairs that can be formed coupling the annotations of gene g_{i1} with those of gene g_{i2}, i.e.

$$s(g_{i_1},g_{i_2}) = \max_{\substack{t_{j_1}=1,\ldots,n_{i_1}\\ t_{j_2}=1,\ldots,n_{i_2}}} \sum (t_{j_1},t_{j_2}).$$

Alternatively, Speer et al. [26] defined the gene functional similarity as the average

$$s(g_{i_1}, g_{i_2}) = \frac{1}{n_{i_1} n_{i_2}} \sum_{t_{j_1}=1}^{n_{i_1}} \sum_{t_{j_2}=1}^{n_{i2}} \sum (t_{j1}, t_{j2}).$$

More complex aggregation functions have been also proposed, e.g. in Schlicker et al. [27], or Tao et al. [28].

8.4 Web-Based Tools for Gene Annotation Analysis

Recently, different tools have been implemented with the goal of automatically analysing and classifying gene lists on the basis of GO terms, and more rarely also of other genomic controlled vocabularies, used to annotate the genes in the lists. Generally, all these tools allow annotating large numbers of biomolecular sequence identifiers with the biomedical information present in heterogeneous and distributed databanks, which they retrieve and integrate by applying information technology approaches. Some of such tools allow classifying genes, or gene products, according to bio-ontological categories (terms), mainly those of the GO, and performing semantic queries on a given gene list. Such queries provide all required semantic categories, and their subcategories, associated with the genes in the given list. Therefore, they enable to identify either how many and which categories are related to a set of genes or how many and which genes of a particular set belong to the same category. Very few more advanced tools allow performing gene classifications also according to some other ontologies or controlled vocabularies besides the GO (e.g. those provided by KEGG, Pfam or OMIM). Some of them also allow analysing statistically the obtained classifications in order to highlight annotation categories (i.e. structural, functional or phenotypic aspects) relevant in the considered set of genes, whose identification might help in unveiling molecular mechanisms involved in complex pathophysiological processes. Towards this goal, different statistical analysis, clustering and knowledge discovery approaches, including the analysis methods previously discussed in Section 3 of this chapter, are being applied. They can be used to support the biological interpretation of high-throughput biomolecular experimental results, for example, generated by means of microarray technologies, which provide numerous lists of genes candidate involved in the biological processes analysed. In fact, in these cases the identified lists need to be annotated with known relevant structural, functional and phenotypic information about each gene in the list, in order to highlight significant features that are common, or sporadic, among the genes in the list. For this aim, it is paramount the role of the gene annotations expressed through controlled vocabularies and ontologies, which allow grouping the genes according to their structural, functional and phenotypic annotation categories that can be statistically analysed [29].

All software tools, most of which are publicly available, that have been developed in the past years to annotate list of genes with controller biomolecular annotations available in different databanks, and analyse and classify the genes according to such annotations, can be grouped into three general categories:

- *Annotation tools* (e.g. EnsMart [30] (http://www.ensembl.org/biomart/martview/) and MatchMiner [31] (http://www.discover.nci.nih.gov/matchminer/index.jsp), which produce only tabular outputs of retrieved gene annotations.
- *Exploratory tools* (e.g. GOSurfer [32] (http://www.bioinformatics.bioen.uiuc.edu/gosurfer/) and MAPPFinder [33] (http://www.genmapp.org/), which provide also annotation browsing functionalities and some form of graphical representation of summarized data.
- *Integrated tools*, which combine annotation and exploration features with statistical analyses and automatic procedures to evaluate the most relevant retrieved annotations for the considered set of genes [34].

The last category tools are clearly the most interesting, although most of them consider only GO annotations. They generally provide an easy-to-use web interface to perform statistical analyses, including those described in the previous S**ect. 3 of this chapter, on the controlled annotations of gene lists. The typical evaluation steps that can be executed with these tools are:

1. *Uploading of the lists* of nucleotide sequence identifiers to be analysed, subdivided into two or more classes (e.g. identifiers of the nucleotide sequences selected as overexpressed or underexpressed in a high-throughput microarray experiment)
2. *Identification of the individual genes* related to the uploaded nucleotide sequence identifiers
3. *Search for the controlled annotations* available for such genes in different biomolecular databanks
4. *Structural, functional and phenotypic categorization* of the considered genes according to the retrieved annotations (e.g. biological processes, molecular functions, cellular components, biochemical pathways, protein domains, inherited disorders)
5. *Numerical and statistical evaluation* (e.g. by enrichment analysis) of the significance of the annotation categories in each class of genes considered compared to the genes in a reference group (e.g. all genes represented by the nucleotide sequences on the microarray used to select the classes of overexpressed and underexpressed genes to analyse)
6. *Tabular and graphical visualization* of the significant structural, functional and phenotypical annotation categories in each of the classes of genes considered; such identified significant categories can help in the biological interpretation of the experimental results that selected the analysed nucleotide sequences.

All these tools have similar functionalities and purposes. Yet, among the currently most relevant tools freely available on the web that implement analysis approaches described in the previous Section 3 of this chapter are *GFINDer* [35–37] and *DAVID Bioinformatics Resources* [38–40]. Besides GO annotations, they consider also other gene and gene product publicly available annotations expressed through other controller vocabularies and ontologies, including those that describe biochemical pathways (KEGG), protein families and domains (Pfam e InterPro), genetics disorders (OMIM), etc. Thus, both of such tools allow analysing list of genes according to their functional and phenotypic features. They provide a very important support to help identifying the biological roles played by the genes selected in functional genomic experiments and translating the massive gene expression and protein data produced into biological knowledge.

8.4.1 GFINDer

GFINDer (http://www.bioinformatics.polimi.it/GFINDer/), the Genome Function INtegrated Discoverer, is a web tool for effective using genomic information available in many heterogeneous databanks accessible via the Internet that allows performing statistical analyses and data mining of functional and phenotypic annotations of gene sets, for instance, identified in high-throughput biomolecular experiments. It automatically retrieves annotations of several functional and phenotypic categories from many different public sources, identifies the categories enriched in each class of a user-classified gene list and calculates statistical significance values for each category. GFINDer also enables gene classification according to functional categories and the statistical analysis of obtained results. It therefore permits better understanding of high-throughput experiment results and mining hidden biomedical knowledge by examining user nucleotide sequence ID lists and applying clustering and statistical analysis methods to their available genomic annotations retrieved from several databanks. The annotations currently considered in GFINDer regard:

- *Biological processes*, *cellular components* and *molecular functions*, provided by the gene ontology
- *Biochemical pathways*, supplied by the KEGG databank
- *Protein families and domains*, by Pfam and InterPro (http://www.ebi.ac.uk/interpro/) [41] databanks
- *Gene expression in human anatomical systems, cellular types, developmental stages, and pathologies*, provided by the eVOC ontologies
- Clinical and phenotypic information (i.e. *Phenotypes* and *phenotype locations* associated with inherited disorders or genetic loci), by the OMIM databank.

The GFINDer system is implemented in a three-tier architecture based on a multi-database structure (Fig. 8.5). In the first tier, the *data tier*, a relational DBMS server manages all different types of provided information, including user uploaded

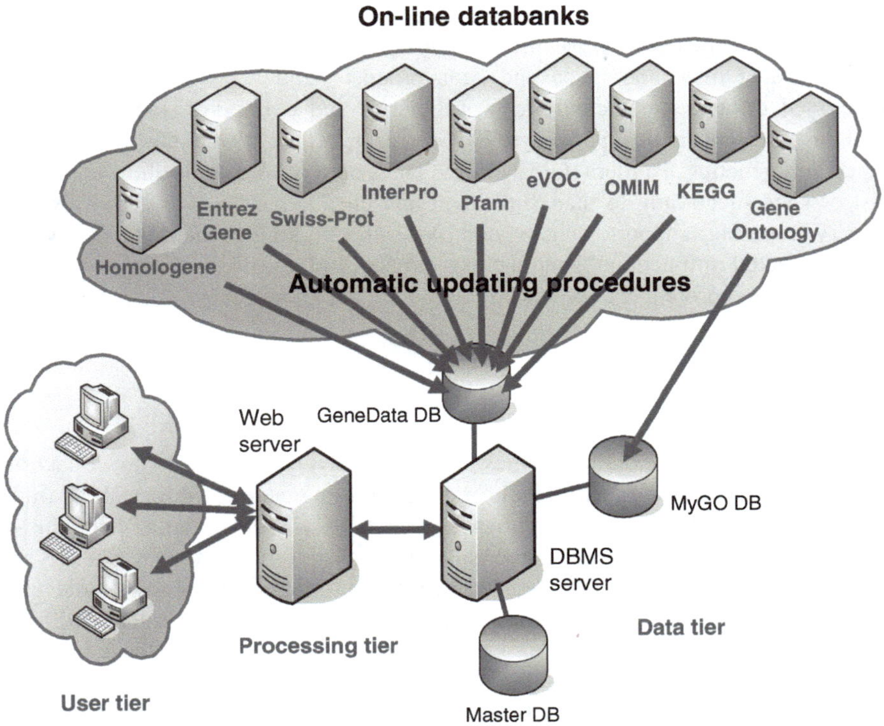

Fig. 8.5 The three-tier architecture of the GFINDer system

lists of classified sequence data, gene annotations and their controlled vocabulary terms and ontological relationships between them. Annotation data integrated in GFINDer data tier are kept updated by software procedures that automatically retrieve them from several public biomolecular and biomedical databanks as soon as new releases become available. In the second tier, the *processing tier*, a web server manages the requests coming from client computers, communicates with the DBMS server on the data layer, and runs all system processing and analyses. The third tier, the *user tier*, is composed of any client computer connected to the web server on the processing tier through an Internet/intranet communication network and loading in its client web browser the GFINDer graphic user interface, implemented as web pages.

The illustrated three-tier architecture enhances the GFINDer system performances by subdividing the required computational power between the two web and DBMS servers. Easiness and friendliness of system usage are busted through the provided common and intuitive web interface, which give access to specific modules that support the computational steps required to evaluate the functional significance of gene lists through statistical indexes. They allow users to study the distribution of different user-selected classes of genes among the several integrated functional and phenotypic annotation categories. Each module supports a specific task, as following described.

- The *Upload* module enables the user to input a plain or classified list of gene identifiers (e.g. GenBank accession numbers, RefSeq IDs, Affymetrix probe IDs, UniGene cluster IDs or Entrez Gene IDs) in the GFINDer web server; classifications can derive from high-throughput experiments (e.g. differential gene expression), from any clustering method applied to such or other gene data, or from different experimental biological conditions.
- The *Annotation* module produces a tabular output of the uploaded gene list enriched with several different annotations integrated in GFINDer data tier and linked to the corresponding original online source in order to allow displaying more information about them and the annotated gene just by clicking on them.
- The *Exploration* modules perform functional and phenotypic categorizations of the input genes according to their annotation categories integrated in the data tier; provided results illustrate the distribution of the considered genes among these functional and phenotypic characteristics. In particular, the *Genetic Disorders* module uses the phenotype and phenotype location vocabularies provided by OMIM, and normalized and structured within the GFINDer data tier, to clearly show how many and which inherited diseases, phenotype locations and specific signs and symptoms are correlated to each considered gene, or how many of the selected genes are associated with each disorder, location or phenotype. Similarly, the *Biochemical Pathways*, *Protein Families & Domains*, *Expression Ontologies*, and *Gene Ontologies* modules do. The latter also provides views based on the GO semantic network to easily and graphically clarify the semantic relationships existing among the represented GO functional categories.
- The *Statistics* modules allow applying easily the statistical tests and corrections described in Section 3 of this chapter in order to analyse the significant enrichment of GO, KEGG, Pfam, InterPro, eVOC and OMIM annotations of the input genes when these are subdivided in different classes, or a reference gene list is also provided (e.g. the list of all genes in the microarray used to select the input genes). This allows highlighting which of the considered functional and phenotypic features each class of the input genes is related to, and with which probability (e.g. significantly over or underrepresented in the user-defined classes of genes). Thus, a plain list of gene identifiers is enriched with biological meaning and statistical significances. All statistical modules show a result table containing, for each functional category associated with the input gene list and the selected gene class, the observed number of input genes, their expected number and the significant *p*-value of the functional category for the selected gene class (Fig. 8.6). Links to the external sources of all annotations analysed for the considered genes are also given.

Based on some of the publicly available genomic resources, GFINDer system effectively supports genomic biomedical investigation through functional annotations and statistical evaluations of the enrichment of different functional and

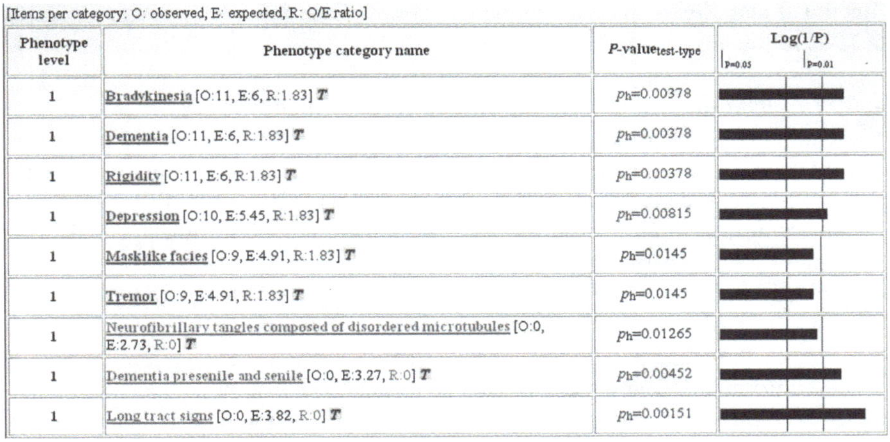
[Items per category: O: observed, E: expected, R: O/E ratio]

Phenotype level	Phenotype category name	P-value$_{test-type}$	Log(1/P)
1	Bradykinesia [O:11, E:6, R:1.83] T	p_h=0.00378	
1	Dementia [O:11, E:6, R:1.83] T	p_h=0.00378	
1	Rigidity [O:11, E:6, R:1.83] T	p_h=0.00378	
1	Depression [O:10, E:5.45, R:1.83] T	p_h=0.00815	
1	Masklike facies [O:9, E:4.91, R:1.83] T	p_h=0.0145	
1	Tremor [O:9, E:4.91, R:1.83] T	p_h=0.0145	
1	Neurofibrillary tangles composed of disordered microtubules [O:0, E:2.73, R:0] T	p_h=0.01265	
1	Dementia presenile and senile [O:0, E:3.27, R:0] T	p_h=0.00452	
1	Long tract signs [O:0, E:3.82, R:0] T	p_h=0.00151	

Fig. 8.6 Example of the use of the *Statistics* module Genetics Disorders of GFINDer: Inherited disorder phenotypes significantly enriched in a list of 18 genes candidate correlated with Parkinson disease (phenotypes in *red*) versus a list of 15 genes candidate correlated with Alzheimer disease (phenotypes in *green*). Phenotype level: level of a given phenotype in the defined Phenotype hierarchy (higher levels correspond to more detailed and specific phenotype descriptions); P-value$_{test-type}$: p-value defining the significance of the enrichment of a given phenotype in a considered class of genes, and initial of used statistical test name (h: hypergeometric distribution test)

phenotypic annotation categories in user-selected classes of genes. Thus, it helps highlighting significant biological characteristics of lists of genes and discovering the relevant involvement of a set of genes in specific biological processes and functions. Among the available tools, GFINDer is the only one that allows analysing also phenotypic annotations (signs and symptoms) in support to the biological interpretation of genes lists (Fig. 8.6). By facilitating a genomic approach to the understanding of the fundamental biological processes and complex cellular pathophysiological mechanisms, GFINDer represents an important aid in biomedical knowledge discovery from high-throughput experiment results.

8.4.2 DAVID Bioinformatics Resources

DAVID (http://www.david.abcc.ncifcrf.gov/), the Database for Annotation, Visualization and Integrated Discovery, Resources, aims to provide functional support to the interpretation of large lists of genes derived from genomic studies. They are based on the *DAVID Knowledgebase*, a backend database that integrates numerous identifiers of genes/proteins and their genomic annotations retrieved from more than 40 publicly available functional annotation sources. Integration is performed around the *DAVID Gene Concept*, a single-linkage method that agglomerates diverse types of gene identifiers belonging to the same gene into one

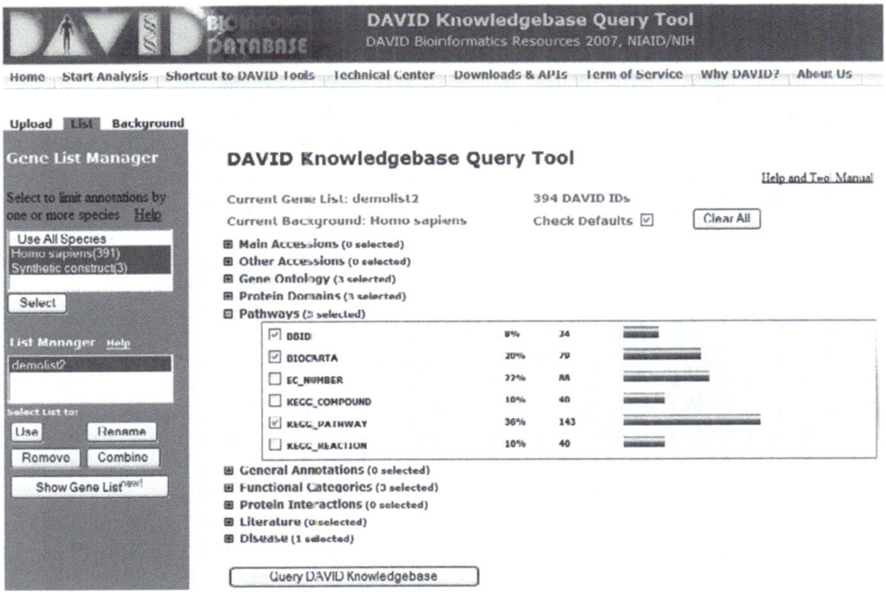

Fig. 8.7 The web-based interface of the DAVID Knowledgebase to query annotations for a given gene list

gene cluster. This method allows large collections of heterogeneous annotations associated with different types of gene identifiers to be comprehensively integrated by a common gene concept. The DAVID Knowledgebase is designed to facilitate high-throughput gene functional analyses, which are enabled through a web interface that allow users querying different types of heterogeneous annotations in a high-throughput manner (Fig. 8.7).

Through such web interface, DAVID also provides a set of analytic tools and functions for gene-term enrichment analysis and quickly grouping of functionally related genes and annotation terms into a manageable number of functional biological modules, in order to support more efficient interpretation of genome-scale datasets. The five main annotation analysis tools that DAVID provides are:

- Gene ID conversion tool
- Gene name viewer
- Functional annotation tool
- Gene functional classification tool
- NIAID Pathogen Genome Browser

Researchers can use such tools to explore their large gene lists in depth from many different biological angles, in order to extract associated biological meanings. For any uploaded gene list, such tools allow users not only to perform the typical gene-term enrichment analysis but also to convert between gene/protein identifiers, visualize many-genes-to-many-terms relationships, dynamically view genes from the list on bio-pathways, search for interesting and related genes or terms, cluster redundant and heterogeneous terms into groups and condense large gene lists into gene functional groups. The latter is accomplished by clustering genes according to their functional similarity computed using the kappa statistics illustrated in Section 3 of this chapter.

The main functionalities provide though the above tools are:

- Identification of enriched biological themes, particularly GO terms
- Discovering of enriched functional-related gene groups
- Clustering of redundant annotation terms
- Visualization of genes on BioCarta and KEGG pathway maps
- Display of related many-genes-to-many-terms on 2D view
- Search for other functionally related genes not in the uploaded list
- Highlight of protein functional domains and motifs
- Listing of interacting proteins
- Linking of gene–disease associations
- Exploration of gene names in batch
- Conversion of gene identifiers from one type to another
- Redirection to related literature

They give investigators the capabilities to interpret the biological mechanisms associated with large gene lists.

8.5 Conclusions

In the post-genomic era, advancements in biomolecular and information technologies provide the opportunity to have both unprecedented amounts of extremely valuable high-throughput experimental nanotechnologydata and the computational capabilities to efficiently manage and effectively analyse them, in order to light the understanding of fundamental biological processes and complex cellular pathophysiological mechanisms and unveil new biomedical knowledge of paramount importance in modern biomedicine and in the health care of the near future. The technological and information resources for knowledge representation and computational analysis, and the software tools implementing them and made easily available through the web, all presented in this chapter, play a very important role towards this goal. They not only allow researchers to describe the current biomolecular knowledge in a standardized and computable form but also to computationally take advantage of such valuable knowledge in order to functionally evaluate experimentally selected lists of genes by means of advanced statistical and information technology approaches. The perspective of such a scenario provided in this chapter and the selected resources here concisely presented show their high relevance for the modern biomedicine and e-health.

References

1. Stevens R, Goble CA, Bechhofer S. Ontology-based knowledge representation for bioinformatics. Brief Bioinform 2000;1(4):398–416.
2. Hill DP, Blake JA, Richardson JE, Ringwald M. Extension and integration of the Gene Ontology (GO): Combining GO vocabularies with external vocabularies. Genome Res 2002;12(12):1982–1991.
3. Hennig S, Groth D, Lehrach H. Automated Gene Ontology annotation for anonymous sequence data. Nucleic Acids Res 2003;31(13):3712–3715.
4. Bodenreider O, Stevens R. Bio-ontologies: Current trends and future directions. Brief Bioinform 2006;7(3):256–274.
5. Kanehisa M, Goto S, Hattori M, Aoki-Kinoshita KF, Itoh M, Kawashima S, Katayama T, Araki M, Hirakawa M. From genomics to chemical genomics: New developments in KEGG Nucleic Acids Res 2006;34(Database issue):D354–D357.
6. Finn RD, Mistry J, Schuster-Bockler B, Griffiths-Jones S, Hollich V, Lassmann T, Moxon S, Marshall M, Khanna A, Durbin R, Eddy SR, Sonnhammer EL, Bateman A. Pfam: Clans, web tools and services. Nucleic Acids Res 2006;34(Database issue):D247–D251.
7. McKusick VA. Mendelian Inheritance in Man and its online version, OMIM Am J Hum Genet 2007;80(4):588–604.
8. Hamosh A, Scott AF, Amberger JS, Bocchini CA, McKusick VA. Online Mendelian Inheritance in Man (OMIM), a knowledgebase of human genes and genetic disorders. Nucleic Acids Res. 2005;33(Database issue):D514–D517.
9. Kelso J, Visagie J, Theiler G, Christoffels A, Bardien S, Smedley D, Otgaar D, Greyling G, Jongeneel CV, McCarthy MI, Hide T, Hide W. eVOC: A controlled vocabulary for unifying gene expression data. Genome Res 2003;13(6A):1222–1230.
10. Ashburner M, Ball CA, Blake JA, Botstein D, Butler H, Cherry JM, Davis AP, Dolinski K, Dwight SS, Eppig JT, Harris MA, Hill DP, Issel-Tarver L, Kasarskis A, Lewis S, Matese JC, Richardson JE, Ringwald M, Rubin GM, Sherlock G. Gene ontology: Tool for the unification of biology. The gene ontology consortium. Nat Genet 2000;25 (1):25–29.
11. Rubin DL, Lewis SE, Mungall CJ, Misra S, Westerfield M, Ashburner M, Sim I, Chute CG, Solbrig H, Storey MA, Smith B, Day-Richter J, Noy NF, Musen MA. National Center for Biomedical Ontology: Advancing biomedicine through structured organization of scientific knowledge. OMICS 2006;10(2):185–198.
12. Rivals I, Personnaz L, Taing L, Potier MC. Enrichment or depletion of a GO category within a class of genes: Which test? Bioinformatics 2007;23(4):401–407.
13. Shaffer JP. Multiple hypothesis testing. Ann Rev Psych 1995;46:561–584.
14. Holm S. A simple sequentially rejective Bonferroni test procedure. Scand Stat 1979;6:65–70.
15. Westfall PH, Young SS. Resampling-based multiple testing. New York: Wiley, 1993.
16. Benjamini Y, Hochberg Y. Controlling the false discovery rate: A practical and powerful approach to multiple testing. J R Stat Soc Ser B 1995;57:289–300.
17. Grossmann S, Bauer S, Robinson PN, Vingron M. Improved detection of overrepresentation of Gene Ontology annotations with parent-child analysis. Bioinformatics 2007;23(22): 3024–3031.
18. Alexa A, Rahnenfuhrer J, Lengauer T. Improved scoring of functional groups from gene expression data by decorrelating GO graph structure. Bioinformatics 2006;22(13): 1600–1607.
19. Günther CC, Langaas M, Lydersen S. Statistical hypothesis testing of association between two lists of genes. Tech Report Preprint Statistics, 1/2006, Department of Mathematical Sciences, NTNU. http://www.math.ntnu.no/preprint/statistics/2006/. Accessed 27 March 2009.
20. Resnik P. Using information content to evaluate semantic similarity in a taxonomy. In: Proceedings of the 14th international joint conference on Artificial Intelligence, IJCAI 95, Montreal, Québec, Canada, 1995 448–453.

21. Zhong J, Zhu H, Li Y, Yu Y. Lecture Notes In Computer Science; Vol. 2393, In: Proceedings of the 10th International Conference on Conceptual Structures: Integration and Interfaces, Springer, London, 2002:92–106.
22. Barutcuoglu Z, Schapire RE, Troyanskaya OG. Hierarchical multi-label prediction of gene function. Bioinformatics 2006;22(7):830–836.
23. Lin D. An information-theoretic definition of similarity. In: Proceedings of 15th international conference on machine learning, San Francisco, CA, USA, 2000:296–304.
24. Jiang JJ, Conrath DW. Semantic similarity based on corpus statistics and lexical taxonomy. In: Proceedings of international conference on research in Computational Linguistics, Taiwan, ROC, 1998:19–33.
25. Lord PW, Stevens RD, Brass A, Goble CA. Semantic similarity measures as tools for exploring the Gene Ontology. Pac Symp Biocomput 2003;8:601–612.
26. Speer N, Spieth C, Zell A. A memetic clustering algorithm for the functional partition of genes based on the Gene Ontology. In: Proceedings of the 2004 IEEE symposium on Computational Intelligence in Bioinformatics and Computational Biology (CIBCB 2004), La Jolla, CA, USA. San Diego, CA: IEEE Press, 2004:252–259.
27. Schlicker A, Domingues F, Rahnenführer J, Lengauer T. A new measure for functional similarity of gene products based on Gene Ontology. BMC Bioinf 2006;7(302): 1–16.
28. Tao Y, Sam L, Li J, Friedman C, Lussier YA. Information theory applied to the sparse gene ontology annotation network to predict novel gene function. Bioinformatics 2007;23(13):529–538.
29. Masseroli M, Pinciroli F. (2006) Using Gene Ontology and genomic controlled vocabularies to analyze high-throughput gene lists: Three tool comparison. Comput Biol Med 2006;36(7–8):731–747.
30. Kasprzyk A, Keefe D, Smedley D, London D, Spooner W, Melsopp C, Hammond M, Rocca-Serra P, Cox T, Birney E. EnsMart: A generic system for fast and flexible access to biological data. Genome Res 2004;14(1):160–169.
31. Bussey KJ, Kane D, Sunshine M, Narasimhan S, Nishizuka S, Reinhold WC, Zeeberg B, Ajay W, Weinstein JN. MatchMiner: A tool for batch navigation among gene and gene product identifiers. Genome Biol 2003;4(4):R27, 1–7.
32. Zhong S, Storch KF, Lipan O, Kao MC, Weitz CJ, Wong WH. GoSurfer: A graphical interactive tool for comparative analysis of large gene sets in Gene Ontology trade mark space. Appl Bioinf 2004;3(4):261–264.
33. Doniger SW, Salomonis N, Dahlquist KD, Vranizan K, Lawlor SC, Conklin BR. MAPPFinder: Using Gene Ontology and GenMAPP to create a global gene-expression profile from microarray data. Genome Biol 2003;4(1):R7, 1–12.
34. Cavalieri D, De Filippo C, Grosu P, Biggeri A. Making sense of whole genome expression data. Application of a universal DNA microarray to cyanobacterial diversity assessment. Minerva Biotecnol 2002;14:291–304.
35. Masseroli M, Martucci D, Pinciroli F. GFINDer: Genome Function INtegrated Discoverer through dynamic annotation, statistical analysis, and mining. Nucleic Acids Res 2004;32(Web Server issue):W293–W300.
36. Masseroli M, Galati O, Pinciroli F. GFINDer: Genetic disease and phenotype location statistical analysis and mining of dynamically annotated gene lists. Nucleic Acids Res 2005;33(Web Server issue):W717–W723.
37. Masseroli M, Bellistri E, Franceschini A, Pinciroli F. Statistical analysis of genomic protein family and domain controlled annotations for functional investigation of classified gene lists. BMC Bioinf 2007;8(Suppl 1):S14, 1–10.
38. Sherman BT, Huang DW, Tan Q, Guo Y, Bour S, Liu D, Stephens R, Baseler MW, Lane HC, Lempicki RA. DAVID Knowledgebase: A gene-centered database integrating heterogeneous gene annotation resources to facilitate high-throughput gene functional analysis. BMC Bioinf 8(426):1–11.

39. Huang DW, Sherman BT, Tan Q, Kir J, Liu D, Bryant D, Guo Y, Stephens R, Baseler MW, Lane HC, Lempicki RA. DAVID Bioinformatics Resources: Expanded annotation database and novel algorithms to better extract biology from large gene lists. Nucleic Acids Res 2007;35(Web Server issue):W169–W175.
40. Huang DW, Sherman BT, Lempicki RA. Systematic and integrative analysis of large gene lists using DAVID Bioinformatics Resources. Nat Protoc 2009:4(1):44–57.
41. Hunter S, Apweiler R, Attwood TK, Bairoch A, Bateman A, Binns D, Bork P, Das U, Daugherty L, Duquenne L, Finn RD, Gough J, Haft D, Hulo N, Kahn D, Kelly E, Laugraud A, Letunic I, Lonsdale D, Lopez R, Madera M, Maslen J, McAnulla C, McDowall J, Mistry J, Mitchell A, Mulder N, Natale D, Orengo C, Quinn AF, Selengut JD, Sigrist CJ, Thimma M, Thomas PD, Valentin F, Wilson D, Wu CH, Yeats C. InterPro: The integrative protein signature database. Nucleic Acids Res 2009;37(Database issue):D211–D215.

Chapter 9
Web-Based Applications in Healthcare

Athina Lazakidou

Abstract Healthcare organizations are undergoing major reorganizations and adjustments to meet the increasing demands of improved healthcare access and quality, as well as lowered costs. As the use of information technology to process medical data increases, much of the critical information necessary to meet these challenges is being stored in digital format. Web-enabled information technologies can provide the means for greater access and more effective integration of healthcare information from disparate computer applications and other information resources. In this chapter, various examples of web-based applications in healthcare area have been described and the core benefits of the web-based applications have been presented.

Keywords: Web-based · social web · web 3.0 · healthcare · handheld devices · quality · performance · security

9.1 Introduction

The Internet's potential is increasingly being harnessed to transform healthcare delivery at the patient level. From growing e-mail use by patients and consumer e-commerce in the drug market to rising electronic procurement by hospitals, Internet diagnosis, and e-Health, the use of the Internet in active healthcare delivery is rapidly gaining ground. Patients create online support communities, search for medical information, and share their experiences, while healthcare professionals get access to the latest information in their field, consult with their colleagues, and communicate with their patients. Indicative of the impact of Internet in healthcare is the fact that almost every healthcare business – from insurers to hospitals to pharmaceutical companies – has a dedicated web site.

A. Lazakidou (✉)
Faculty of Human Movement and Quality of Life Sciences, Dept. of Nursing, University of Peloponnese, Sparti General Hospital Building Complex, GR-23100 Sparti, Greece
e-mail: lazakid@uop.gr

A. Lazakidou (ed.), *Web-Based Applications in Healthcare and Biomedicine*, Annals of Information Systems 7, DOI 10.1007/978-1-4419-1274-9_9,
© Springer Science+Business Media, LLC 2010

Recent web-based technologies have created completely new possibilities for various medical information systems. Web-based applications have come a long way and now offer competitive advantages to traditional software-based systems, allowing businesses to consolidate and streamline their systems and processes and reduce costs.

9.2 Web Mobile-Based Applications for Healthcare Management

Healthcare organizations are constantly designing effective systems aiming to help achieve customer satisfaction. Web-based and mobile-based technologies are two forms of information technologies that healthcare executives are increasingly looking to merge as an opportunity to develop such systems. Web mobile-based applications for healthcare management address the difficult task of managing admissions and waiting lists while ensuring a quick and convincing response to unanticipated changes of the clinical needs. Web mobile-based applications for healthcare management tackle the limitations of traditional systems and take into consideration the dynamic nature of clinical needs, scarce resources, alternative strategies, and customer satisfaction in an environment that often imposes unexpected deviation from planned activities.

The World Wide Web Consortium's goal of integrating web-based with mobile-based technologies is "to make browsing the Web from mobile devices a reality". These technologies, however, do not routinely reduce costs, improve quality, or achieve customer satisfaction unless they create, from the customer's perspective, a value-added service. From the healthcare angle, these emerging technologies considerably improve three critical value-added service dimensions in relation to information flow between hospital personnel as well as between hospitals and patients. These dimensions are timeliness, accessibility, and mobility. The third dimension is the result of integrating mobile-based applications with web-based systems.

- Timeliness: a reference to how up-to-date information is with respect to information system users' needs. It reflects also how fast the information system is updated after the state of the represented hospital system changes. Accurate but out-of-date information may have no value for the decision-making process. Difficulties in updating the information in a timely fashion make the system less valuable. Timeliness also requires real-time information flow between various functions of healthcare organizations.
- Accessibility: The availability of relevant and complete information when needed is one of the key issues that drive healthcare executives to allocate a considerable portion of their budgets to installing advanced information systems. The flow of healthcare information is restricted and governed by legislation. This raises the issue of security. Accordingly, the acceptability of a system is directly related to the consistency between accessibility and security issues. Accessibility and

timeliness form key drivers for adopting web-based systems. Accessibility and timeliness allow local, state, or even national authorities to receive up-to-date information from all or designated hospitals to guide the authority in emergencies at the national level. A system with adequate accessibility and timeliness of the flow of information can be used to exchange information at the international level to combat the international spread of SARS (severe acute respiratory syndrome), bird flu, or any other infectious diseases that may pose a serious threat to global health security.

- Mobility: The ability to move. In mobile-based computing, mobility refers to the capability of a device (e.g., a mobile phone) to handle information access, communication, and business transactions whilst in a state of motion. Mobility causes mobile-based applications to differ from web-based applications at two levels:

  1. *The communication level*: Web services are connected with wired channels to the external environment, whereas mobile services (m-services) are connected with wireless channels.
  2. *The computation-location level*: Web services are executed on the service side. M-services are executed on the client side after being transferred from the server side.

9.3 A Web-Based Electronic Health Record: The IZIP System

IZIP is an electronic health record (EHR) system with Internet access, currently in operation in the Czech Republic. The EHR includes relevant information about all contacts of the citizen with healthcare services, compiled from regular GP visits, dental treatments, laboratory and imaging tests, and healthcare provided by hospital services. Through software modules within the electronic systems of these diverse healthcare providers, interoperability with the IZIP system is assured, and during each visit with a single "click" new data can be uploaded to the central system.

With the consent of the patient, the IZIP system allows doctors to access the central EHR at the time and point of care, so that each doctor can resume treatment where the previous doctors have stopped.

The principal role of IZIP is to provide both the technical and the service infrastructure for this comprehensive record integrating medical data from individual healthcare professionals and healthcare provider organizations (HPOs), and assuring full control by the insured citizen. They have the right to access and read their own EHR, but they cannot change them. They can authorize healthcare professionals to view and update their data, converting citizens to an active participant in the healthcare system. They are thus better placed to make responsible decisions about their health, cooperate better with healthcare providers, and gain a picture of the technical, resource, and financial possibilities and limitations of the proposed or available services and procedures. This is a basic change compared to the conventional system of health record administration, where the HPO, not the citizen, had the power to disclose information.

The Internet health files comprise structured parts of the medical documentation. Only healthcare professionals are authorized to insert data into the IZIP system. Records in the IZIP system contain:

- Anamnesis
- Results of examinations performed by a GP or specialist, in chronological order
- Results of laboratory tests and examinations
- A list of prescribed and issued medicines and drugs
- X-rays, scans, and other images
- Reports on hospitalizations
- Vaccination history
- Information on other treatments, including type and location. (http://ec.europa.eu/information_society/activities/health/docs/events/opendays2006/ehealth-impact-7-5.pdf).
- Core impact:
  - √ Empowering citizens – they are the gatekeepers to information about their own health
  - √ Instant access to comprehensive patient information independent of the location of the citizen at the time of care, even abroad
  - √ Full interoperability of core patient data and information among all healthcare providers
  - √ Improved communication between healthcare providers and support for continuity of care
  - √ Significant reduction in duplicative examinations and tests
  - √ Positive net economic benefit to society.
- Main beneficiaries:
  - √ Citizens have control over the information on their health history and access to it at the point of need
  - √ Doctors and other healthcare providers have access to the full medical account of the patient, including examination results and full list of medications at the point and time of care. This leads to better quality care and time savings
  - √ Insurance companies and the healthcare system as a whole benefit from the costs avoided by avoiding duplicative tests and unnecessary treatment.
- Economic results:
  - √ First year of annual net benefit, i.e., when annual benefits exceed annual costs: 2005, year 7
  - √ Estimated annual net benefit for the year 2008: approximately € 60 million
  - √ First year of cumulative net benefit: 2006, year 8
  - √ Estimated cumulative benefit by 2008: approximately € 180 million
  - √ Cumulative investment costs, including operating expenditure, by 2008: approximately € 90 million
  - √ Estimated productivity gain, measured in decrease in e-Health cost per patient: 74%
  - √ Distribution of benefits to 2008: citizens – 10%; HPOs – 37%; insurance company – 53%

9.4 A Web-Based Diabetes Patient Data Management System for Epidemiological and Clinical Analysis

Diabetes being a multifactorial disorder, a diabetes patient needs to be monitored for a number of clinical parameters such as blood sugar, cholesterol, insulin, blood pressure and environmental parameters such as stress, diet, exercise, etc. The diabetes patient data management system [1] was developed using Oracle 8 and ASP 3.0 (Active Server Pages) to enable efficient management of the voluminous data generated during treating a diabetes patient. With a view that the medical specialist can access the patient data from any geographical location, this system was developed using a web-based approach. This web-enabled software gives the authorized health provider an access to the entire treatment and response history of the patient at a given instance. Thus it takes care of the security issue as accession authority is checked for every web page for that particular session. This system is form-based, menu-driven and the data could be entered into the system by filling in the forms, e.g., patient's personal details, medical check-up details, which includes information about the patient's condition, treatment rendered, pathological test details such as blood sugar, urine sugar, lipid profile, routine urine test, etc. The system has provision to print the prescription and the pathological test reports, which could be given to the patients. The database system is fully searchable through the search options which are developed using SQL (Structured Query Language). Interactive, form-based web pages were developed for querying the database online.

This system, apart from managing the day-to-day data of the diabetes patient, can be used for epidemiological and clinical research. It could also find application in the comparison between the patients under similar ailments, drug therapy, biochemical and genetic/familial backgrounds, etc. It can be used for a comparative analysis of the diabetes patients, involving various criteria such as age of onset, sex, symptoms, type of diabetes, and associated diseases. Such study will generate valuable insights into the pattern of disease, response of the patients to medical treatment, and will provide prognostic and diagnostic parameters. It can be also used for keeping the follow-up of group of patients for selected parameters for a longer duration and generate reports with the help of query system, which in turn can be used for further research. It can form a base for pharmaceutical industry in the field of clinical trials. Moreover, as the system has the potential to store and retrieve data of a large population, it has application in clinical areas through data mining.

9.5 A Web-Based Application with Digital Signature for Drugs Dispensing Management

The result of an information technology research project, based on the utilization of a web-based application for managing the hospital drugs dispensing, is the wHospital system [2]. Part of this web-based application (wHospital) back bone and its key distinguishing characteristic is the adoption of the digital signature system, initially deployed by the Government of Lombardia, a Northern Italy Region, throughout the distribution of smart cards to all the healthcare and hospital staffs.

The main advantage of a web-based application is indeed the easiness of delivering applications through a hospital pre-existent information system: only a *web* browser is needed by the client host. The disadvantage of web architecture is the difficulty in the software programming and implementation of client procedures, such as the one implied with the digital signature.

The developed system is a web-based application with a proposed Health Records Digital Signature (HReDS) handshake to comply with the national law and with the Joint Commission International Standards. The prototype application, for a single hospital Operative Unit (OU), has focused on data and process management, related to drug therapy.

Amongst the most challenging project activity was the staff training, especially in using the TabletPC and PDA. The choice to develop a prototype of the system in order to carry out the staff training helps for both training and user requirements analysis. Every new developed software modules was indeed viewed and approved by the OU staff. With this approach, even the first initial application utilized by the staff had minor impacts on the working process.

Moreover, during the shadowing sessions, it was immediately possible to estimate a work reduction of about 30 min per nurse in the time dedicated to the transcription from the therapies plan sheet to the working sheet. Qualitatively, when this activity is automated with wHospital, the related clinical risk will reduce.

Other clinical risks, such as the one related to drug dispensing errors, i.e., from incorrect preparations of the drug dosage, can only be minimized and overcome through the implementation of an automatic dispensing system. A complete quantitative and qualitative analysis of the benefits that wHospital delivers, considering the clinical risk reduction, the working process optimization, as well as the consequently increased care and attention provided to the patient, requires a wider sample of case.

9.6 A Web-Based Application for Prioritization Public Health Resources

Although setting priorities is an important step in making public health policy, the benefit of using epidemiology to prioritize scarce public health resources has not been fully recognized. This situation is mostly due to the complexity of proposed models for setting priorities. The authors [3] describe a public health priority setting model, Missouri Information for Community Assessment Priority Setting Model (Priority MICA), which uses epidemiologic measures available in most surveillance systems across the United States. Priority MICA uses data from birth and death certificates, hospital discharges, emergency departments, risk factors from the Behavioral Risk Factors Surveillance System, and eight epidemiologic measures to construct six priority criteria: size (the number of emergency department visits, hospitalizations, and deaths), severity (number of deaths of people younger than

65), urgency (trends in deaths and hospital morbidity), preventability (evidence-based score), community support (score of social support for preventive action), and racial-disparity (race comparison through death and morbidity rate ratio).

Priority MICA is part of a web-based interactive tool that makes available data from a wide variety of surveillance systems (http://www.dhss.mo.gov/MICA). The top 10 priority diseases determined by Priority MICA were compared to a more traditional method of ranking diseases by mortality rates. Using the additional criteria in Priority MICA identified four more priority diseases than were identified using just mortality while the ranking of the other six priority diseases differed between methods.

9.7 A Web-Based GIS for Healthcare Decision Support

Epidemiological changes of end-stage renal disease (ESRD) during the past decade showed an increasing incidence and prevalence. However, the magnitude of this phenomenon was not precisely known in France. A Renal Epidemiology and Information Network (REIN) was then built to face this poor epidemiological knowledge of ESRD. A Multi-Source Information System (MSIS) was then set up. This web-based application integrates a tool dedicated to improving our knowledge of demand and supply of care for ESRD. This project involves research units (Universities Paris 5 and Grenoble, INSERM), professionals (Société de Néphrologie, Société francophone de dialyse, Société française de Transplantation), state Agencies (Agence de Biomédecine, Institut de Veille Sanitaire, Caisse Nationale d'Asssurance Maladie, Direction de l'Hospitalisation et de l'Organisation des Soins), and patient representatives.

The project team implemented a Geographical Information System (GIS) to support public health decision-making for ESRD. SIGNe (Système d'Information Géographique pour la Néphrologie) was dedicated to dynamically visualize and analyze ESRD demand and supply of care. It was developed according to web-GIS, data warehouse, and data mining technologies, aiming to analyze ESRD epidemiology in order to improve access to care, improving public health decision-making [4].

SIGNe offers a dynamic interface for accessing and contributing to healthcare information concerning ESRD. It allows the representation of the demand as well as the supply of care. Moreover, it helps describe the current match between the location of care and the place of residence of ESRD patients. It is thus a support to healthcare decision-making.

9.8 A Web-Based System for Distributed Healthcare Cooperative Work Support

Healthcare is characterized by close collaboration and information sharing among many distinct actors, who cooperate for the patient care in different temporal moments, also at a distance. In this context, availability to care givers of all relevant patient health data and of specific healthcare co-operative work supporting tools is fundamental for best patient treatment. The authors [5] designed and implemented He@lthCo-op, a web-based modular system supporting cooperative work and patient information secure sharing among healthcare personnel also from remotely located sites. He@lthCo-op enables easily gathering, storing, and accessing patient clinical and personal data anytime and from anywhere an Internet connection is available.

9.9 A Web-Based System for Healthcare Activity Monitoring and Prediction

The UK National Health Service is subject to variation in demand for medical services, particularly during the winter. The system developed assist with hospital bed management in NHS Scotland by monitoring and predicting activity within hospitals and the primary care sector [6]. System Watch gathers daily hospital numbers of emergency admissions and beds occupied by emergencies. It uses this and other information to model long- and short-term demand for emergency bed admissions and present predictions in a graphical form through a web-based user interface. The article evaluates the accuracy of predictions and the initial experience of the use of System Watch by bed managers. The results indicate that System Watch's accuracy is sufficient for planning purposes at both health board area and hospital level. Finally, additional possible uses of System Watch are described and future developments outlined.

9.10 A Web-Based Monitoring System for Home-Based Rehabilitation with Stroke Patients

Research on developing low-cost home-based rehabilitation systems aim to provide support for the rehabilitation of post-stroke patients in the home environment to promote/aid functional recovery and ultimately enhance their quality of life (QoL). A web-based system has been proposed for monitoring the home-based rehabilitation and providing both therapeutic instruction and support information. The system [7] will support specific rehabilitation interventions, provide a three-dimensional (3D) visual output, and measure the effectiveness of the resulting actions undertaken by the participant. Information regarding process can be reviewed and accessed by the patient and health professionals.

Current development has produced a web-based tool that allows the healthcare professional the ability to view the patient's rehabilitation history and provide feedback to the patient. The monitoring system consists primarily of three modules, a backend database module, data processing module, and 3D rendering module.

SMART project is funded by EPSRC EQUAL (enhance QoL) initiative. The project aims to examine the scope, effectiveness, and appropriateness of systems to support home-based rehabilitation programs for the elderly and their caregivers. The system offers different levels of user access – (1) health care rehabilitation professionals and (2) patients and their caregivers. The professionals have full access to all information/data relating to their patients, those patients who belong to a clinic or hospital not affiliated with the healthcare professional will be inaccessible. However, a consultancy tool is available whereby a professional can request support from another colleague. This consultancy process may only be instigated by the professional who belongs to the same clinic/hospital as the patient, in this case information about a particular patient can be shared across hospitals. Patients and their caregivers are only granted access to their own data whereby they can review the rehabilitation process and progress and get feedback from the professionals.

Many of the rehabilitation systems currently available in laboratory environment only provide stick diagram visualization, which can be difficult to interpret. The main aim of developing the 3D rendering module is to improve upon the stick diagram, easing the level of interpretation. The web-based monitoring system proposed provides an important platform in the home-based rehabilitation system. Patients and their caregivers and rehabilitation professionals can access and review the information regarding rehabilitation process and adjust their movement during rehabilitation.

9.11 A Web-Based Healthcare Screening Tool for Seniors

MySeniorCare is an essential tool for organizations that deliver or facilitate healthcare to the elderly, such as retirement communities, assisted living facilities, nursing homes, and other medical practices. Today, many senior living facilities and eldercare healthcare providers are experiencing shortages in caregiver staff and primary care physicians; and daily care staff members are often unfamiliar with what constitutes the aging process. For staff that has little or no expertise in recognizing the common ailments of aging, MySeniorCare automates the geriatric screening process and provides the tools necessary to detect these common geriatric syndromes in the early treatable stages.

By using MySeniorCare, healthcare organizations can:

- Mitigate liability – meet targeted state regulatory and licensing requirements, leverage reporting of screening data to show treatment-plan progress, reduce liability by mitigating medical errors
- Increase efficiency and save time – obtain early, accurate at-risk diagnoses faster through automated screening processes; conversion from paper to electronic processes saves time, money, and paperwork
- Reduce cost – mitigate chronic healthcare cost due to missed diagnoses; save money by maximizing staff expertise
- Improve quality of care – customize care treatment plans based on screening data and reporting for individuals and populations

- Leverage existing staff – reduce staff hours needed for screenings and maximize physician visits and staff daily care regimens
- Improve decision-making – improve decision-making by tracking at-risk diagnosis over time
- Identify need for ancillary therapies – Improved diagnostics provides evidence-based data to support the need for ancillary therapies (http://www.prweb.com/releases/caredatatrak/03302009/prweb2273264.htm)

9.12 A Web-Based Approach to HIS with Handhelds

Clinical requirements like bedside patient data capture and access in healthcare bring up new demands to Hospital Information Systems (HIS). The most suitable solutions are applications for mobile devices. The technological basis (PDA, WebPad, Wireless LAN, Bluetooth) of mobile computing in healthcare has developed rapidly over the past years.

This stimulated the development of numerous applications suitable for different fields of medicine.

Mobile devices used in healthcare can basically divided into two groups: firstly offline applications running autonomously on a mobile device. The second group comprises online applications, loading up data via different hardware interfaces, and after processing loading them down back to the leading application.

Most offline applications are solely information systems using databases (i.e., medication, dictionaries, catalogues) or small applications as, for example, formula calculators. In general, this allows only a restricted use in special fields and yields limited benefits in clinical routine.

Online applications, on the other hand, are able to upload data or applications from an already existing system using hardware interfaces (docking cradle, infrared, bluetooth, or wireless LAN). After processing or simply presenting the data, the results are then downloaded back to the leading application. However, this approach often requires the implementation of additional features, or the re-implementation of existing ones, in order to make the feature suitable for a new device. In both cases data are provided by a software interface, which requires the additional implementation of an import/export interface in the non-mobile application.

The basis of IS-H*MED is an advanced *n*-tier architecture separating data, application, and presentation layers. This architecture combined with further SAP components allow a web-based user interface (GUI) instead of the standard desktop presentation.

The central component is the Internet Transaction Server (ITS), which connects the application layer of IS-H*MED with a standard web server. Requests from web sites are sent to the ITS by the web server, which calls IS-H*MED transactions via RFCs or BAPIs. The results are then returned to the ITS using the same interfaces. Using pre-defined templates, ITS generates HTML pages, which are made available at the web server for browser presentation.

Moreover, ITS provides a gateway which checks access authorization based on the ISH*MED's security settings. This secures exclusive access to IS-H*MED data and functions via web applications for authorized users only. This guarantees a secure access to IS-H*MED data and functions using any common web browser.

In cooperation with T-Systems (Vienna) and SAP AG (Walldorf) has been developed an application in order to exemplify optimal support of clinical staff using the technology described above combined with wireless LAN. This was specified for a surgical consultation service enabling full access to a HIS using a pocket PC.

The first step was to analyze the typical workflow of a surgical consultant, which allowed us to identify information and function required for the specific clinical situation. On this basis has been defined suitable HTML pages, which served as prototype for the verification of the design model for data presentation and navigation. The application is implemented in the integrated development environment of IS-H*MED, the so-called workbench.

The following services should be offered to the surgical consultant:

- An easy personalized authorization
- Task lists
- Work lists
- Current consultation request
- Patients and case information
- Medical documents as findings and reports
- Plain bed scheduling
- Standard services, e.g., SMS
- Exemplary access to Internet and intranet (http://subs.emis.de/LNI/Proceedings/Proceedings15/GI-Proceedings.15-17.pdf)

In front of the patient's room, the consultant can look up details via his work list, particularly information on the request (e.g., the medical problem or a brief medical history), on the patient (e.g. personal data, attending doctors), or on the case (e.g., admission or transfer data, prior cases). Additional medical documents can be displayed, if available in IS-H*MED or any other connected source. Exemplarily, this is implemented for laboratory findings. First, the doctor gets a list of existing laboratory finding documents, which he/she can look up in detail on a tip. This provides the surgeon with all necessary – and moreover up to-date – information for the consultation. Frequently, the situation demands a transfer to the consultant's department for further diagnosis or treatment. Therefore, the application includes a plain bed scheduling service, which supplies a current list of available beds in the consultants department. Detailed information on the respective bed can be obtained and pre-reservations can be made by tipping a button. The upcoming transfer of a patient is announced instantly to the receiving ward, thus reducing organizational expenses. Finally, the doctor can finish the consultation, which is then removed from his current work list.

9.13 Benefits of Web-Based Applications

Web-based applications have evolved significantly over recent years, and with improvements in security and technology, there are plenty of scenarios where traditional software-based applications and systems could be improved by migrating them to a web-based application.

Below are some of the core benefits of web-based applications:

- Cross-platform compatibility. Most web-based applications are far more compatible across platforms than traditional installed software. Typically, the minimum requirement would be a web browser of which there are many (Internet Explorer, Firefox, Netscape, etc.). These web browsers are available for a multitude of operating systems and so whether the users use Windows, Linux, or Mac OS, they can still run the web application.
- More manageable. Web-based systems need only be installed on the server placing minimal requirements on the end user workstation. This makes maintaining and updating the system much simpler as usually it can all be done on the server. Any client updates can be deployed via the web server with relative ease.
- Highly deployable. Due to the manageability and cross-platform support, deploying web applications to the end user is far easier. They are also ideal where bandwidth is limited and the system and data are remote to the user.
- Secure live data. Typically, in larger more complex systems data are stored and moved around separate systems and data sources. In web-based systems, these systems and processes can often be consolidated, reducing the need to move data around. Web-based applications also provide an added layer of security by removing the need for the user to have access to the data and back end servers.
- Reduced costs. Web-based applications can dramatically lower costs due to reduced support and maintenance, lower requirements on the end user system, and simplified architecture.

9.14 Conclusion

Web-based information systems with clinical guidelines are becoming increasingly necessary as the amount and depth of information needed to respond to patients have increased. Hospitals need to adapt not only to deliver this information to healthcare providers, but also to help them synthesize this information.

Web-based applications have come a long way and now offer competitive advantages to traditional software-based systems, allowing businesses to consolidate and streamline their systems and processes and reduce costs. Ensuring the security and privacy of sensitive information is a critical prerequisite to creating public trust for web-based applications that aim to improve patient's care in a reliable and cost-effective way.

References

1. Ranade S, Deobagkar DN, Deobagkar D. Application of the web-based diabetes patient data management system for epidemiological and clinical analysis. Indian J Med Inform 2007;2(1):3–3, ISSN 0973-9254.
2. Rossi L, Margola L, Manzelli V, Bandera A. wHospital: a web-based application with digital signature for drugs dispensing management. Proceedings of the 28th Annual International Conference of the IEEE (EMBS' 2006), 2006:6793–6796.
3. Simoes EJ, Land G, Metzger R, Mokdad A, Prioritization MICA: a web-based application to prioritize public health resources. J Public Health Manag Pract 2006;12(2):161–169.
4. Richard J-B, Toubiana L, Le Mignot L, Ben Said M, Mugnier C, Le Bihan-Benjamin C, Jaïs J-P, Landais P. A web-based GIS for health care decision-support 2005.
5. Masseroli M, Visconti A, Bano S, Pinciroli F. He@lthCo-op: a web-based system to support distributed healthcare co-operative work. Comput Biol Med 2006;36(2):109–127.
6. Brown H. A web-based system to monitor and predict healthcare activity. Health Inform J 2005;11(1):63–79.
7. Zheng H, Davies RJ, Black ND. Web-based monitoring system for home-based rehabilitation with stroke patients. IEEE CBMS 2005, 2005;419–424.

Chapter 10
Evaluation for Web-Based Applications

Anastasia N. Kastania and Stelios Zimeras

Abstract Web applications are of the following categories: document-centric, interactive, transactional, workflow-based, portal-oriented, collaborative, social web, ubiquitous and semantic web. The web application modelling methods (content, hypertext, presentation, customization) and architectures (layered or data-aspect) influence the quality of a web application. Technology-aware web application design involves presentation, interaction and functional design. Testing involves planning, preparing, performing, reporting and agile approaches. In this chapter a model is proposed to evaluate web applications.

Keywords: Usability · Culture and communication · Graphical user interfaces · Quality · Performance · Security

10.1 Introduction

Web applications include product, usage and development characteristics and are subjected to continuous evolution. Requirements engineering methods need adaptation when dealing with web applications development. The present work is focused to exploit various aspects aiming to contribute to the design and development of web applications certification frameworks and various web quality seals (Fig. 10.1).

Web sites can bee classified [8] using three classes: (a) *The web typology or digital business models*: In this class the web site is analysed using specific types of web models and is characterized as one of them. A representative in electronic business models [32] describes 11 ways to conduct e-commerce according to the innovation degree and the functional incorporation [1, 17, 19, 33]. (b) *The* "stages of development models": In this class the models distinguish different development stages

A.N. Kastania (✉)
Department of Informatics, Athens University of Economics and Business, Patission, Athens 10434, Greece
e-mail: ank@aueb.gr

A. Lazakidou (ed.), *Web-Based Applications in Healthcare and Biomedicine*,
Annals of Information Systems 7, DOI 10.1007/978-1-4419-1274-9_10,

© Springer Science+Business Media, LLC 2010

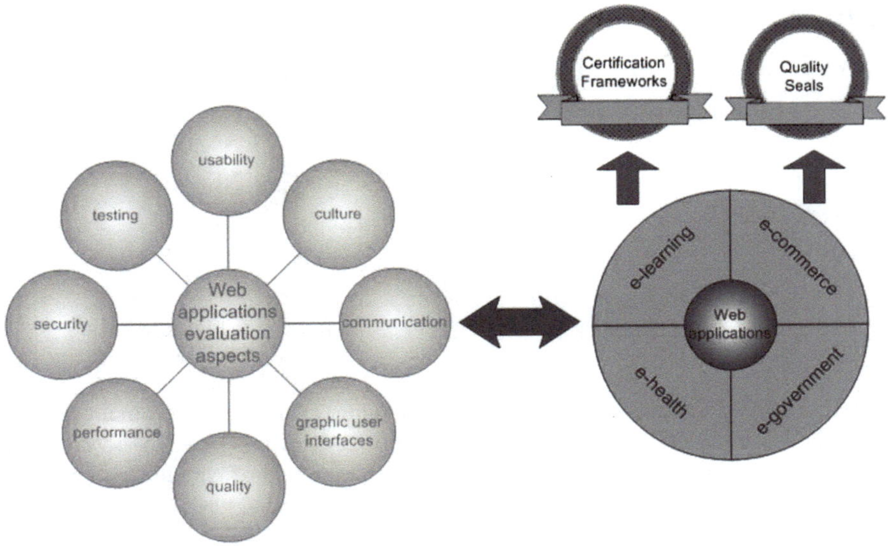

Fig. 10.1 A model to evaluate web applications

according to the functionality of the web site. As an outcome, the web site is categorized according to its functionality. Representatives of this class [7] have performed a research on hundreds of web sites from 18 different sectors and have classified them according to their functionality for information provision, order processing, multimedia use and e-mail use. Another representative [14] performed classification in 12 groups using a matrix having in one dimension the aim (presentation, delivery, processing) and in the other the value (timeliness of information, provision, processing, logistic support, visual impression). Another important model is the Extended MICA [6] that distinguishes three stages of wide functionality (presentation for basic or complete information provision, delivery of interaction expressed in various levels and processing). (c) *The use of a Scoring system*: Specific characteristics of the web site are scored. According to the total score, the web site can be compared to other web sites. Eliot uses binary scoring [10] giving one mark for each one of five functionality levels assigned in six categories (information and business operations, information and marketing of products/services, transactions, customer services, ease of use and innovation). Gartner [12] developed a scoring system for evaluating 76 characteristics of a web site coded in Likert Scale (from 1 to 9) organized in sections (web site design, web site functionality, web site value for the customer), with different weighting scores per section and subsection and with different characteristics per sector. An interesting web site evaluation framework is the Extended Web Assessment Method – WAM [28] which measures the degree of proper adoption of e-commerce applications in some sectors (music, consumer goods, e-banking). It is a useful instrument for evaluating e-commerce applications per sector and evaluates the web site considering only the customer view [29].

10.2 Usability

Usability is a fundamental characteristic of software quality. The international standard ISO/IEC 9126 defines usability as "the set of characteristics of a software product that are related to use and evaluates use by a predetermined set of users". Usability is characterized by the ease of use, understanding the necessary actions, the use functionality and the presentation attractiveness. Another international standard, ISO 9241-11, defines usability as "the extend to which a product can be used by predefined users to fulfil specific aims with efficiency, efficacy and in a satisfactory degree within a specific environment of use". Factors influencing the degree of usability are the effectiveness of actions, the efficiency of resources, the user's satisfaction and the environment of use. The difference in the second previously mentioned international standard is that it has many conditions (who is the user, which are the user goals, how it is indented to use the product) which allow to overcome lack of definition existing in ISO/IEC 9126. Turner reports that to increase the number of visitors in a web site the usability is necessary [34]).

Apart from the usability principles [23, 24], metrics also exist that measure usability. According to Nielsen [23] usability is related to the following characteristics: (a) ease of learning to use the system; (b) good performance in the operation of commands; (c) maintenance of using capability in the frame of time; (d) few errors in operation and ways to correct them; and (e) user satisfaction according to subjective criteria.

Usability of web applications is characterized by response times, interaction efficiency, colours, text layout, page structure, navigation structure, multiculturalism, confidence-generating measures and meta-design criteria [14].

Methods to evaluate usability are divided into three general categories: (a) *Exploratory methods:* The goal is to record user opinion for the experience gained in the web site about preferences, needs and problems. These methods are research based on the content (the evaluators use interviews based on exploratory dialogues and not structured questions), ethnographic studies (users are observed by the evaluator), interviews and focus groups (to collect answers about user experience), research focused on randomized interviews (based on a list of questions), questionnaires (with questions given to the user to record the degree of satisfaction) and recorded sessions (the user exploits the system where actions are recorded automatically). (b) *Analytic methods:* These are used in usability laboratories without user participation. The goal is to exploit the degree the interfaces are consistent with the proper design rules. The evaluators have relative knowledge and skills. These methods are heuristic evaluation (the evaluator exploits the successful application of design principles checking language comprehensiveness, ease of remembering actions, presentation consistency, feedback capability, clear and easy error handling, comprehensive error messaging and error avoidance), knowledge tracing (user exploits user interaction through a simulation process), official usability inspection (combining heuristic evaluation and knowledge tracing), multiple tracing (users and experts discuss all interface elements to reveal all possible problems), consistency inspection (the homogeneity of the interface and the consistency of functioning is exploited) and finally audit based on standards (conformity with industry standards). (c) *Experimental methods:* A requirement is user participation in a usability laboratory. A representative user sample performs various tasks using the interface, and the degree of usability is examined. The real user behaviour and system performance are recorded. These methods include: the protocol of the speaking subject (the subject records opinions during the experiment), the multiple investigation method (users perform together their different activities to develop products that demand user groups and collaboration), questionnaire protocol (the designers question the users during testing) and performance measurement (quantitative performance measurements are extracted during testing based on predefined actions).

Usability evaluation methods [5] are based either on the participation or on the absence of participation of real users. The difficulty to select a proper user group is a weakness of the exploratory and experimental methods. The possibility of user training to gain the skills for usage is also limited. Simulation with real user experience is also difficult. The exploratory and experimental methods have the weakness the user focuses on the symptoms and not on problem causes and have increased demands in time and cost. On the contrary, analytical methods allow diagnosing problem causes. The strength is the participation of fewer and most relevant users with the subject. The weakness is the greater dependency from the subjectivity of the evaluation and possibly the wrong estimate of user problems. It is proposed [27] combining the three methods to extract valid and precise results.

Web usability engineering trends include usability patterns, mobile usability and accessibility (for people with different kinds of disabilities).

10.3 Culture and Communication

The cultural identity in its subjective dimension is to feel belonging in a society. Designing and setting up web sites apart from the successful user interface directed to a wide audience with various national origins and cultural identities, another aspect that should be considered, is the cultural interface [11].

There is research exploiting how the cultural dimension affects the user of a web site and how the form of the web site overcomes possible obstacles because of cultural differences. Researchers have tried to conduct this research based on Hofstede classical classification of cultural profiles [16] with various results.

It is not accidental the fact the preferences, prejudices and symbolisms that are determined by the cultural frame are considered in the design and implementation of web sites with elements (like the relationship with the colour, the visual impression for graphics, the orientation of elements in the web page) that influence the user. These are associated with the degree of usability of each web site [2].

The rapid technological advances and the emersion of the Internet as a new field to conduct interpersonal, public and intercountry communication cause new questions on effects and changes in various levels. An interesting subject is to study the role and the relationship of the Internet with the national conscience and national identity.

Various user classifications can be extracted using their national origin or their culture. Also various communication issues arise related to the visitor/user of a web site because of the fact the receiver of a message is characterized with a personal way of engagement and interpretation of the various accepted messages. On the message receiving and decoding process, the main challenge is to detect the contribution of the receiver in the constitution of the message meaning.

Good knowledge of the cultural particularities of the potential visitors and the likely interjection of other factors (demographic characteristics, linguistic media-tion) are essential for the successful constitution of a web presence because of the fact the media are characterized by many dimensions such as their direction (one-way or bidirectional), user activity (passive or energetic), the distribution (frequency, sound, text), the audience (a lot, few, one) and the most important dimension which is the communication goal.

10.4 Graphic User Interfaces

Graphic user interfaces are designed to allow the web site visitor to use easily a computer system. The four principles of a good user interface design [24] are visibility, conceptual model, mapping and feedback. The following design principles [34] should be followed to have a successful design of the user interface: selection of the alignment type, existence of tables, selection of the font types to be used (few are advised), use of the blue colour and underline style to be limited only for the hyperlinks and spelling correctness of the text.

Nielsen suggests few more characteristics for graphic user interfaces quality [23]: (a) avoidance of complex images in the background which make difficult the reading of a page; (b) avoidance of animation use which disturbs and extracts the attention; (c) when use of video is indented, it is necessary to provide information for loading time; (d) use of thumbnails is advised when using photos; (e) avoidance to open many different windows; and (f) provision of a "friendly printing" choice or creating Acrobat PDF files for the content the user wishes to print. The most important advice is to test the web site under difficult circumstances (with slow connection at an ordinary computer). Another important element is navigation (selection of the navigation system). The navigation used widely is the hierarchical one.

According to a theoretical framework [32], the categories for the quality of information included in a user interface are: (a) *Internal:* The information must be of "quality", that is to say valid; otherwise the source that broadcasts information loses reliability; (b) *Content*: The information must be relevant, complete and in the right proportion; and (c) *Representative*: The way information is provided must be reliable, consistent, concise and easily comprehensible.

10.5 Quality

Quality is the notion of transcendental in Aristotle. There are many definitions of quality.Quality is the synthesis of all the characteristics of a product or service (including performance) that fully satisfies stakeholders (customers, actors, owners) expectations. It is a holistic idea that incorporates the properties and elements of innovative vision, marketing, design, construction and maintenance to assure compliance of a product or service to stakeholders' specific requirements and needs. Aspects characterizing quality are improvement, stakeholder satisfaction and survival (or growth). Quality dimensions are the operational characteristics, reliability and resistibility, conformity to requirements, duration of life and modifiability, service before and after product delivery, aesthetics and appearance, and finally perception (transcendental, objective, subjective).

Ten quality principles related to cultural web sites are transparency, effectiveness, maintenance, accessibility, user centred, responsiveness, multilingualism, interoperable, managed, and preservance [22].

The six software quality characteristics described in ISO/IEC standard 9126 are functionality, reliability, usability, efficiency, maintainability and portability.

WebQual [20] is an evaluation instrument to measure web site quality designed to evaluate and detect features that influence and determine if the user will visit again the web site. The WebQual approach evaluates a web site from the client perspective (how the client-user engages the informative content, the web site presentation and the characteristics that are related and are addressed to the user). WebQual places emphasis to (a) the importance of quality of the web site's informative charge using the theoretical communication model of Shannon & Weaver [30] (possible difference between the transferred and the engaged message so they are not always identical) and (b) the theoretical framework and the practical implementation of quality function deployment process.

SERVQUAL [25] approach consists of five dimensions (tangibles, reliability, responsiveness, assurance and empathy) which have been consistently ranked by customers to be most important for service quality across all industries.

Content quality is of fundamental importance, especially in the communication frame that is shaped in the Internet where communication between the transmitter and the receptor is currently bidirectional and interactive. Data quality [36] has been exploited and a framework was developed that captures the aspects of data quality that are important to data consumers. In the Technology Acceptance Model (TAM), scales have been developed and validated for perceived usefulness and perceived ease of use [9]. SITEQUAL is an instrument that allows getting user feedback (consumer's expectations and perceptions) on the overall quality of B2C electronic commerce web sites.

Models also exist to evaluate quality of portals and e-services [13, 21, 26].

10.6 Performance

Performance indicators of a web application are the response time, the throughput and utilization. Performance analysis is necessary to determine the relationship between performance indicators and the workload. Analytical techniques can be adopted (operational analysis, queuing networks, simulation and measuring approaches). Performance optimization methods [18] aim to improving the performance of web applications. These are: (a) acceleration within a web application (load balancing between the client and server, embedding server side applications, pregenerating web content, adapting HTTP responses to client capabilities); (b) reduction of transmission time (web caching, content pre-fetching, web server replication, load balancing); and (c) server tuning.

10.7 Security

Web application security has certain characteristics that demand adoption of security techniques. Issues about security are confidentiality, authorization, authentication, accountability, integrity. Web application security [37] needs to be assured (a) on the client (desktop security, security of personal data), (b) during request/responses (network security, secure message exchange, non-repudiation), and (c) at the service provider (host-security, service availability). Usage of encryption, digital signatures and certificates is a need as well as secure client–server interaction.

10.8 Testing

Methods, techniques and tool classes for web applications testing [31] include functionality (suitability, accuracy, interoperability, compliance, security), reliability (maturity, fault tolerance, recoverability), usability (understandability, learn ability, operability, attractiveness), efficiency (timing behaviour) and resource utilization.

There are several automatic web testing tools for accessibility testing and repair, usability testing, performance testing, security testing, analysing web servers' logs and classifying a web site after learning the classification criteria from other web sites [4]. Further, the W3C has published a Quality Assurance Activity Statement [35].

10.9 Discussions and Conclusion

In this chapter a model is proposed for evaluating web applications. The aspects presented are usability, culture and communication, graphical user interfaces, quality, performance and security. These aspects are expected to contribute in the design and development of web applications certification frameworks and various web certification quality seals.

10.10 Terms and Definitions

Usability: set of attributes that bear on the effort needed for use, and of the individual assessment of such use, by a stated or implied set of users [3].

Communication: the process by which information is exchanged between individuals or computers through the use of a commonly accepted set of symbols [3].

User Interface: the part of the computer system that communicates with the user. It is the part of the system with which the user comes into contact physically, perceptually and cognitively [3].

Quality: is the synthesis of all the characteristics of a product or service (including performance) that fully satisfies stakeholders (customers, actors, owners) expectations.

Performance: is the process of determining the effectiveness of a software application, a network or hardware.

Security: the combination of availability, confidentiality and integrity. Availability relates to ensuring that information and vital services are available to users when required. Confidentiality refers to the protection of sensitive information from unauthorized disclosure. Integrity means safeguarding the accuracy and completeness of information and computer software [3].

References

1. Afauh, A. and Tucci, C. (2001) Internet Business Models and Strategies: Text and Cases, MacGraw-Hill/Irwin
2. Badre, A. (2000) The Effects of Cross-Cultural Interface Design Orientation on World Wide Web User Performance, GVU Tech Reports
3. Beolchi, L., Loeurng, F., Fitzgerald, M., and Fatelnig, P. (1999) European Telemedicine Glossary, Office for Official Publications of the European Communities, ISBN 92-828-7147-9
4. Brajnik, G. (2002) Quality Models Based on Automatic Webtesting, CHI2002 workshop: Automatically evaluating usability of Web Sites, Minneapolis, USA
5. Bowman, D., Gabbard, J., and Hix, D. (2002) A survey of usability evaluation in virtual environments: Classification and comparison of methods, Presence: Teleoperators and Virtual Environments, Vol. 11, No. 4, 2002, pp. 404–424
6. Burgess, L. and Cooper, J. (2000) Extending the Viability of Model of Internet Commerce Adoption (MICA) as a Metric for Explaining the Process of Business Adoption of Internet Commerce, paper presented at the 3rd International Conference on Telecommunications and Electronic Commerce, Dallas, TX
7. Cockburn C. and Wilson T.D. (1996) Business use of the World Wide Web, Information Journal of International Management, Vol. 26, No. 2, pp. 83–102
8. Davidson, R. (2002) Development of an Industry Specific Web Site Evaluation Framework for the Australian Wine Industry, School of Commerce Research Paper Series: 02-9, ISSN: 1441-3906
9. Davis, F.D. (1989) Perceived usefulness, perceived ease of use, and user acceptance of information technology, MIS Quarterly, Vol. 13, pp. 319–340
10. Elliot, S. (2002) Electronic Commerce B2C Strategies and Model, John Wiley & Sons, UK
11. Fasouli, A. (2007) Evaluation of Websites of the Secreteriats General of Communication and Secreteriats General of Information for fifteen countries of the European Union, Diploma Thesis, National School of Public Administration, Greece
12. Gartner (2002) Gartner Web Site Evaluation Application
13. Halaris, C., Magoutas, B. Papadomichelaki, X., and Mentzas, G. (2007) Classification and synthesis of quality approaches in e-government services, Internet Research Journal, Vol. 17, No. 4, pp. 378–401

14. Hitz, M., Leitner, G., and Melcher, R. (2006) Usability of web applications. In Kappel, G., Proll, B., Reich, S., and Retschitzegger, W. (Eds.), Web Engineering, John Wiley & Sons Ltd
15. Ho J. (1997) Evaluating the WWW: A global study of commercial sites, Journal of Computer Mediated Communication, Vol. 3, No. 1, June
16. Hofstede, G. (1980). Culture's Consequences: International Differences in Work-Related Values, Sage, Beverly Hills, CA, USA
17. Hoger, E.A., Cappel, J.J., and Myerscough, M.A. (1998) Navigating the web with a typology of corporate web users, Business Communication Quarterly, Vol. 61, No. 2, June, pp. 39–47
18. Kotsis, G. (2006) Performance of web applications. In Kappel, G., Proll, B., Reich, S., and Retschitzegger, W. (Eds.), Web Engineering, John Wiley & Sons Ltd
19. Lawrence, E., Corbitt, B., Tidwell, A., Fisher, J., and Lawrence, J.R. (1998) Internet Commerce: Digital Models for Business, John Wiley & Sons, Sydney
20. Loiacono, E.T., Watson, R.T., and Goodhue D.L. (2007) WebQual: An instrument for consumer evaluation of web sites, International Journal of Electronic Commerce, Vol. 11, No. 3, pp. 51–87
21. Magoutas, B., Halaris, C., and Mentzas, G. (2007) An ontology for the multi-perspective evaluation of quality in e-Government services. In Electronic Government, Lecture Notes in Computer Science, Springer Berlin/Heidelberg, pp. 318–329
22. Minerva e-Europe European Cultural Website Quality Principles (2004) Available: http://www.minervaeurope.org/userneeds/qualityprinciples.htm
23. Nielsen, J. (1999) Designing Web Usability: The Practice of Simplicity, New Riders Publishing Thousand Oaks, CA, USA
24. Norman, D. A. (1988) The Design of Everyday Things, Doubleday, New York
25. Parasuraman, A., Zeithaml, V.A., and Berry, L.L. (1988) SERVQUAL: A multiple item scale for measuring consumer perceptions of service quality, Journal of Retailing, Vol. 64, No 1, pp. 12–40
26. Papadomichelaki, X., Magoutas, B., Halaris, C., Apostolou, D., and Mentzas, G. (2006) A review of quality dimensions in e-Government services. In Electronic Government, Lecture Notes in Computer Science, Springer Berlin/Heidelberg, pp. 128–138
27. Pappakou, N.-A. (2006) Comparative evaluation of the Ministries of Foreign Affairs Websites for fifteen countries of the European Union, Diploma Thesis, National School of Public Administration, Greece
28. Schubert, P. (2002) Extended Web Assessment Method (EWAM): Evaluation of electronic commerce applications from the customer's viewpoint, International Journal of Electronic Commerce, Vol. 7, No. 2, pp. 51–80
29. Schubert P. and Dettling W (2001) Web Site Evaluation: Do Web Applications meet user applications? Music, Consumer Goods and e-Banking on the Test Bed, in the Proceedings of the 14th Bled Electronic Commerce Conference, Bled, Slovenia, pp. 383–403
30. Shannon, C.E. and Weaver W. (1949) A Mathematical Model of Communication, University of Illinois Press, Urbana, IL, USA
31. Steindl, C., Ramler, R., and Altmann, J. (2006), Testing web applications. In Kappel, G., Proll, B., Reich, S., and Retschitzegger, W. (Eds.), Web Engineering, John Wiley & Sons Ltd
32. Timmers, P. (2000) Electronic Commerce: Strategies and Models for Business-to- Business Trading, John Wiley & Son
33. Turban, E., King, D., Lee, J., Warkentin, M., and Chung, H.M. (2002) Electronic Commerce 2002: A Managerial Perspective, Prentice-Hall, Englewood Cliffs, NJ, USA
34. Turner, C. (2000) The Information E-Conomy – Business Strategies for Competing in the Global Age, First published Kogan Page Limited: London and Milford
35. W3C Quality Assurance Activity Statement http://www.w3.org/QA/Activity.html

36. Wang, R.Y. and Strong D.M. (1996) Beyond accuracy: What data quality means to data consumers, Journal of Management Information Systems, No. 12, April, pp. 5–34
37. Wimmer, M., Kemper, A., and Seltsam, S. (2006) Security for web applications. In Kappel, G., Proll, B., Reich, S., and Retschitzegger, W. (Eds.), Web Engineering, John Wiley & Sons Ltd

Chapter 11
Web-Based Communities for Lifelong Medical Learning

Iraklis Varlamis and Ioannis Apostolakis

Abstract The exponential growth of medical information, the increased demands for expertise and the limited time that people have to spend for self-improvement create the need for delivering the appropriate knowledge to the appropriate people in the minimum of time. Traditional learning and training approaches are inadequate to fulfil the needs of doctors and medical practitioners, who need always to get informed on new technologies, devices and products and seek for solution in specific problems. Open educational programs and e-learning solutions usually fail to adapt to the emerging needs. The only viable solution seems to be education on demand and communities offer good ground for this. This work examines web-based medical communities as means for delivering education on demand whilst in the same time allowing participants to contribute their expertise. Successful community paradigms are reviewed and the structure of a community for medical learning is detailed. The community tools increase the synergy among industry, practitioners and scientists and allow information sharing, "on the spot" advices and collaborative knowledge building. In the same time, patients receive valuable consults and industry disseminates information on new products and devices and promotes professional excellence. This work summarizes the benefits from the use of communities in deploying medical education to professionals and students, discusses best practices and pitfalls that should be avoided and gives a sketch of the community structure and tools to be employed.

Keywords: Web-Based Learning Communities · Virtual Community · Lifelong Learning · Medical Education · Web 2.0

11.1 Introduction

The aim of education is to provide the basis for lifelong learning and improvement. Universities offer standard curricula aiming to cover the fundamental needs of their students in a few years scope. On the other side, institutes and companies

I. Varlamis (✉)
Department of Informatics and Telematics, Harokopio University of Athens, Athens, Greece
e-mail: varlamis@hua.gr

A. Lazakidou (ed.), *Web-Based Applications in Healthcare and Biomedicine*,
Annals of Information Systems 7, DOI 10.1007/978-1-4419-1274-9_11,

© Springer Science+Business Media, LLC 2010

offer lifelong education in order to improve specific skills and competencies in a short period of time. In a similar manner, medical education comes in two variations: (a) medical studies offered by universities and schools of medicine, where students follow predefined curricula and receive support from their professors and other academics, (b) lifelong education of physicians, continuing training on their field of expertise and learning through reading and practicing.

Mainly in the second case, the aims, capabilities and availability of attendants vary significantly, since they usually have to cope with their morning work and their family duties. As a matter of fact, several issues, such as the limited duration of training programs, the loaded schedule of trainees, the inevitable absences due to other obligations, the multitude of topics to be covered, the variance of attendants' interests and needs, have to be considered in order to create a competitive training program that will fit everyone's needs.

Community approaches have several advantages that can be exploited in favour of medical doctors and students. Since a single institute is not always capable in coordinating such a composite effort, we capitalize on the building of a virtual community for education. The community should use all available tools in order to support attendance and inform people on the topics, requirements and aims of programs, in order to deliver information, training material, and support on demand, in a daily basis. The community should comprise training institutes, educators and trainees, who will interact and cooperate in order to achieve maximum gain and flexibility.

The educational role of the community is strengthened by a multitude of ways: (a) the use of asynchronous and many-to-many communication and collaboration tools, facilitates and increases the participation of members to the activities of the community; (b) the dynamic role assignment to members, allows them to be educators and trainees in the same time, and increases their awareness on the community activities; (c) the content repository of the community is continuously enriched with new content such as reading material, assignments, self-assessment tests, members' communication logs, thus creating a common community knowledge, which can be valuable for future members.

In the following section, we refer to other works that attempt to offer education on a medical community. In Section 11.3 we give an overview of the communication and knowledge management tools that can support the medical community. In Section 11.4 we present the structure of the medical community. In Section 11.5 we illustrate the expected merits of the suggested approach and discuss the issues that need special attention. Finally, in Section 11.6 we present our conclusions and give our thoughts for future work.

11.2 Related Work on Medical Education and the Web

The aim of web-based learning communities is to collaboratively improve knowledge in the field of expertise of the community. In the case of open learning communities, everyone is allowed to participate and either offer or consume the collective knowledge [1]. As a result, the members of a web-based learning community vary from the non-experienced learner to the subject matter expert inside and outside of the community. The core activity of virtual learning communities is writing. People exchange messages with a shared goal of building understanding produce an information base, which is available to future members of the community [2]. Learning is no longer a transmission of knowledge from a teacher to a student, but a process of knowledge construction in which each participant contributes and benefits from the ideas shared by the group. Useful knowledge sources comprise: questionnaires addressed to patients and their families, personal reflections of patients, discussion forum logs, virtual interviews of doctors and experts, etc.

Virtual learning communities are emerging everyday in many health-related domains. All these communities functioning today can be divided in four types of communities, classified by the intended members [3]. Virtual healthcare delivery teams in which healthcare providers of different disciplines (such as physicians, nurses, social workers, physical therapists) create a team to combine their knowledge and expertise in order to provide a comprehensive plan of care [4]. An example is the virtual medical teams for the continuous treatment of home care patients, developed by Pitsillides et al [5]. The second type of healthcare communities comprises the virtual research teams, where healthcare researchers and professionals employ new ICT technologies in order to communicate and exchange information. An example is The Virtual Radiopharmacy (VirRAD) [6] eLearning program. The third type comprises healthcare communities that support virtual disease management as a means of enhancing the care plan and the provider–patient relationship, while emphasizing on the prevention of deterioration through the delivery of practical guidelines. An example is the home asthma telemonitoring (HAT) system presented in [7]. Finally, another category of virtual communities comprises support groups, where people with interests gather "virtually" to share experiences, ask questions or provide emotional support and self-help [8]. As of April 2004, Yahoo! Groups listed at least 25,000 electronic support groups in health and wellness sections.

More and more, physicians browse web information in order to stay current in many areas of medicine. However, it is physically impossible to gather and absorb all the available data on research findings, new medications and legislative changes affecting medicine. In order to facilitate the continuing learning process, several organizations have developed web sites that collect, filter, organize and redistribute medical information [9]. These sites use a credit-based system that enforces physicians to attend courses successfully.

Another aim of learning communities is to replace Internet as an information source for patients [4]. A common scenario wants patients to spend hours in collecting information from the Internet before visiting their doctors [8]. Such information can be misleading and confusing and is better to be filtered before visiting the doctor). Such filtering can be performed inside a learning community [10].

For example, MedConnect [11], which is affiliated with the HealthAtoZ Professional and the University of the Sciences in Philadelphia, offers text- and graphic-based case presentations, and several types of educational opportunities on primary care issues. Similarly MedScape's site [12] for continuing education (for professionals and patients) offers the ability to subscribe for monthly newsletters and alerts, to browse various medical education modules, to perform self-assessment and gain credits or even receive an instant certificate. CME [13] is another source for continuing medical education; it is owned by American Health Consultants and offers for a small fee a larger variety of CME courses than most web pages.

An interesting community approach for providing education and support in rehabilitation issues is WheelchairNet [6], which has been developed in cyberspace by the University of Pittsburgh. As part of the community activities, the Wheelchair University offers academic and continuing education programs on rehabilitation and wheeled mobility areas. Research is a continuing and joint work of clinicians, manufactures, scientists, patients and transporters. However, web sites are the only means of virtual communication, which lack interactive services (i.e. forums).

Sermo [14] is another community approach, targeted to physicians. It works as a forum, allowing physicians to post observations and questions about clinical issues and hear other doctors' opinions. The closed nature of the site has led some sources to refer to Sermo as a "MySpace for Physicians".

In a project developed at St George's, University of London, UK, named Clinical Skills Online (CSO) [15], online videos demonstrate core clinical skills common to a wide range of medical and health-based courses in higher education. The video courses are categorized by topic, by user's expertise and occupation and are available to the public. The option of user feedback is available through a questionnaire and a free text comments form.

What is obvious, from all the previous examples, is that an organization (i.e. university, hospital or company) is necessary for the coordination of the educational process, for the design of programs, modules and educational solutions and for the certification of the acquired knowledge. Lifelong medical education is currently delivered in the form of information updates, reading or viewing material in electronic format or traditionally in classrooms and laboratories. What is missing is the ability to identify students' needs and design custom solutions for them. What is also missing is a flexible environment that will allow communities to evolve, community members to help and get help on everyday issues [16] and at the end of the day to assess and certify their knowledge.

In order to build this environment, we suggest the full exploitation of virtual communities and their tools. In the following section, we present the architecture of a community for medical education and discuss the critical issues for a smooth and successful operation.

11.3 A Virtual Community for Medical Education

Virtual communities gather people with common interests and practices. Community members communicate regularly and for some duration in an organized way over the Internet, using a common platform or set of tools [11]. In virtual learning communities, learning is the common interest, Internet is the carrier and network technologies are the supporting infrastructure. Anyone interested in learning is a potential member for the community, and is likely to communicate their opinion to other community members.

A review of the existing solutions in education reveals the power and flexibility of communities [3]. The undeniable gain from using communities in education springs from the increase in membership. Continuity is another important issue for any virtual community. From a technical point of view, continuous system maintenance is necessary for the stability of the community infrastructure. Moreover, a reputation system may help to elicit good behaviour, encourage knowledge sharing among individuals and strengthen members' bonds to the community.

However, increased participation results in augmented administrational and operational costs and risks. Since the members carry all community tasks, the definition and assignment of roles, duties and rights to members is crucial. In opposition to virtual enterprises and organizations, the definition of rights and responsibilities in a community is not strict and changes according to members' need and participation.

11.3.1 Members

Potential members of a medical community for education are medical students, nurses and doctors that need medical training, trainers and tutors, researchers seeking to exchange knowledge, universities and institutes that offer training and companies that produce medical solutions and educational material on them.

Students or trainees are the building blocks of the community. They join the community in order to attend an educational program and obtain knowledge. They request for training and receive support and guidance by other community members or experts. Student-members should provide their educational profile in detail in order to be accepted. A pre-evaluation procedure will give educators a better view on members' knowledge and skills.

Universities and medical schools are the community motors. They assemble educational modules into classes and then targeted programs and guide students and trainees to improve skills. They undertake the administration of the community and in parallel monitor and facilitate members. They study the members' needs, design and offer courses and direct members to the appropriate knowledge. Individual educators and researchers are able to offer their expertise to the community, always under the administrators' control. The anatomy of a learning community is depicted in Fig. 11.1 and explained in the following.

In complement to the community members, several people, in the community background, guarantee the smooth operation of the community and the uninterrupted delivery of services. The IT staff that technically supports the community, the employees of the telecommunication services provider and the directors of the

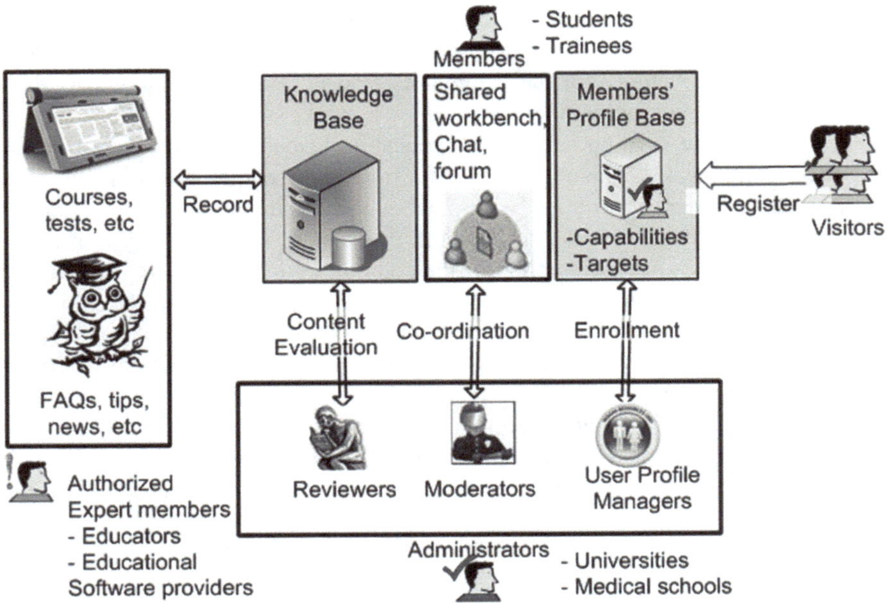

Fig. 11.1 A community for medical education

organization, company or hospital that hosts the virtual community are persons that do not actually participate in the community but play a key role in its secure operation.

11.3.2 Roles

Administrators and moderators are the two most important roles in any virtual community [17]. Administrators are selected from the educational institutions and are responsible for managing members' profiles and evaluating content. Tutors are assigned with the task of producing new educational material upon request. The same people carry out a moderator role in the community services. Additional material can be obtained from volunteers out of the community borders.

Apart from the educational subjects, community members need technical support on the use of the community services. The technical staff of the institutes will initially become the community facilitators [6]. However, regular community members with technical expertise can be accredited this role. The role tasks comprise the editing of help files or user manuals, the answering of frequently asked questions and the response to members' requests for help. Facilitators will help new members, either students or tutors, to get accustomed to the community services and take full advantage of them.

A hierarchical structure of roles, an accreditation and a reputation system will encourage members' participation and contribution [18]. Active and capable members of a community are promoted or assigned new roles. Members that do not contribute are restricted, demoted and set aside by other members.

11.3.3 Supportive Structures

The building blocks of a virtual community are its members and an initial content. The collaboration of members, inside a secure and trustful community environment will increase content, will assist members to ameliorate their profiles and will attract new community members. In order for the community to thrive, the harmonic cooperation of all members must be achieved.

The primary aim of members of the learning community is to improve skills and competencies. As a consequence, the community should consider the particular needs and targets of lifelong learners [2], which in the case of medical communities comprise among others: medical theory, nursing theory, management, patient psychology, health regulation, prevention, emergency handling, trauma management, rehabilitation, etc. The community should be able to adapt content and courses at any time, in order to capture changes in the work environment and follow the rapid technological advances. A profile base where members' skills, needs and educational targets are recorded is very useful in the design of new courses or seminars. The analysis of members' profiles will give better educational solutions and create competitive groups of learners.

A "knowledge base" [19] will contain educational material organized by topic, course scenarios, educational solutions, program evaluation reports, answers to users' requests, etc. Additionally, it should offer self-assessment solutions to trainees and exam scenarios that will lead to certification. The educational content will be enriched during the community lifecycle, with new study material, tests and activities. Educational programmes must comprise reusable learning objects that can be easily recomposed or transformed to fit individual needs. The use of learning objects facilitates the monitoring of content, since it is easier for institutions to rate the quality and suitability of content uploaded by educators. Additional training material can be added by authorized members, only after evaluation.

The success of a health-related virtual community is based on the frequency and quality of members' contribution. A trust management mechanism [1] that keeps record of the members' reputation inside the community and continuously updates it by analyzing other members' feedback can be useful for encouraging members' contribution and increasing members' awareness on faulty consultation and fraud. The reputation management module will gather members' opinions on other members, will process data and provide each user x with a reputation score for any other community member y. This score will be based on the community reputation for this member y (what others think of y) and the direct trust towards this member (what x thinks of y). This mechanism will encourage members' contribution to the community and in the same time will discourage malicious behaviour since it will lead to decrease of trust.

In addition to the members' reputation mechanism and the content evaluation process, the community must develop a mechanism that acquires and processes user feedback on the educational process as a whole. User polls, complaint forms, and user-feedback forums will facilitate community designers to locate the platform errors and the points where the educational process can be improved.

Finally, the power of the community resides in the ability of members to collaborate. It is essential in this case to build a collaboration environment and encourage members' interaction through group activities. In such activities, distant members of a virtual class are forced to communicate, participate in synchronous activities, split composite activities into tasks and work in subgroups, etc.

In the following section, we present how the available community tools can be combined in favour of the medical community.

11.4 A Prototype Community Structure

11.4.1 Services

The community must build a gateway for people or companies outside its borders that wish to cooperate with the community. Information services are the front-end of a community. A web site with informative material on the community activities, sample courses, contact information and a feedback form will allow companies or individuals to offer content and potential students to reach and join the community. The community site should be simple and provide support to the community members. This can be established by providing informative material to members (online tutorials, manuals, frequent questions and answers, etc.) and by assigning guidance roles to selected existing members (facilitators, moderators, etc.).

Communication services (synchronous or not, private or public) are vital to all community members: to educators for coordinating their collaborators, guiding and supporting their students, to students for discussing about assignments and requesting help on activities.

Collaboration services are very useful when they are coupled with educational activities. A group project turns autonomous learning into a collective activity and helps students to improve their analytical and collaboration skills.

11.4.2 The Assembly of Web and Web 2.0 Tools

The nucleus of the virtual community should be equally accessible to members and visitors.

A web site is necessary to welcome web visitors and guide potential members into joining the community. The site should provide informative content on the community aim and structure and can be created as a joint effort of the universities or educational institutes that support the community. The web site will advertise the educational programs and will provide information concerning every day activities of each course, news and announcements of interest to the students.

The web site administration should be performed by technical staff from the educational partners of the community (i.e. the university). Coordination tasks will be held by the registrar office that will be responsible for the members' accounts, their participation in virtual classes, etc.

A smart and cost-free solution for the web site is presented in [20]. There, the web site was a blog, created by the university. The blog was visible to anyone, but practically only registered community members were allowed to update content or comment. In an effort to delegate administration tasks, a "weblog umbrella" was created (see Fig. 11.2).

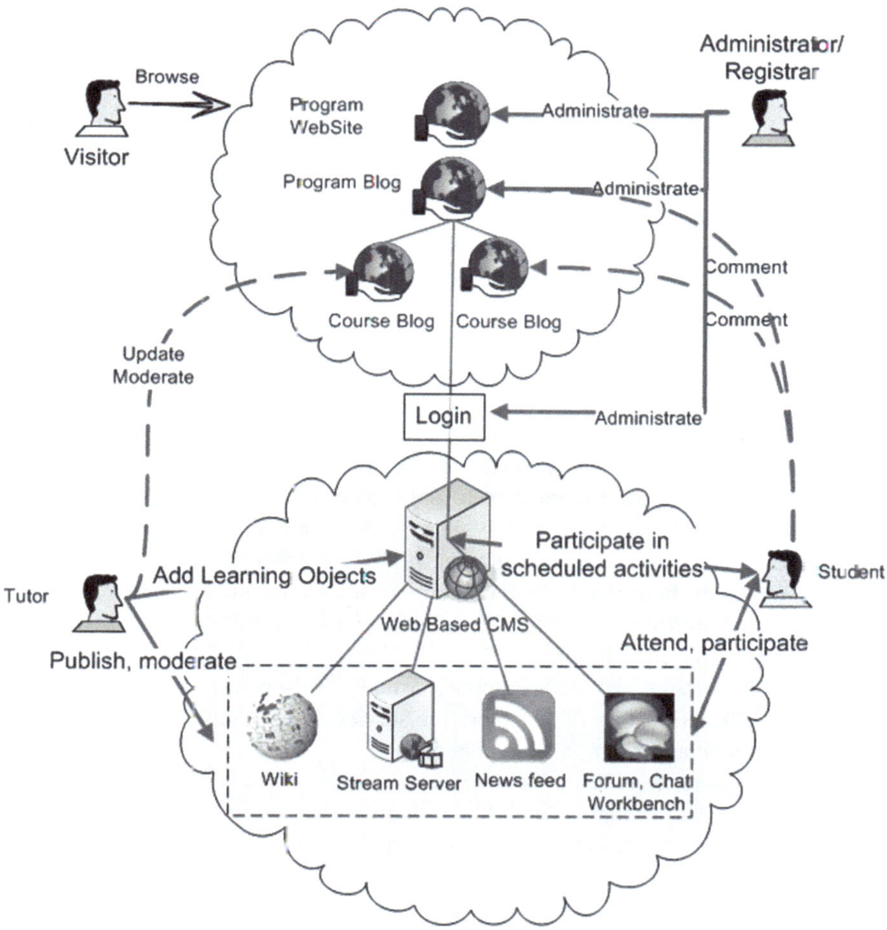

Fig. 11.2 The blogs on top of the community

Blogs (or web logs) are easily updatable web sites where administrators can post messages by filling a few forms and without special knowledge on web design technologies. Separate blogs for each course allow course tutors to better organize their courses, to add or drop material, to add short notices or announcements and manage the comments or posts of the community members. The students were permitted to comment on the tutor notices, thus providing them with useful feedback. Weblog visitors were able only to read announcement or comments. On the top of this set of weblogs we created an additional weblog for the whole program, in which community members were able to post messages. The program web log was accessible for the program web page and provided links to all program courses.

Below this umbrella that provides general information on the program lies the main educational activities of the community. These activities can be ideally supported by a web-based course management system (i.e. Moodle, eFront, Claroline, Blackboard, Atutor, etc). Such systems are specialized in managing and delivering on line courses, and assemble various community tools such as forums, wikis, etc.

In the majority of courses, tutors use the community application solely for provided reading material to students. However, in several cases, students and professors need the forum, chat and other services in order to coordinate their actions. When an integrated course management system is not available, the community can still be operational by combining various open source tools.

Computer-mediated chat, discussion forums and newsgroups can be formed and supported by the community administrators. Such forums will host discussions focused on the class learning goals [17] and will be used from tutors for guiding their students. Mailing lists and web feeds can be in assistance of the tutor for the coordination of a course. For example, the tutor will be able to inform students on an upcoming examination or assignment.

When there is need for building collaborative knowledge and making it available to medical students and practitioners, wikis are a cost-free open source solution. A wiki is the collaborative coverage of a topic from the members of a community. Any member can contribute or modify the content under conditions (proper reason, provide references, etc.). The vast number of medical wikis currently available [21] is an indication of their popularity and their importance for medical matters. A wiki can be created and moderated by the domain experts in order to quickly build a terminology source for students.

Other collaboration services comprise, virtual workbenches, virtual blackboard, etc. The results and history of collaboration services are usually stored and used as a reference by other community members. Such applications usually require specialized software and dedicated sources and thus are not widely used for medical education. The educational potential of virtual worlds has attracted the interest of medical communities and created new opportunities for medical education in the cyberspace [14, 22].

When a teleconference room is available, distant courses can be performed from the joint institutes. Tutors and students communicate using real-time video over a streamed media server. Educational multimedia content (i.e. medical videos from surgeries, recorder sessions or courses, etc.) can be stored in media repositories and made available to community members. Free video hosting servers can be used for this task; however, bandwidth and storage limitations, restricted access and other issues should be considered.

The applications presented in the bottom section of Fig. 11.2 can be accessible both to students and tutors; however, the degree of participation increases for students as moving from left to the right. All these services (i.e. wikis, streaming media, news feed, forum, chat, workbench, etc.) can be offered through separate tools and platforms or ideally through the same web-based CMS.

The next section illustrates the gains for individuals, companies, organizations and biomedical science in general.

11.5 Expected Results From the Community Approach

The educational role of the medical learning community is jointly supported by more than one community services and structures. According to [15], the educational solutions that can be offered by the educational community comprise autonomous courses, complete course series, complete programs, standalone teaching or teaching associate with study material, training programs targeted to special groups of trainees, programs that lead to certification, etc. In a medical learning community, members chose any of the above solutions and employ one or more of the following learning methods in order to achieve their common aims: they study the related educational material, attend seminars and lectures, examine related clinical case studies and participate on medical meetings.

Table 11.1 presents how the aforementioned learning methods are supported by the community services and structures.

A side role of communities apart from the education of doctors and students is the increase of synergy between companies, experts and clients. Doctors can join

Table 11.1 Learning Methods and Community Services

	Study theory	Attend seminars	Examine cases	Medical meetings
Knowledge base	Study material	Online seminars, audiovisual content	Clinical case databases	Minutes of meetings are added to the repository
Collaboration tools	Collaboratively collect reading sources (in a wiki)		Simulation environments	Synchronous and asynchronous services, telemedicine
Communication services		Userfeedback and online questions		Teleconferencing

the community and share their knowledge with other colleagues. Communities also support the exchange of empirical knowledge that is more focused to patients' and doctors' needs than theoretical knowledge. Participation in forums allows patients to ask questions and doctors and engineers to increase the consultation time. Finally, when communities are open to the industry, they can receive information on new products and devices, thus promoting professional excellence of engineers. The result is that community members will work smarter that harder, will communicate expertise to the new members and acquire maximum benefits. The benefits from the use of communities are the main motive behind the participation.

The benefits for practitioners range from the alleviation of their everyday tasks to the development of their skills and professional profile. Professionals share their knowledge voluntarily with other members, invite new members and contribute on the expansion and guidance of the community. Active personal contributions to the community is a long-term investment and leads to recognition (awards, fellowships). Through the community, doctors and nurses can be informed and trained on tools and techniques of their field of expertise. Training can be delivered by specialized institutes and lead to professional certifications. The community can be a vault to their career, as new job opportunities emerge from the professional network. The ability to remotely collaborate with other community members increases job flexibility (contingent workers, freelancers etc.)

The benefits for the medical industry are mostly organizational and strategic. Firms have the ability to define key knowledge areas, and cover their needs for expertise by directly contacting doctors through the community. They can also define the strategic resources and the core competencies of medical industry and target research to this direction. Organizational restructuring allows companies to expand their borders and to better organize and monitor the production lifecycle. They are able to advertise their products easier and with minimum cost and increase their potential markets.

The gains for research institutes, universities and scientific organizations comprise interaction with industry and consequently applied research, increase of basic research through the collaboration of researchers worldwide. Universities can act as focal points of the community of practice by providing support and guidance to enterprises and education and training to engineers. Moreover, through the cooperation with industry, research increases funding and gains access to empirical data.

11.6 Conclusions and Future Work

The gains from the use of virtual learning community are many for universities, students and professionals. Students exchange empirical knowledge and carry out learning activities. Tutors increase their consultation time and contribute to the guidance of members more easily.

The benefits from the use of communities are the main motive behind the participation. The benefits for the educational institutes are mostly organizational and strategic.

It is in our next plans to increase the activities of our community and create new educational scenarios that fully exploit the community infrastructure. We already set up a community using open source tools and software and we intend to analyse the users' behaviour inside the community in order to detect what is attractive and what is not for the students, what possible flaws in courses result in decreased participation. Finally, it is our aim to design an evaluation framework, which will be used to assess the usability of the provided services and interfaces and to judge on the educational value of the community approach in medical education.

References

1. Kommers P, Rödel S, Luursema JM, Geelkerken B, Kunst E. Learning surgical interventions by navigating in virtual reality case spaces. Int Conf Comput Sci 2003;1015–1024.
2. Harasim L. What makes online learning communities successful?: The role of collaborative learning in social and intellectual development. In: Vrasidas C, Glass GV (eds.), Distance Education and Distributed Learning. Greenwich, CT: Information Age Publishing, 2002: 181–200.
3. Papadopoulou A, Varlamis I, Apostolakis I. Models and practices for the development of e-learning communities in healthcare. In Proceedings of 5th ICICTH, Samos, Greece, 2007.
4. Demiris G, The diffusion of virtual communities in health care: Concept and challenges. Patient Educ Counsel 2006;62(2):178–188.
5. Pitsillides A, Pitsillides B, Samaras G, Dikaikos M, Christodoulou E, Andreou P, Georgiadis D. DITIS: a collaborative virtual medical team for home healthcare of cancer patients. In: Istepanian R, Laxminarayan S, Pattichis C (eds.), M-Health: Emerging Mobile Health Systems. New York: Kluwer Academic/Plenum Publishers, 2006.
6. VirRAD – The Virtual Radiopharmacy – a Mindful Learning Environment (2007), Retrieved May 4, 2007 from http://community.virrad.eu.org/.
7. Finkelstein J, O' Connor G, Friedmann RH. Development and implementation of the home asthma telemonitoring (HAT) system to facilitate asthma self-care. In Proceedings of the 10th Med Info Conference, London, UK, 2001.
8. Eysenbach G, Powell J, Englesakis M, Rizo C, Stern A. Health related virtual communities and electronic support group: systematic review of the effects of online peer to peer interactions. Br Med J 2004;328:1166–1172.
9. Allen JW. The Internet for Surgeons, New York: Springer, 2002.
10. Moon J. Discussing health issues on the Internet. In: Dasgupta S (ed.), Encyclopedia of Virtual Communities and Technologies. USA: George Washington University, 2005.
11. MedConnect website. 2008-04-01. URL:http://www.medconnect.com. Accessed: 2008-04-01. (Archived by WebCite® at http://www.webcitation.org/5WkmyPQCa).
12. MedScape website. 2008-04-01. URL:http://www.medscape.com. Accessed: 2008-04-01. (Archived by WebCite® at http://www.webcitation.org/5Wkn2l56Y).
13. CME website. 2008-04-01. URL:http://www.cmeweb.com. Accessed: 2008-04-01. (Archived by WebCite® at http://www.webcitation.org/5WkmvRHDS).
14. Sermo website. 2008-04-01. URL:http://www.sermo.com. Accessed: 2008-04-01. (Archived by WebCite® at http://www.webcitation.org/5Wkn4URn6).
15. Barker K. Canadian Recommended E-Learning Guidelines, FuturEd and CACE (Canadian Association for Community Education), January 2002. Retrieved March, 5, 2009 from http://www.col.org/SiteCollectionDocuments/CanREGs_Eng.pdf.

16. Varlamis I, Apostolakis I. The educational role of communities of practice in biomedical engineering. 5th European Symposium on Biomedical Engineering, Patras, Greece, 2007.
17. Apostolakis I, Varlamis I, Papadopoulou A. Electronic Learning Communities, in Greek. Athens: Papazisis, 2008.
18. Shek SPW, Sia CL. Using reputation system to motivate knowledge contribution behavior in online community. Pacific Asia Conference on Information Systems 2007 Proceedings. Paper 125. http://aisel.aisnet.org/pacis2007/125.
19. Sampson DG. Enhancing educational portals through capturing collective knowledge of web-based learning communities. Int J Web Based Commun 2006;2(3):260–272 (doi: 10.1504/IJWBC.2006.011758).
20. Varlamis I, Apostolakis I. A framework for building virtual communities for education. First European Conference on Technology Enhanced Learning (EC-TEL 2006) Joint Workshop on Professional Learning, Competence Development and Knowledge Management, 2006.
21. Medical Wiki's list. 2008-04-01. URL:http://davidrothman.net/list-of-medical-wikis/. Accessed: 2008-04-01. (Archived by WebCite® at http://www.webcitation.org/5Wkn0VMg6).
22. Antonacci DM, Modaress N. Second life: the educational possibilities of a massively multiplayer virtual world (MMVW). Presented at Southwest Regional Conferences, 2005. Accessed: 2008-03-17. (Archived by WebCite® at http://www.webcitation.org/5WORXSGL5).

Chapter 12
Evaluation of Wikis Exploited for Medicine Courses Teaching

Georgia Lazakidou, Konstantinos Siassiakos, Athina Lazakidou, and Christina Ilioudi

Abstract Implementing the principles of constructivist approaches to learning Wiki systems are being utilized for various purposes, one of which concerns the education of medical and nursing students. Their use in medicine courses enhances a plethora of issues, most of which are related to the learning effectiveness and their integration into the course from an instructional perspective. The present chapter reviews numerous research studies focusing on the evaluation issues such as the variables and techniques that have been used. Also, related issues regarding the problems that arise from the evaluation methods and the priorities that should be taken are discussed under the scope of fully utilizing the potential of social software.

Keywords: Learning Wiki Systems · Medicine Courses · Web 2.0 · Collaboration Tools · Communication Services

12.1 Introduction

Web-based collaborationware (alternatively known as Web 2.0 tools) have been the focus of educational research as they carry the potential of complementing, improving and adding new collaborative dimensions to the many web-based medical/health education [1]. They afford users the added advantage of reducing the technical skill required to exploit these tools by allowing users to focus on the information and collaborative tasks themselves.

Wikis are gaining ground as a learning tool especially in higher education. In higher education relatively little is known about their use in the context of a course. According to Elgort [2], there are two common ways that Wikis are used: as social software and as a tool that provides support for group projects and activities, with the former usually associated with open access and the latter associated with restricted access. In both cases, Wikis demand a kind of self-regulation in order to be used, and as a result they are extremely recommended for the higher education purposes

G. Lazakidou (✉)
Department of Technology Education and Digital Systems, University of Piraeus, Karaoli and Dimitriou, GR-18534 Piraeus, Greece
e-mail: glazak@unipi.gr

A. Lazakidou (ed.), *Web-Based Applications in Healthcare and Biomedicine*, Annals of Information Systems 7, DOI 10.1007/978-1-4419-1274-9_12,

© Springer Science+Business Media, LLC 2010

in which students are adults. Current research [3, 4] that has been carried out has shown many examples of using Wikis for medical/healthcare education purposes, but most of them mainly research the possible result they may have in learning process or outcomes and substantially the reason for including Wikis in educational process.

Having many researchers exploited the Wikis for the medical/healthcare education purposes numerous questions have been arisen especially around the issue of making full use of the potential of Wikis. Having no clear answer –yet – about the reason of integrating Wikis in educational process, it is necessary to attempt a review of present studies and make the associated conclusions while discussing parallel issues. The present study reviews the related studies and focuses on the evaluation methods and techniques that are used to measure the extent Wikis have been correlated to the learning process and performance. Inevitably, most studies research variables common in nature with the feature of Wikis – namely, the social aspects, motivation and usefulness. However, neither of them can directly answer if Wikis are finally effective for healthcare/medical courses.

12.2 Wikis

The term "wiki" is derived from the Hawaiian phrase, wiki-wiki, which means quick. A wiki is a collaborative web site whose content can be edited by visitors to the site, allowing users to easily create and edit web pages collaboratively [5]. In essence, a wiki is a simplification of the process of creating HTML web pages in combination with a system that records each individual change that occurs over time, so that at any time a page can be forced to revert to any of its previous states [6]. A wiki may also provide tools that allow the user community to monitor the constantly changing state of the wiki and discuss the issues that emerge. Some wikis restrict access to a group of members, allowing only members to edit page content although everyone may view it. Others allow completely unrestricted access, allowing anyone to both edit and view content [7]. Wikis can be used as a source of information and knowledge, as well as a tool for collaborative authoring. Wikis allow visitors to engage in dialog and share information among participants in group projects or to engage in learning with each other by using wikis as a collaborative environment in which to construct their knowledge [1]. Among its advantages belong its simplicity, openness and lack of structure [8].

In recent years wikis are being used for various teaching and learning purposes. They have been utilized in many areas of education including composition, literature, distance education, philosophy, design engineering, symbolic logic and mathematics [6]. In some circumstances there is an attempt to utilize wikis for medicine courses facilitating the burden and complexity of medical studies. They have been used in various ways such as for classroom activities (information distribution, collaborative artefact creation, discussion, review, as a tool for building e-learning content, icebreakers for online groupwork, etc.).

In higher education wikis have been used in various ways, too [9, 10]. Par examples, Wikis have been developed as a course that revolves around lectures such as those at Harvard Law School (http://cyber.law.harvard.edu/cyberone/wiki/Main_Page). Also, they have been developed to provide collaborative content management in the context of teaching and learning to the University of Calgary community (http://wiki.ucalgary.ca/page/Main_Page). In Neurobiology Great Controversies is a course Wiki that includes students' projects.

12.3 Healthcare and Wikis

In healthcare the use of wikis could take place not only in medical schools and courses but also patients could create dynamic web pages like wikis. In this case we have two kinds of users: that user who selects to participate actively (by creating a site, posting comments, searching for sites of interest) and that one who selects to participate passively (by reading sites only). The scope is to exchange information between patients affected by illness, physicians and public. In particular, patients could keep something like diary about their disease state, progress and setbacks. Also family, friends even physicians from remote areas have the opportunity to "visit" people who are affected and learn about them. Through sites patients may provide their personal experience to people with the same medical problem. The above are some of the social aspects which follow wikis and how effective and efficient tools could be for healthcare.

The patients' wikis creation is a special case that we often observe at a university level. Wiki is a collaborative web site in which the content can be edited by anyone who has access to it. The most popular wiki is Wikipedia. Educators in medical and nursing schools believe that the use of such technologies lead students to learn and perform best. But also wikis can solve problems like lifelong learning, especially for those who live in remote areas. Wikis make obtainable the training from the large central hospitals and academic centres of excellence in the main cities. The use of wikis web sites by tutors can provide their students with necessary support during their studies. Such technologies can contribute to the creation of dynamic learning communities, to support continuing medical education/professional development (CME/CPD) and patient education and can be useful on the long run for virtual collaborative clinical practice and learning based on the currently available initial online medical/health-related examples and literature about these tools.

Wikis can also be used by health librarians. Wikis support the principles of collaboration, knowledge sharing and socialization. They are easy to use, interactive and built on open platforms. Also they give teaching opportunities for health librarians. At this moment wikis are used for a lot of projects. But very important is the use of wikis in libraries. More specific, librarians use wikis to build repositories (portfolio) and create dynamic content for web sites. Below we mention wikis applications that are taking place in medicine:

- Ask Dr. Wiki (http://www.askdrwiki.com) is a web site which serves medical information. This site is for physicians and medical students.
- Ganfyd (http://www.ganfyd.org) is a medical knowledge base and has restricted editorial policies.
- PubDrug (http://www.pubdrug.org/) is an information database intended for use of pharmacists and other health professionals.

Wikis could give the opportunity to health librarians to collaborate with physicians and other health professionals.

12.4 Aim of the Study

While Wikis are currently being used in several ways all over the world for educational purposes, it is necessary to investigate their real significance and relation to the learning process and performance. The present study aims to review those works that refer to the utilization of Wikis for healthcare/medical education purposes. Reviewing the related works, we aim to reveal to what extent the Wikis have been already exploited and which aspects of their use need to be researched under the scope of learning process in higher education.

12.5 Method of the Study

The relevant literature for the present review is found in many disciplines: in journals, in www, in communications, in all grades of education, in educational technology, as well as in the subject disciplines. Many articles advocate in favour of use of Wikis in higher education via collaborative activities in educational procedure.

The primary sources of literature were followed by ERIC (a search engine) searches using keywords from the articles identified in the journals articles. Yet, the theoretical foundations and researches on Wikis use were included in the studied literature. This is not a complete review of all Wikis uses, but our review has been limited to those studies that concern the higher education and the healthcare/medical courses. What was examined in this review is how much closed or not from establishing a full utilization of the Wikis potential for healthcare/medical courses in higher education. Wikis utilization reviewed here will be discussed in two main fields: the evaluation variables and the evaluation techniques that have been used during the research efforts to incorporate Wikis potential into higher education procedure. The selection of the following research studies has been done according to the Web 2.0-related research references.

12.6 Description of Other Distinguished Research Studies

Boulos et al. [1] conducted a study to explore how Web 2.0 (wikis, blocks and podcasts) applications could help for virtual collaborative practice and learning. The study concerned students in higher education and specific medical and nursing students. For the survey the researchers did not use any evaluation technique, but it was based only on the currently available initial online medical/health-related examples and literature. These kinds of technologies are proposed as effective because they can support mobile learning. Students are now more mobile than ever, and often find themselves multitasking, working in part-time jobs, or located some distance from a parent institution on professional practice placement. A similar situation is faced by clinicians in remote areas, who often lack training and proper academic support because of their geographic situation from the large central hospitals and academic centres of excellence in the main cities. Also, wikis and blogs encourage learners and give them the motivations actively involve in their own construction of knowledge. According to the authors a social aspect of these technologies has the potential to both liberate and tie learners together creating dynamic learning communities. The result is that it is still in progress the best way of use of these tools for teaching and learning productivity and support continuing medical education/professional development and patient education.

Ebner et al. [11] conducted a study that its results contrast to others [12, 13], which report the success of Wikis use in education. Their study concerns the use of wikis by higher education students in order to research the potential of utilizing a wiki system for supporting learning and collaboration. About 152 students participated in two case studies while they were supposed to use the wikis to collect knowledge during one semester. For this purpose the researchers used a pre/post questionnaire and the method of semi-structured interview. In the first case study the number of participants was 152 (included students who answered the questionnaire and the semi-interview) from whom 8 were female and 69 male (only 77 students answered the questionnaires). The youngest student was aged 21 and the oldest 36. The evaluation variables at the beginning of the semester concerned prior knowledge about structural concrete, use of wikis in general, and teamwork for learning. At the end of the semester the use of BauWiki was evaluated. The result from the first case study was that during the semester, none of 152 students actively created a new article or edited an existing one on the wiki. Also from the questionnaire concluded that the 61% of students reported to have accessed BauWiki at least once during the semester for learning or retrieving information and 39% of students reported that they did not use the provided articles at all. Combining the results from the questionnaire and the semi-interview concluded that 38% of students reported technical difficulties as major reasons for not using BauWiki, and 57% reported reasons related to a lack of motivation. In the second case study 135 students participated and 88 questionnaire answers were collected. Here, the ages ranged from 19 to 24. The studied variables were the same as in the first case study. The percentage of students who passively accessed articles of the Wiki was, in contrast to the first case study, significantly higher. The analysis of questionnaires revealed that 95% of students accessed an article at least once during the semester, and 5% reported that they never accessed articles. A remarkable finding is that the access rate significantly decreased in the learning phase for the exam. Moreover, the participated students reported – during the semi-structured interview – the ease-to-use of the BauWiki as well as its usefulness for collaborative learning. Finally, the researchers drew the conclusion that the problems of not using the wikis were not technological in nature but rather sociological and psychological. They suggest that the future research must reveal those socio-motivational and psychological aspects that lead to the use of wikis in education in order to provide improvements of learning and collaborative purposes.

Sandars et al. [3] studied the usefulness of social software such as wikis in first-year medical students. For this purpose 212 students participated in and a structured self-administered questionnaire survey was used. The questionnaire included questions about blogs, messaging and social networking sites as well as wikis. The analysed results for the wikis found that a fifth of male students used them to contribute information. Female students did not show any statistically important finding. The study identified that the use of social software like wikis advances the collaboration between medical students, the communication and sharing knowledge. The conclusion drawn in this study concerns the future of wikis use by the medical students. Specifically, it is referred that they should maintain the informality and privacy of these platforms. Yet, it is proposed that the medical educators should consider how to integrate social software into current curricula and institutional virtual learning environments. The latter is considered important for young people – as the medical students – who are at ease with the technology of social software and choose to publicly share the content they attain with older people or other students all over the world.

One year earlier Sandars and Morrison [4] conducted a survey on first-year medical and psychology students to study their methods of learning. The population goal was students who were born between 1982 and 1991 as they are considered to be constantly exposed to computer-based technology. The "Net Generation" is considered to be the challenge for medical schools and universities. They intended to track down their learning needs and how they should be included in the undergraduate curriculum. The researchers used a questionnaire that included questions about the usefulness of wikis in learning process and the students' familiarity with technologies such as wikis and blogs. The results confirmed the researchers' initial hypotheses as the majority of participants entered the university with adequate experience in online systems and social software and thus positive attitude towards them.

A different research study was conducted by Alonso et al. [14], who utilized Wiki logs to investigate the effectiveness, motivation and social aspects such as the participation, cooperative efforts, and communication. In their study, first-year students participated to and they were asked to use the Wiki in order to create Wiki groups working on a scientific topic. The participated teachers went periodically to groups' wikis and evaluated the students' learning process. After a Wiki article was categorized, the students looked to the category's description to see what it was their error and tried to correct them. Remarkably self-learning was part of this process by the way of auto-evaluation. Two main categories were also used to give a general indicator to students' performance and guided their learning ("Need to improve" and "Good progress"). Finally, the researchers concluded that Wikis facilitate the knowledge sharing and the attainment of necessary – for collaboration – transversal skills.

Harris and Zeng [15] conducted a survey focused on a case study about the use of wikis in an Online Record Documentation Systems Course. In particular, he used a wiki named Confluence in which two collaborative pages for each of the groups (two classes, we will explain below) are created and used by the groups for the group project. The participants were students from two consecutive classes, 2006 and 2007, in a health information management baccalaureate online course. The 2006 class contained 12 groups consisting of 52 students. The 2007 class contained six groups consisting of 30 students. For the research, questionnaire and a last open-ended question were used. The results showed that 44% of the students in 2006 and 50% in 2007 agree Confluence is a tool for facilitating learning; also, half of the participants in both classes agree it is a tool for student activities and for reflective group interaction; one third of them want to see its application in other courses. The conclusions that the researcher make are that the use of wikis could enforce educational procedure and wikis can be considered an effective tool for supporting online teaching.

12.7 Conclusions

Reviewing the above research studies and the results of our comparative study in terms of the studied evaluation variables and the techniques that have been used it is well concluded that Wikis have not been fully researched. Motivation, social aspects and usefulness belong to the most researched variables in terms of the use of Wikis for healthcare/medical purposes and this is reasonable as they are common in nature of Wikis philosophy. The effectiveness of Wikis use is less studied than the above variables and this can be attributed, on the one hand, to the complexity that the effectiveness – as a concept – concerns and, on the other hand, to the measurement difficulty. The latter is obvious in the fifth study [14] in which the researchers utilized the log files (Table 12.1) in order to conclude the effectiveness of Wikis use in higher education.

Table 12.1 The Comparative Synopsis of the Reviewed Studies

Researchers's Study	Population Goal	Evaluation Variables	Evaluation Techniques
1 Boulos et al. (2006)	Higher Education Students	Effectiveness, Motivation, Social aspects	
2 Ebner et al. (2008)	Higher Education Students	Usefulness, Motivation Social Aspects	Pre/Post questionnaire, Semi-standardized Interview
3 Sandars et al. (2008)	Higher Education Students	Usefulness	Questionnaire
4 Sandars and Morrison (2007)	Higher Education Students	Usefulness, Motivation	Questionnaire
5 Alonso et al. (2007)	Higher Education Students	Effectiveness, Motivation, Social Aspects	Log Files Analysis
6 Harris (2008)	Higher Education Students	Usefulness, Social Aspects	Questionnaire

Moreover, reviewing the above studies it seems that most researchers prefer using questionnaires for the studied variables to log files or interviews. Actually, log files are utilized in only one study. Semi-standardized interview is recorded in one study [1], too. This may be attributed to the complexity that quantitative research includes as well as the difficulty (or incompatibility) of log files extraction and utilization.

12.8 Discussion

The upper goal of this study was to review the evaluation variables and techniques that are studied in some of the research studies about the Wikis use for healthcare/medical course purposes. We aimed to reveal those aspects of the research about the Wikis use in healthcare/medical course that need further study in order to fully utilize its potential.

The growing development of social software, in which Wikis belong, has turned our attention to the social aspects of learning and the related learning pedagogy has been enhanced (see constructivism). All grades of education has been dramatically affected by that, but especially higher education still searches for that technology that relates to the related population-goal as well as their needs under the scope of the future citizen.

Wikis, as genuine social software that addresses to self-regulated adults, seem to be the probable answer to that request. In healthcare/medical courses Wikis have been exploited, especially by innovative institutes and research centres, most of which with great success. The relative studies that have been conducted show an interesting impact of Wikis on learning usefulness, motivation and collaboration among the participants. The latter is obvious as Wikis are considered the shared repositories of knowledge. However, researchers have not definitely decided yet their learning effectiveness. Moreover, their integration into higher education curriculum has not shown any best practice. Thus, it is not clear yet why they should be integrated into the learning tools of higher education.

It is worth mentioning that the studied evaluation techniques here could be considered restricted by the existing capabilities of Wikis. On the one hand, in few studies Wikis are referred as an assessment tool. On the other hand, questionnaires are mostly used evaluation techniques. Taken into account that questionnaires have caused many doubts about the objectivity they may ensure, it is justifiable why we do not consider this technique reliable enough to end up that Wikis are proposed for healthcare/medical courses. We propose that further research needs to be carried out to this direction, but evaluation techniques should be enriched. A mixed evaluation study could give a "safe" answer to the question of worthy use of Wikis for higher education courses.

References

1. Boulos MK, Maramba I, Wheeler S. Wikis, blogs and podcasts: a new generation of web-based tools for virtual collaborative clinical practice and education. BMC Med Educ 2006, 6:41, Available at: http://www.biomedcentral.com/content/pdf/1472-6920-6-41.pdf.

2. Elgort I. Using Wikis as a learning tool in higher education. In ICT: Providing choices for learners and learning. Proceedings ASCILITE, Singapore, 2007.
3. Sandars J, Homer M, Pell G, Croker T. Web 2.0 and social software: the medical student way of learning. Med Teach 2008;14:1–5.
4. Sandars J, Morrison C. What is the net generation? The challenge for future medical education. Med Teach 2007;29(2–3):85–88.
5. Chao J. Student project collaboration using Wikis. Proceedings of the 20th Conference on Software Engineering Education and Training (CSEE&T 2007), Dublin, Ireland, July 3–5, 2007.
6. Parker KR, Chao JT. Wiki as a teaching tool. Inter J Knowl Learn Objects 2007;3: 57–72.
7. Olson G. New tools for learning. Retrieved November 2006, Available at: http://faculty.eicc.edu/golson/tools.htm.
8. Honegger BD. Wikis – a rapidly growing phenomenon in the German-speaking school community. Proceedings of the 2005 International Symposium on Wikis, San Diego, CA, USA, October 16–18, 2005;113–116.
9. Bower M, Woo K, Roberts M, Watters PA. Wiki pedagogy – a tale of two wikis. Paper presented at the 7th International Conference on Information Technology Based Higher Education and Training (ITHET' 06), Sydney, Australia, 2006.
10. Choy SO, Ng KC. Implementing wiki software for supplementing online learning. Aust J Educ Technol 2007;23(2):209–226.
11. Ebner M, Kickmeier-Rust M, Holzinger A. Utilizing Wiki-systems in higher education classes: a chance for universal access? Universal Access Inf Soc 2008;7(4): 199–207.
12. Guzdial M, Rick J, Kehoe C. Beyond adoption to invention: teacher-created collaborative activities in higher education. J Learn Sci 2001;10(3):265–279.
13. Raitman R, Augar N, Zhou W. Employing Wikis for online collaboration in the E-learning environment: case study. In Proceedings of the third International Conference on Information Technology and Applications, IEEE Computer Society, July 4th to 7th 2005, Sydney, Australia 2005;142–146.
14. Alonso I, Alcalá F, Fernández BV, Brugos JAL, Wiki use in learning for topography Spanish students. EUROCAST 2007, 2007;423–430.
15. Harris ST, Zeng X. Using Wiki in an online record documentation systems course, Perspect Health Inf Manag 2008;5:1.

Chapter 13
Computer-Based Oxygen Transport Scenario Analysis: A New Web-Based Medical Education Resource

D. John Doyle

Abstract This report describes a simple interactive HTML/JavaScript-based educational resource aimed at educating physiology students, medical students and physicians on the field of oxygen transport physiology. It can be run on almost all personal computers with a web browser that supports JavaScript.

Keywords: Medical computing · oxygen transport modeling · physiological simulation · web-based medical education

13.1 Introduction

Although students of physiology and medicine are exposed to the importance of oxygen at numerous points in their training, the information they receive may sometimes be so abstract that the clinical significance of what they are taught may not be fully understood. As a result, training on this important topic may be suboptimal, with students possessing an incomplete understanding and even frank misconceptions concerning some of the issues regarding oxygen transport physiology.

This report describes a simple interactive HTML/JavaScript-based educational resource aimed at educating physiology students, medical students and physicians on the field of oxygen transport physiology. It can be run on almost all personal computers with a web browser that supports JavaScript.

13.2 What the System Does

The system allows individuals to look at changes in oxygen transport parameters (e.g., arterial oxygen tension, arterial oxygen saturation, etc.) as a result of choices of parameters such as cardiac output and hemoglobin concentration.

D.J. Doyle (✉)
Professor of Anesthesiology, Cleveland Clinic Lerner College of Medicine of Case Western Reserve University, Staff Anesthesiologist, Department of General Anesthesiology, Cleveland Clinic Foundation, 9500 Euclid Avenue, E31 Cleveland, OH 44195, USA
e-mail: doylej@ccf.org

A. Lazakidou (ed.), *Web-Based Applications in Healthcare and Biomedicine*, Annals of Information Systems 7, DOI 10.1007/978-1-4419-1274-9_13,

© Springer Science+Business Media, LLC 2010

Table 13.1 Input Parameters

PAO_2 (mmHg)	Alveolar oxygen tension
Shunt (fraction)	Qs/Qt expressed as a fraction
Hb (g/dL)	Hemoglobin concentration
VO_2 (mL/min)	Oxygen consumption rate
CO (L/min)	Cardiac output
P_{50} (mmHg)	Oxygen tension for 50% saturation

Table 13.2 Output Parameters

PaO_2 (mmHg)	Arterial oxygen tension
SaO_2 (fraction)	Arterial oxygen saturation
CaO_2 (vol%)	Arterial oxygen content
PvO_2 (mmHg)	Mixed venous oxygen tension
SvO_2 (fraction)	Mixed venous oxygen saturation
CvO_2 (vol%)	Mixed venous oxygen content

That is, based in the inputs listed in Table 13.1, the system computes the outputs listed in Table 13.2.

13.3 System Objectives

Based on a review of the literature and discussions with colleagues and students (see the Needs Analysis presented in Appendix 13.2), the following objectives were established for the project.

13.3.1 Objective 1

Provide brief information for medical students and residents on various aspects of oxygen transport:

- Oxyhemoglobin dissociation curve
- Oxygen attached to hemoglobin
- Oxygen dissolved in plasma
- Oxygen content equation
- Pulmonary shunt equation
- Oxygen transport equation

13.3.2 Objective 2

Provide students with an understanding of the importance of the following oxygen transport parameters in influencing tissue oxygenation:

- Alveolar oxygen tension
- Shunt fraction

- Hemoglobin concentration
- Oxygen consumption rate
- Cardiac output
- Oxygen tension for 50% saturation (P_{50})

13.3.3 Objective 3

Develop an interactive mathematical model of oxygen transport that medical students and residents can use to ask “what if” questions concerning oxygen transport physiology. This model would incorporate a Computational Engine based on JavaScript that would run on recent vintages of Microsoft Internet Explorer, with parameters entered using the “form” capabilities of HTML. This was to be the *primary objective* of the project, since excellent resources already exist to allow students to meet Objectives 1 and 2 above. It was also turned out to be the most difficult and most technical aspect of the project, as it required skill in JavaScript programming.

13.4 Using the System

One starts the system by double-clicking on the main file called *Index.htm*. Upon doing this one’s web browser will be launched and an image similar to that shown in Fig. 13.1 appears on the screen, with a menu with six self-explanatory options.

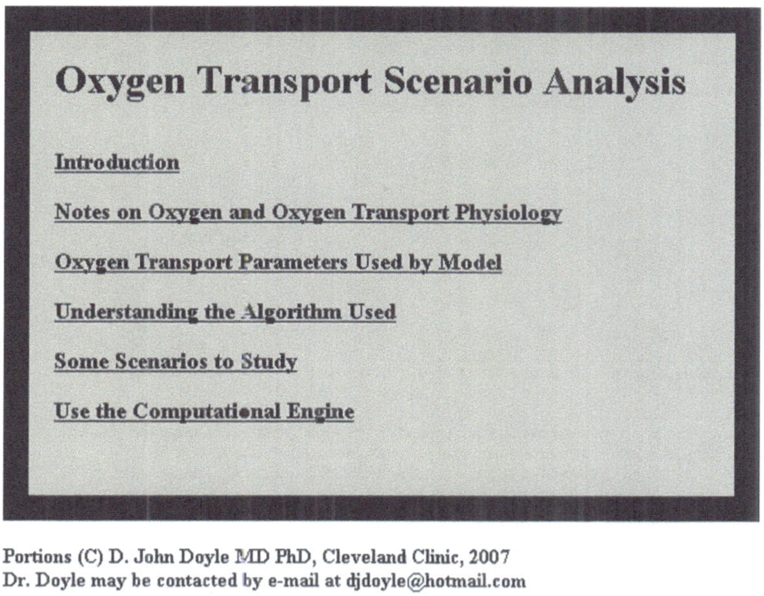

Fig. 13.1 The opening menu

To use the system one then merely clicks on the menu option desired. The last option (Use the Computational Engine) is the main selection; every other selection is merely supportive to this.

When the Computational Engine is run, the warning shown in Fig. 13.2 may appear, depending on the security options selected in your web browser settings. This warning appears because of the use of JavaScript in the system. Select *Yes* to proceed. The screen similar to that shown in Fig. 13.3 then appears. Then enter some sample data (Fig. 13.4) and click on the "COMPUTE" button (Fig. 13.5).

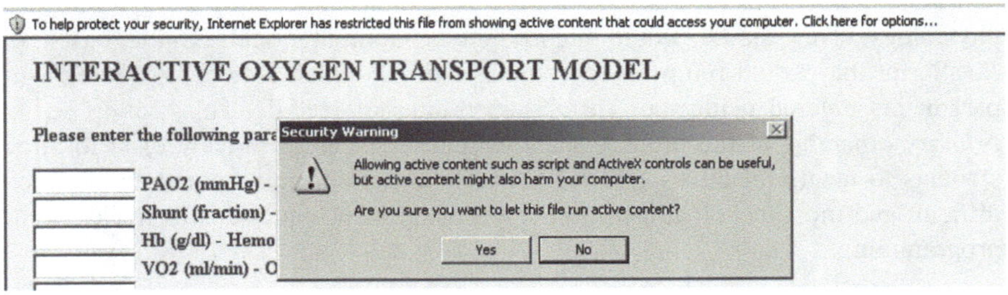

Fig. 13.2 A popup security warning may occur when the program is launched. Click for options where indicated, then select *Yes* to proceed. The result will be something similar to Fig. 13.3

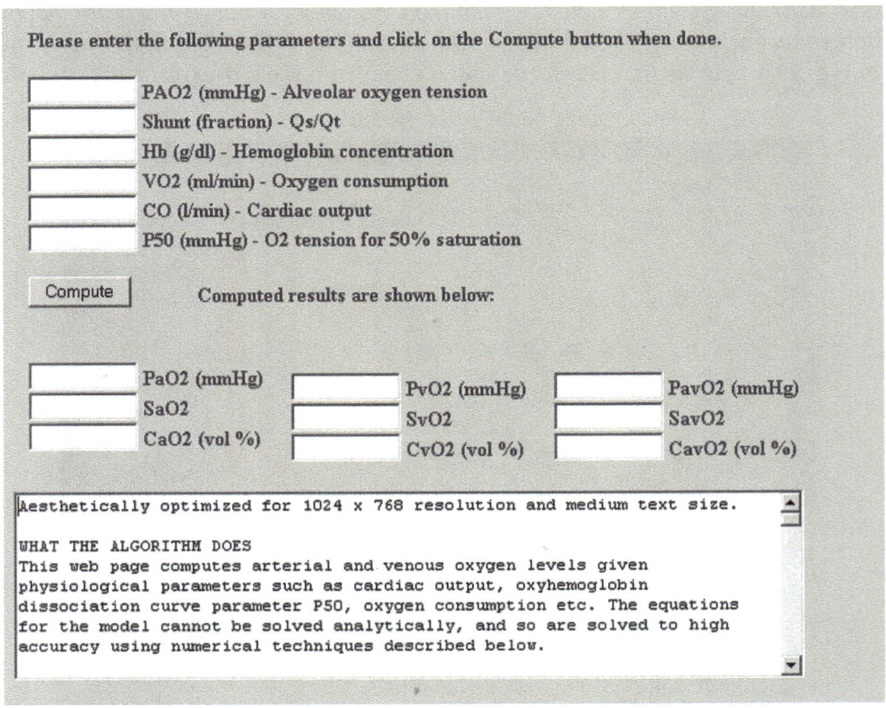

Fig. 13.3 The system is now ready to accept data. Note also the scrolling text box that explains how the algorithm works

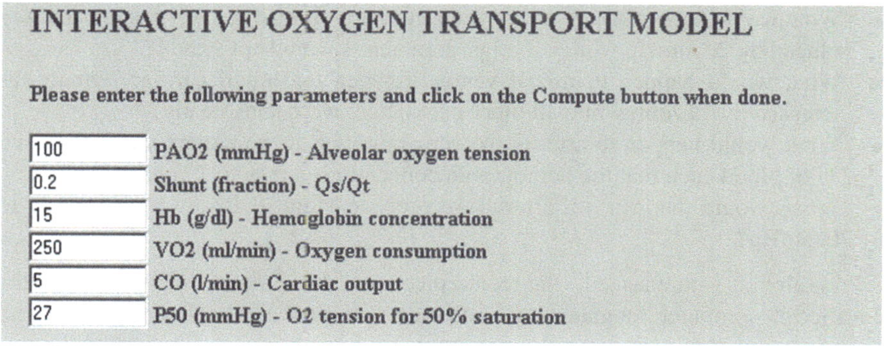

Fig. 13.4 Sample data entered. The calculated results are shown in Fig. 13.5

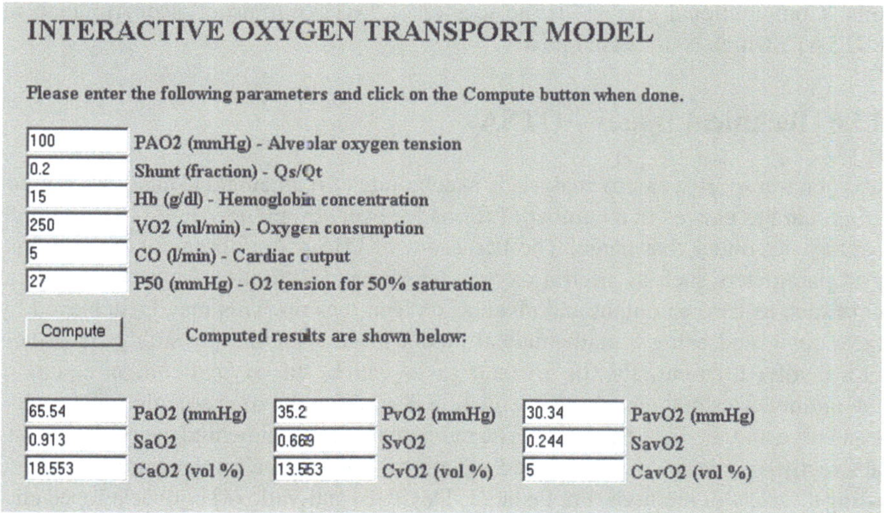

Fig 13.5 After the "COMPUTE" button is clicked, the computed results are displayed

13.5 Discussion

The project involves two main components: (1) a number of didactic small elements on the physiology of oxygen transport suitable for use in medical education (meeting Objectives 1 and 2) and (2) an interactive mathematical module of oxygen transport physiology that could be used to ask "what if" physiological questions (meeting Objective 3).

The "what if" physiological questions concerning oxygen transport physiology would be questions of the following form:

- "What would happen to arterial oxygen tension if cardiac output was reduced by 50% while all other parameters were kept steady?"

- "What would happen to arterial oxygen saturation if inspired oxygen tension was reduced by 20 mmHg while all other parameters were kept steady?"
- "What would happen to mixed venous oxygen tension if cardiac output was increased by 1 L/min while all other parameters were kept steady?"
- "What would happen to arterial oxygen saturation if the patient was transfused 2 U of blood such that the hemoglobin concentration rose to 12 g/dL?"
- "What would happen to arterial oxygen tension if P_{50} were lowered to 20 mmHg?"

As already emphasized, the centerpiece of the project involves uses the JavaScript computer language to implement the mathematical model involved. And as noted above, in using the system, users ask physiological "what if" questions by entering physiological parameters such as cardiac output or hemoglobin concentrations to obtain computed parameters such as arterial oxygen. Central to this "Computational Engine" is the science of "oxygen transport scenario analysis (OTSA)", which is discussed next.

13.6 Technical Issues – OTSA

Oxygen transport scenario analysis is a technique of mathematical analysis or modeling that has existed in a number of forms for over several decades [1–4], although usually not under that name. The basic aim of OTSA is to predict oxygen transport parameters such as arterial oxygen tension and saturation from physiological data such as cardiac output and alveolar oxygen tension. This may be achieved by developing and using a mathematical model to describe the physiological principles involved (essentially, the alveolar gas equation, the oxygen content equation, the pulmonary shunt equation, an equation describing the oxyhemoglobin dissociation curve and the Fick equation). The mathematical model behind everything exists abstractly as a series of interrelated equations, but may be implemented or solved using a variety of methods. For instance, Doyle [3] and Vaile [4] both developed custom software for their OTSA model, while earlier investigators resorted to algebraic and graphical techniques to solve the equation set without computer programming. In most cases the software involved has not been made widely available for a number of reasons, such as the need for the person who runs the software to know how to edit the software as the scenario parameters are changed, and the lack of simple means of distributing the software (such as the Internet).

Basically, the Computational Engine is a JavaScript-powered web page that computes arterial and venous oxygen levels from a set of physiological parameters such as cardiac output, oxyhemoglobin dissociation curve parameter P_{50}, oxygen consumption. In essence, system uses the parameters in Table 13.1 to calculate the oxygenation parameters in Table 13.2.

The equations involved in the model are nontrivial, even difficult, and cannot be solved analytically. Rather, they must be solved to high numerical accuracy using special heuristic techniques. The details by which the applicable equations can be solved are a complex technical issue that is discussed next.

13.7 Understanding the Equations

We now present the mathematical basis for the computational process that must be understood for the implementation of the "Computational Engine" section of the project in JavaScript.

The pulmonary shunt equation is used as a foundation upon which arterial oxygenation and gas exchange indices can be studied. It may be expressed as:

$$\frac{Qs}{Qt} = \frac{Cc'O_2 - CaO_2}{Cc'O_2 - CvO_2}, \tag{1}$$

where

$Cc'O_2$=end-pulmonary capillary oxygen content,

CaO_2=arterial oxygen content,

CvO_2=mixed venous oxygen content,

and where the CxO_2 terms above are defined by the *oxygen content equation:*

$$CxO_2 = 1.34 \times HbSxO_2 + 0.0031 \times PxO_2,$$

where x is one of a, v or c′ and where Hb is the blood hemoglobin concentration.

Specifically, this gives us the following full set of equations for oxygen content in the arterial, venous and end-pulmonary capillary settings:

$$Cc'O_2 = 1.34 \times HbSc'O_2 + 0.0031 \times Pc'O_2,$$

$$CaO_2 = 1.34 \times HbSaO_2 + 0.0031 \times PaO_2,$$

$$CvO_2 = 1.34 \times HbSvO_2 + 0.0031 \times PvO_2,$$

where

SxO_2 is the blood oxygen saturation,

PxO_2 is the blood oxygen tension,

and where x is one of a, v or c′.

We next direct our attention to the shunt equation. By algebraic manipulation of the shunt equation, it is possible to relate arterial oxygen tension to its influencing factors:

$$PaO_2 = PAO_2 - \left[Ca - vO_2 \times \frac{(Qs/Qt)}{(1 - Qs/Qt)} - 1.34 \times (Sc'O_2 - SaO_2) \times Hb\right] / 0.0031, \tag{2}$$

where Qs/Qt is the shunt fraction, PAO_2 (units of mmHg) is the alveolar oxygen tension, $Ca\text{-}vO_2$ (units of vol%) is the arterial/mixed-venous oxygen content difference $(Ca\text{-}vO_2 = CaO_2 - CvO_2)$, $Sc'O_2$ is the end-pulmonary capillary fractional saturation, SaO_2 is the arterial saturation and Hb is the blood hemoglobin concentration (units of g/dL).

The alveolar gas equation is next used to determine PAO_2:

$$PAO_2 = (PB - PH_2O) \times FIO_2 - PaCO_2 \left[FIO_2 + \frac{(1 - FIO_2)}{R} \right], \tag{3}$$

where PB is the barometric pressure (assumed to be 760 mmHg), PH_2O is the patient's water vapor pressure (assumed to be 47 mmHg), $PaCO_2$ is the arterial CO_2 tension (usually assumed to be 40 mmHg), FIO_2 is the fraction of inspired oxygen, and R is the gas exchange ratio (usually assumed to be 0.8).

Note that Equation (2) does not explicitly show the influence of the parameter P_{50} on arterial oxygen tension; such influences are mediated indirectly, principally through the SaO_2 term. To make explicit the influence of PaO_2 and P_{50} on SaO_2, we use the relationship given by Hill:

$$SaO_2 = \frac{PaO_2^n}{PaO_2^n + P_{50}^n}, \tag{4}$$

where n is an empirical constant (generally taken as 2.65). A similar expression relates PAO_2, P_{50}, and $Sc'O_2$.

The arterial oxygen tension as well as the alveolar/arterial oxygen tension difference and the arterial/alveolar oxygen tension ratio can then be obtained using Equations (2)–(4) for specific choices of physiological variables. Unfortunately, Equation (2) is not easily solved because it requires the solution of two simultaneous nonlinear equations [i.e., Equations (2) and (4)].

To solve these equations, an inelegant but effective brute-force computational strategy was employed, although more advanced computational methods based on successive approximation methods might be more appealing to those more skilled than I in the art and science of numerical analysis.

13.8 Sample Clinical Scenarios

13.8.1 Case 1

Mr. Jones has severe adult respiratory distress syndrome (ARDS), with a parameter set with respect to Table 13.1 of 600, 0.45, 10, 200, 5, and 27, and for which he gets a resulting arterial oxygen tension of 57 mmHg. Consideration is given to increasing his hemoglobin concentration to 15 from 10 by transfusion. All else being equal, how much would this improve his oxygenation?

13.8.2 Case 2

Repeat Case 1 under the assumption that as a result of the heart doing more work to take care of the additional blood transfused, the patient's oxygen consumption goes up by 100–300 mL/min.

13.8.3 Case 3

Repeat Case 1, except instead of transfusing blood consider an infusion of dopamine (an inotrope) to increase cardiac output to 7 L/min. Assume that as a result of the increased cardiac effort the patient's oxygen consumption goes up by 100–300 mL/min. What would be the net effect on oxygenation?

13.8.4 Case 4

Mr. Smith, a smoker, wants to know what kind of oxygen levels he could expect at high altitude. His current parameter set is 100, 0.1, 15, 250, 5, and 27, for which his arterial oxygen tension is 79 mmHg. What would be the expected oxygen tension, all else being equal, if the alveolar arterial tension fell to 50 mmHg during a mountain ascent?

13.8.5 Case 5

Repeat Case 4 under the additional assumption that, as a result of altitude acclimatization, the oxyhemoglobin dissociation curve shifts to the left, resulting in a P_{50} of 19 mmHg.

13.8.6 Case 6

Mr. Wong has severe sepsis syndrome, with a parameter set of 600, 0.4, 12, 250, 3.5, and 27, and for which he gets an arterial oxygen tension of 47 mmHg. Consideration is given to doubling his cardiac output to with hemodynamic tuning. All else being equal, how much would this improve his oxygenation?

13.8.7 Case 7

Repeat Case 6, assuming that as a result of the increased cardiac effort the patient's oxygen consumption goes up by 100–350 mL/min. What then would be the net effect on oxygenation?

13.8.8 Case 8

Dr. Price, an altitude physiologist, wants to know what kind of oxygen levels he could expect at high altitude if he could shift his oxyhemoglobin dissociation curve to the right to a P_{50} of 35 mmHg. His current parameter set is 100, 0.1, 15, 250, 5 and 27, for which his arterial oxygen tension is 79 mmHg. What would be the expected oxygen tension, all else being equal, if the alveolar arterial tension fell to 50 mmHg during a mountain ascent? Do the calculation for both P_{50} values to find the best one in this setting.

Appendix 1 – Algorithm Details

What the Algorithm Does

This algorithm computes arterial and venous oxygen levels given physiological parameters such as cardiac output, oxyhemoglobin dissociation curve parameter P_{50}, oxygen consumption. The equations for the model cannot be solved analytically, and so are solved to high numerical accuracy using numerical techniques described below.

Parameters Needed

PAO_2 (mmHg)
  Alveolar oxygen tension
  Normal is about 100 on room air
Shunt (fraction)
  Qs/Qt expressed as a fraction
  Normal is 0.1 or less
Hb (g/dL)
  Hemoglobin concentration
  Normal is 12 to 16
VO_2 (mL/min)
  Oxygen consumption rate
  Normal is 150 to 500 or more
CO (L/min)
  Cardiac output
  Normal is 3 to 10 or more
P_{50} (mmHg)
  Oxygen tension for 50% saturation
  Normal adults have a P_{50} of 27

Parameters Calculated

PaO_2 (mmHg)
  Arterial oxygen tension
SaO_2 (fraction)
  Arterial oxygen saturation
CaO_2 (vol%)
  Arterial oxygen content
PvO_2 (mmHg)
  Mixed Venous oxygen tension
SvO_2 (fraction)
  Mixed Venous oxygen saturation
CvO_2 (vol%)
  Mixed Venous oxygen content

Algorithm Variables and Pseudocode for Arterial Oxygenation Calculations

For algorithm details, see [3].

Variables for Arterial Oxygenation Calculations

N is the iteration counter
Minimum is initially set to any very large number
PSTART is the starting trial oxygen tension
P is the trial oxygen tension
PSTEP is the step size between iterations
PAO_2 is the alveolar oxygen tension
PA is P^2.65
P_{50}A is P_{50}^2.65
CO is cardiac output
CAV is the arteriovenous oxygen content difference
CAV = VO_2/(10 * CO)
Z is the shunt fraction (*Qs*/*Qt*)
S is the trial oxygen saturation
PO_2 is the best estimate of the arterial oxygen tension so far
SO_2 is the best estimate of the arterial oxygen saturation so far
PO_2 is the best estimate of the arterial oxygen content so far

Pseudocode for Arterial Oxygenation Calculations

```
Starting with a low value of P and working your way
up, find the value of P that best matches the equations
involved in a minimum error sense.
BEGIN
Minimum = any large number
for (N = 0; N < 10000001; N++)
  {P = PSTART + N* PSTEP ;
  if (P > PAO2) {break ; //go to the end and print out
PO2, SO2 and CO2}
  PA = P ^2.65 ; S = PA/(PA + P50A) ;
  PP = PAO2 - (CAV * (Z/(1-Z)) - 1.34 * HB * (SCO2 - S))/
0.0031
  Error = absolute value of (P - PP) ;
  if (Error < Minimum)
    {Minimum = Error ;
    PO2 = P ; SO2 = S ;
    CO2 = 1.34 * HB * S + 0.0031 * P ;
    }
  }
END
```

Pseudocode for Venous Oxygenation Calculations

```
Venous calculations are done after the arterial
calculations.
Thus,
PO2 is known (arterial oxygen tension)
SO2 is known (arterial oxygen saturation)
CO2 is known (arterial oxygen content)
PVO2 is to be determined
SVO2 is to be determined
BEGIN
CVO2 = CO2 - CAV
Minimum = any large number
for (N = 0; N < 10000001; N++)
  {P = PSTART + N * PSTEP ;
  if (P > PO2) {break ; //go to the end and print out
PVO2, SVO2 and CVO2}
  PVA = P^2 .65 ; SV = PVA/(PVA + P50A) ;
  CVO2CALC = 1.34 * HB * SV + P*0.0031
  Error = absolute value of (CVO2 - CVO2CALC) ;
```

```
  if (Error < Minimum)
    {Minimum = Error ;
    PVO2 = P ; SVO2 = SV ;
    }
  }
END
```

Appendix 2 – Needs Analysis

As a faculty member for over 20 years, first at the University of Toronto and now at Case Western Reserve University, the author has had frequent occasion to work with medical students, interns and residents in a didactic capacity. Usually, this is in the context of informal one-on-one teaching sessions in the Operating Room or in the Intensive Care Unit, both settings where disturbances of patient oxygenation can have catastrophic consequences. As a result, issues related to oxygen transport physiology are frequent didactic topics in these settings.

As a result of this experience in clinical teaching, it eventually become apparent that the current methods of teaching the principles of oxygen transport do not always confer a satisfactory degree of understanding, and the notion that students might better come to understand the oxygen transport physiology if they had some sort of interactive computer model to use was entertained. Such a model would allow students to explore the effects of clinical interventions such as changing oxygen concentrations or transfusing blood without putting patients at risk. This was the first indication for a need for the proposed initiative.

With time the author had the opportunity to discuss with a number of colleagues the potential value of an interactive computer model to teach oxygen transport physiology. These colleagues agreed that such a tool could be valuable, not only for medical education but possibly also as an aid to clinical decision-making. Their discussions confirmed that there was a need for the proposed initiative, but they also pointed out that the project might be far from straightforward.

Another source of insight concerning the need for the proposed initiative was from informal discussions with medical students and residents, who almost universally agreed that such a resources could be a valuable teaching tool if it were (1) easy to use, (2) easy to access and (3) inexpensive or free.

Encouraged by these developments, a Medline search of the medical literature from 1966 to 2006 was conducted to see if anyone had written about the problems of teaching oxygen transport physiology and what solutions might be considered. Unfortunately, while there was much material found concerning clinical trials and other matters related to oxygen transport physiology, there was nothing to be found specifically dealing with the challenges of teaching this topic.

Based on this informal (but nonetheless helpful) needs assessment, I set about to establish the objectives for this project. Once again, this process proceeded informally based upon conversations with colleagues and students and with reference to standard textbooks of physiology and critical care medicine. The result of this process is the present project.

References

1. Torda TA. Alveolar-arterial oxygen tension difference: A critical look, Anaesth Intens Care 1981;9:326–330.
2. Schnider AJ, Stockman JA, Oski FA. Transfusion nomogram: An application of physiology to clinical decisions regarding the use of blood. Crit Care Med 1981;9:469–473.
3. Doyle DJ. Arterial/alveolar oxygen tension ratio: A critical appraisal. Can Anaesth Soc J 1986;33:471–474.
4. Vaile JP, Carlisle CJ, Annat G, Rousselet B, Motin J. Arterial-alveolar oxygen partial pressure ratios: A theoretical reappraisal. Crit Care Med 1986;14:153–154.

Chapter 14
Development of an Educational Web Site to Assist in Learning Clinical Airway Management

D. John Doyle

Abstract This report describes the planning, implementation, trials, and tribulations in an ultimately successfully effort to develop and launch a web-based medical education resource dealing with clinical airway management. The resource, aimed primarily at medical students, can be accessed online at www.airwayeducation.net.

Keywords: Clinical airway management · educational web pages · medical education

14.1 Introduction

Clinical airway management is one of the cornerstones of acute care medicine and as such is important to emergency room physicians, anesthesiologists, paramedics, and many other healthcare providers. In recent years, there has been a virtual explosion of new information in the field of clinical airway management, with new algorithms, new technologies, and new procedures being described in the medical literature or promoted by medical societies. This enormous growth in information, however, has lead to problems in making this information available to clinical practitioners in a form that is useful to them.

Fortunately, because of the web, access to medical information resources throughout the world has never been greater or easier. There is thus an ongoing need for making new information available thus via the web. The project was undertaken to address this challenge, focusing particularly on the needs of medical students and starting residents in learning the fundamentals of clinical airway management. The result was an airway education web site that can be accessed online at http://airwayeducation.net. From the onset of the project, the primary goal was

D.J. Doyle (✉)
Professor of Anesthesiology, Cleveland Clinic Lerner College of Medicine of Case Western Reserve University, Staff Anesthesiologist, Department of General Anesthesiology, Cleveland Clinic Foundation, 9500 Euclid Avenue, Cleveland, OH 44195, USA
e-mail: doylej@ccf.org

A. Lazakidou (ed.), *Web-Based Applications in Healthcare and Biomedicine*, Annals of Information Systems 7, DOI 10.1007/978-1-4419-1274-9_14,
© Springer Science+Business Media, LLC 2010

to provide information in a format that would be clear, succinct, and definitive, and offering generous use of graphical illustrations and summary tables.

14.2 Beginnings

The start of the project began several years ago with a perception that there was a need for a readily accessible high-quality web-based resource on clinical airway management aimed at medical students and junior residents. This issue arose on a number of occasions at the annual meetings of the Board of Directors of the Society for Airway Management, where it was repeatedly suggested that, of the various methods of education available, the use of the web offered special promise in terms of wide accessibility and low cost, especially compared to more traditional methods of medical student and physician education such as didactic lectures, maintaining a speakers bureau, producing educational videos for distribution as DVDs or video cassettes, or producing and distributing glossy brochures.

A number of formal needs assessment survey instruments were considered for the project (e.g., surveying people at medical conferences, using a postal survey, using an Internet-based survey). However, although the technology associated with conducting such a survey may be easier than ever (especially with the advent of web-based survey systems such as www.surveymonkey.com), regulatory barriers were identified that were potentially problematic, such as the need for formal institutional approval by an ethics committee, with its associated bureaucracy.

As a result, it was decided to rely solely on informal methods for conducting the needs analysis, such as conducting a Medline search of the medical literature, conducting informal discussion with colleagues, residents, and medical students, as well as conducting informal discussion with nationally recognized exports. This process occurred over a 2- to 3-year period as the author met informally at conferences with individuals interested in clinical airway management or had contact with medical students and residents in the course of teaching.

14.3 Methods

For some time there has been an interest in the medical community in using web-based methods for medical education. Web pages are a particularly useful means of providing information of almost any kind. They are easily accessed and relatively easily updated. Linkages to other documents are easily provided, and support for tables, graphics, and even multimedia features like audio and video can be built in without enormous training and expertise. While my early efforts in web page development were relatively primitive undertakings based on hand-coding in the HTML language, I soon found myself exploring a variety of software packages to make the task easier. Over time I tried out and mastered Netscape Composer, Microsoft FrontPage, Net Objects Fusion and several other less known packages available as shareware. Later, when I tried out Macromedia Dreamweaver, it eventually became apparent that the richness and complexity of the latest professional packages were unsuitable for dilettantes like me – their steep learning curve left me focusing more on the software than on the content I wanted to show to the world. In due course I came to learn and love a less well-known web page development system known as Homestead (www.homestead.com). It is reasonably powerful, yet is particularly easy to use. As a result I ended up using it for this project.

From the onset of the project, consideration was given to the use of appropriate design principles for the web page construction, so as to avoid a garish result. In this respect I particularly took guidance for a marvelous but dated book by Flanders and Willis entitled "*Web Pages That Suck: Learn Good Design by Looking at Bad Design*" (1998).

A substantial amount of time was devoted to content development: writing paragraphs and figure legends, finding images suitable to illustrate a teaching point, finding external web resources to link to, etc. To a substantial degree I was able to rely on content developed earlier, but with modifications to make the islands of material more self-contained and better illustrated. A good deal of time was also spent searching for images that would best compliment the text in each island of material. This task was greatly simplified by the availability of a number of images search engines. All of the clinical images used in the project were tagged with an image credit line giving the address where the image was obtained.

14.4 Practical Issues

Some of the theoretical issues concerned with web site development were discussed earlier. I would now like to comment on some of the practical issues encountered. My original plan was to develop a series of "learning objects" and then use them to construct a number of "islands" of information in web page format. This initiative thus began by using Microsoft Word to produce a series of text-only stand-alone documents that would form learning objects on their own. When complete, these Microsoft Word files were then made into pure ASCII text files to form a similar series of stand-alone learning objects in pure text format.

Once the text material was completed, attention was directed at establishing a series of graphic images that could both stand on their own or be incorporated into a composite learning object in conjunction with one of the text-only learning objects described above. In either case, associated with each graphic image would ordinarily be a both a figure legend to help explain the meaning of the image as well as an "image credit" explaining where the image came from.

A third type of learning object entity, hypertext links to external materials, was also collected with a view to incorporating them into the various web pages. This external material consisted mostly of scientific review articles in PDF format as well as some educational videos.

With this material at hand, construction of the various web pages comprising the site began. Although Homestead offers a number of template pages that can be used

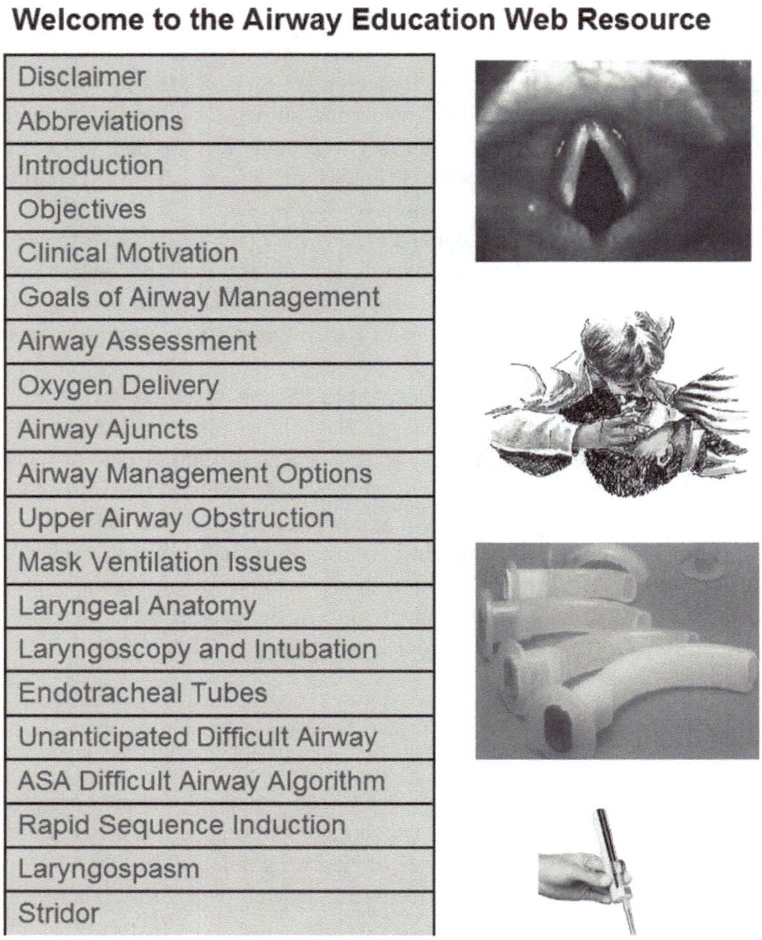

Fig. 14.1 Partial screen capture of the main menu for the project web site

to produce a consistent "look and feel" across a site, I found none that appealed to my conservative and minimalist tastes, and I eventually decided to start each web page "from scratch", relying on a simple brownish yellow background (color #F4CE53) for each pages backdrop. To this background was added text material from one of the pure text learning objects developed earlier, as well as zero or more graphic images with their associated figure legends (Figs. 14.1 and 14.2).

Following the importation of these learning objects, in order to produce an aesthetically pleasing result, it was necessary to format each web page using Homestead's various controls. Not infrequently, this was followed by an inevitable compulsion to re-edit the text component, now making it slightly different from the original learning object from which the text was based. This, of course, resulted in a lack of direct correspondence between the web page and the learning objects upon

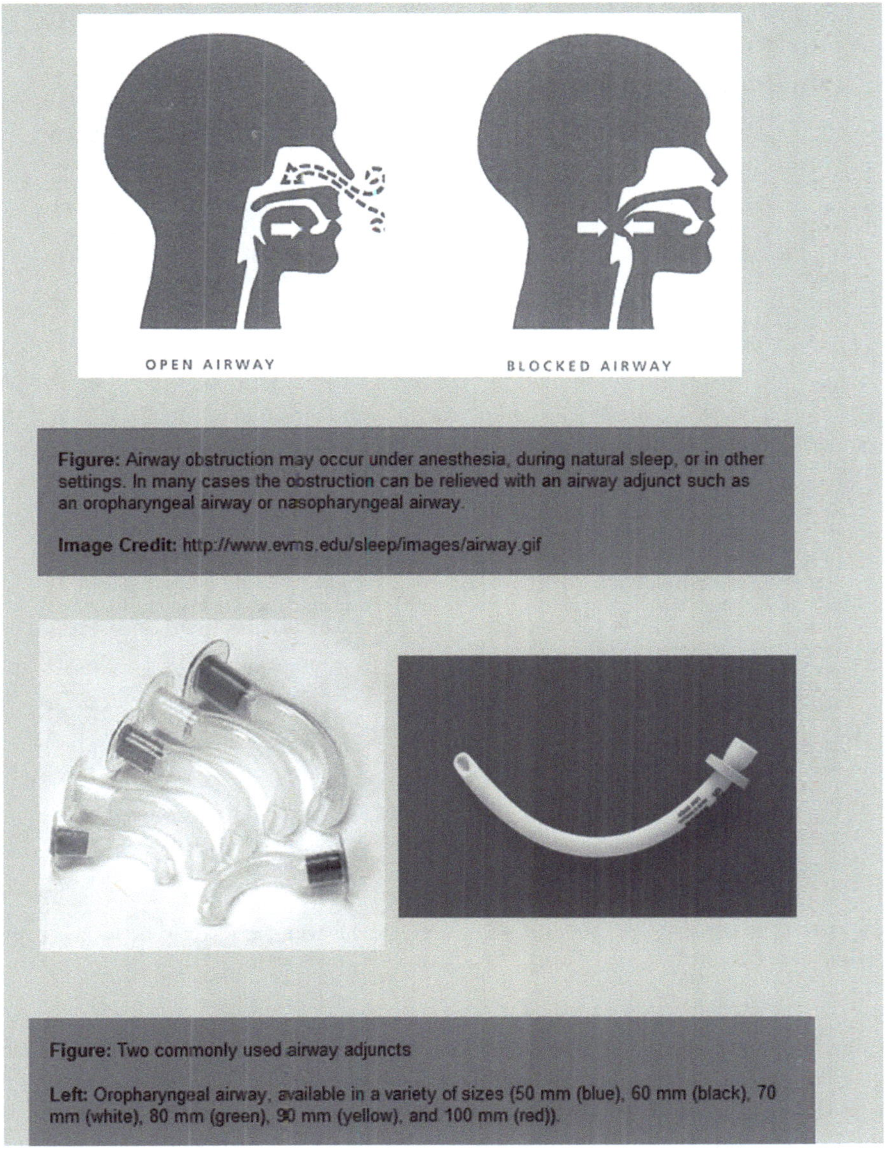

Fig. 14.2 Screen capture of one of the islands of information from the project web site

which it was originally based, with the result that all of the learning objects had to then be reconstructed to reflect the further editing that all writers are by nature drawn to (Fig. 14.3).

At one point I thought that might be a good idea to "polish" the source code produced by the Homestead software system with a view to improving upon it. This

Clinical Case 1

A Newspaper Clipping Tells it All

A newspaper clipping tells the tragic story (Montreal Gazette Feb. 1994): "The death of a woman during childbirth at LaSalle General Hospital could have been avoided if doctors had checked her respiratory tract before anesthetizing her for a caesarean birth, a coroner says." According to the coroner "the woman died of asphyxiation and heart failure during surgery because doctor hadn't checked to see whether she would be able to breathe while unconscious". According to the newspaper account, the patient had a rare condition where the back of her tongue covered "nearly all her throat" and noted that the patient "was unable to breathe through the face mask" applied to her face. After the doctors "tried several times to give her oxygen through tubes" (but failed because they were all too large), a surgical airway was attempted, but cardiac arrest occurred before the airway could be secured, and the patient died.

Discussion

Hypertrophy of the lingual tonsils is an unusual condition that may cause complications such as airway obstruction, abscess, sleep apnea, and recurrent epiglottitis. While some lesions are visible at the bedside (e.g. while checking the Mallampati classification of the patient's oropharynx), many others may not be visible at all without special tools generally used only by ENT specialists. In this respect, the coroner may have been unfair in his judgment. A similar tragedy involving a 24-year-old woman whose markedly hypertrophied lingual tonsils prevented intubation after anesthetic relaxation during preparation for appendectomy has been reported by Cohle et al (1993). The huge hypertropic tonsils totally obstructed the glottic aperture after induction, resulting in a "can't intubate/can't ventilate situation". A recent review of the literature has been published by Ovassapian et al. (2002).

References

Cohle SD, Jones DH, Puri S. Lingual tonsillar hypertrophy causing failed intubation and cerebral anoxia. Am J Forensic Med Pathol 1993 14:158-61

Ovassapian A, Glassenberg R, Randel GI, Klock A, Mesnick PS, Klafta JM. The unexpected difficult airway and lingual tonsil hyperplasia: a case series and a review of the literature. Anesthesiology. 2002;97:124-32.

Fig. 14.3 The web page for Clinical Case 1. Compare this with the source code for this page, shown in the next figure

turned out to be a bad idea. It turns out that the source code produced by Homestead is not optimized to allow human optimization, as the sample code shown in Fig. 14.4 (the source code for Case 1) illustrates. Furthermore, if the Homestead system is used a further time to make further changes to the web page in question, any hand editing will be lost anyway. As a result, my attempts to "hand polish" the source code ended up being rather short-lived.

Another issue with Homestead that presented some difficulty was in attempting to produce a version of the project to run on a CD-ROM or USB flash drive. Thus far, attempts to use the **File – Save As** command in Internet Explorer to save the web site onto a local drive have resulted in fatal errors. However, a number of "work arounds" may still be available, such as downloading the materials using Firefox or another web browser, or using a utility such as

```
<!DOCTYPE HTML PUBLIC "-//W3C//DTD HTML 4.01 Transitional//EN">
<html>
        <head>
                <!-- <hs:metatags> -->
                <meta http-equiv="Content-Type" content="text/html; charset=ISO-8859-1">
                <meta name="generator" content="Homestead SiteBuilder">
                <!-- </hs:metatags> -->

                <!-- <hs:title> -->
                <title>Case1</title>
                <!-- </hs:title> -->
                <script type="text/javascript">
                        <!--
                                                function reDo() {
                                                    top.location.reload();
                                                }
                                                if (navigator.appName == 'Netscape' && parseInt(navigator.appVersion) <
5) {
                                                    top.onresize = reDo;
                                                }
                                                dom=document.getElementById
                                        //-->
                </script>
                <link type="text/css" href="http://www.homestead.com/~media/elements/Text/font_styles_ns4.css" rel="stylesheet">
                <style type="text/css">
                        @import url(http://www.homestead.com/~media/elements/Text/font_styles.css);
                </style>

        </head>
        <body onunload="" onload="" id="element1" link="#3333CC" bgcolor="#FFFFFF" scroll="auto" vlink="#6633CC">
                <noscript>
                        <img alt="" src="http://www.homestead.com/~media/elements/shared/javascript_disabled.gif" height="40" border="0"
width="373">
                </noscript>
                <!-- <hs:element2> -->
                <div style="position: absolute; top: 32px; left: 30px; width: 589px; height: 609px; z-index: 0;" id="element2"><div style="height:
609px; padding: 15; border-width: 0; border-color: #000000; border-s tyle: solid; background-color: #F4CE53;"><div><font face="Helvetica, Arial, sans-serif"
class="size10 Helvetica10" color="#000000"><b>Clinical Case 1</b ><br></font></div><div><font face="Helvetica, Arial, sans-serif" class="size10
Helvetica10" color="#000000"><br></font></div><div><font face="Helvetica, Arial, sans-serif" class="size12 Helvetica12" color="#000000"><b>A Newspaper
Clipping Tells it All   </b><br></font></div><div><font face="Helvetica, Arial, sans-serif" class="size10 Helvetica10"
color="#000000"><br></font></div><div><font face="Helvetica, Arial, sans-serif" class="size10 Helvetica10" color="#000000">A newspaper clipping tells the
tragic story (Montreal Gazette Feb. 1994): &#8220;The death of a woman during childbirth at LaSalle General Hospital could have   been avoided if doctors
had checked her respiratory tract before anesthetizing her for a  caesarean birth, a coroner says.&#8221; According to the coroner &#8220;the woman died of
asphyxiation and heart failure during surgery because doctor hadn&#8217;t checked to see whether she would be able to breathe w  hile
unconscious&#8221;. According to the newspaper account, the patient had a rare condition where the back of her tongue covered & #8220;nearly all her
throat&#8221; and noted that the patient &#8220;was unable to breathe through the face mask&#8221; applied to her face. After t he doctors &#8220;tried
several times to give her oxygen through tubes&#8221; (but failed because they were all too large), a surgical airway was attempted, but cardiac arrest
occurred before the airway could be secured, and the patient died. <br></font></div><div><font face="Helvetica, Arial, sans-serif" class="size10 Helvetica10"
color="#000000"><br></font></div><div><font face="Helvetica, Arial, sans-serif" class="size10 Helvetica10" color="#000000"><b>Discussion 
</b><br></font></div><div><font face="Helvetica, Arial, sans-serif" class="size10 Helvetica10" color="#000000"><br></font></div><div><font
face="Helvetica, Arial, sans-serif" class="size10 Helvetica10" color="#000000">Hypertrophy of the lingual tonsils is an unusual condition that may cause
complications such as airway obstruction, abscess, sleep apnea, and recurrent epiglottitis. While some lesions are visible at t he bedside (e.g. while checking
the Mallampati classification of the patient&#8217;s oropharynx), many others may not be visible at all without special tools g enerally used only by ENT
specialists. In this respect, the coroner may have been unfair in his judgment. A similar tragedy involving a 24-year-old woman whose markedly
hypertrophied lingual tonsils prevented intubation after anesthetic relaxation during preparation for appendectomy has been rep orted by Cohle et al (1993)
The huge hypertropic tonsils totally obstructed the glottic aperture after induction, resulting in a &#8220;can&#8217;t intubat e/can&#8217;t ventilate
situation&#8221;.  A recent review of the literature has been published by Ovassapian et al. (2002).<br></font></div><div><font face="Helvetica, Arial
sans-serif" class="size10 Helvetica10" color="#000000"><br></font ></div><div><font face="Helvetica, Arial, sans-serif" class="size10 Helvetica10"
color="#000000"><b>References</b></font><font face="Helvetica, Arial, sans-serif" class="size10 Helvetica10" color="#000000"> 
<br></font></div><div><font face="Helvetica, Arial, sans-serif" class="size10 Helvetica10" color="#000000"><br></font></div><di  v><font face="Helvetica,
Arial, sans-serif" class="size10 Helvetica10" color="#000000">Cohle SD, Jones DH, Puri S. Lingual tonsillar hypertrophy causing failed intubation and
cerebral anoxia. Am J Forensic Med Pathol 1993 14:158-61<br></font></div><div><font face="Helvetica, Arial, sans-serif" class="size10 Helvetica10"
color="#000000"><br></font></div><div><font face="Helvetica, Arial, sans-serif" class="size10 Helvetica10" color="#000000">Ovassapian A, Glassenberg
R, Randel GI, Klock A, Mesnick PS, Klafta JM.   The unexpected difficult airway and lingual tonsil hyperplasia: a case series and a review of the
literature. Anesthesiology. 2002;97:124-32.<br></font></div></div></div>
                <!-- </hs:element2> -->
                <!-- <hs:realtracker> -->
                <script type="text/javascript">
                        <!--
                                        var id='';var res='';var partnerid=90006;
                                        var user='1750604906';
                                        var pp='Case1';
                                        function f(s){f2(s)};
                                        function f2(s){document.write('<img alt="" src="'+s+'" height="1" width="1" border="0"/>')};
                                //-->
                </script>
                <script
src="/~site/Scripts_ExternalRedirect/ExternalRedirect.dll?CMD=CMDGetJavaScript&amp;H_SITEID=RTK1&amp;H_AltURL=%2F%7Esite%2Frealtracker%2
Frt_s90022.js&amp;HSGOTOURL=http%3A%2F%2Flayout1.realtracker.com%2Fincludes%2Frt_s90022a.js" type="text/javascript">
                </script>
                <script type="text/javascript">
                        <!--

        f('/~site/Scripts_ExternalRedirect/ExternalRedirect.dll?CMD=CMDGotoURL&H_SITEID=RTK1&H_AltURL=%2f%7esite%2ftp.gif&H_HSGOTOU
RL=http%3a%2f%2fweb4.realtracker.com%2fnetpoll%2fimulti.asp&use r='+escape(user)+'&pn='+escape(partnerid)+'&pp='+escape(pp)+'&js=1&to=-
360&userurl='+escape(location.href)+res);
                                //-->
                </script>
                <noscript>
                        <img alt=""
src="/~site/Scripts_ExternalRedirect/ExternalRedirect.dll?CMD=CMDGetGif&amp;H_SITEID=RTK2&amp;H_AltURL=%2F%7Esite%2Ftp.gif&amp;H_HSGO
TOURL=http%3A%2F%2Fweb4.realtracker.com%2Fnetpoll%2Fimulti.a sp%3Fuser%3D1750604906%26pn%3D90006%26pp%3DCase1%26js%3D0%26b%
3D0%26to%3D-360" height="1" border="0" width="1">
                </noscript>
                <!-- </hs:realtracker> -->
        </body>
</html>
```

Fig. 14.4 The source code corresponding to the web page for Clinical Case 1

WebWhacker (http://www.bluesquirrel.com/products/webwhacker/), **WebReaper** (http://www.webreaper.net), or similar utility (Fig. 14.3).

14.5 Quality, Effectiveness, and Dissemination Issues

As indicated earlier, the primary goal of the project was to provide introductory information about clinical airway management to medical students and residents in a format that was clear, succinct, and definitive, and offering generous use of graphical illustrations and summary tables.

In the early days of the project, draft materials were shown to selected interested individuals for informal commentary. Later this process became more formal, and once the first formal draft of the web site was completed, anesthesiologists in our department with a special interest in education were asked to review the site from both clinical and pedagogic perspectives, using the evaluation rubric provided in Table 14.1. This resulted in a number of suggestions that were subsequently implemented.

Following this internal review, a letter requesting reviewers was sent to all members of the Discussion List of the Society for Airway Management, an electronic

Table 14.1 The Suggested Evaluation Rubric for the Web Site

Please use your experience and judgment in evaluating this medical education web site. Some of the criteria you may choose to employ in your evaluation are provided below. In addition, you may have evaluation criteria not explicitly indicated below that you may wish to utilize in your evaluation

Writing
- The text follows basic rules of grammar, spelling, and composition
- The writing style is appropriate to the intended audience

Content
- The purpose of the site is clear
- The information will be useful to its intended audience
- The information presented is accurate

Authority
- The author is clearly identified
- The author is qualified to write on the topic
- The author provides a clear way to be contacted

Currency
- The site indicates the date of the last revision
- The site has been updated recently

Accessibility
- You can connect quickly to the site
- The site is free
- The site loads quickly

Organization
- The type styles and background make the pages clear and readable
- The links work, are easy to identify, and are logically grouped
- The layout is clear and easy to follow, and is consistent from page to page

discussion forum. Following further changes, dissemination of information concerning the web site was achieved informally through personal contacts made at national and international annual meetings (such as those of the Society for Airway Management, the American Society of Anesthesiologists, the Canadian Anesthesiologists' Society), as well as formally via e-mail notices.

14.6 Reflective Critique

If we had to do things again, next time around I would start by taking a more focused approach to the project. In retrospect, considerable time was spent evaluating a number of wWeb page production packages that might have been better spent focusing

Table 14.2 Synopsis of the Health on the Net Code of Conduct

1. Authority
Any medical or health advice provided and hosted on this site will only be given by medically trained and qualified professionals unless a clear statement is made that a piece of advice offered is from a non-medically qualified individual or organization
2. Complementarity
The information provided on this site is designed to support, not replace, the relationship that exists between a patient/site visitor and his/her existing physician
3. Confidentiality
Confidentiality of data relating to individual patients and visitors to a medical/health web site, including their identity, is respected by this web site. The web site owners undertake to honor or exceed the legal requirements of medical/health information privacy that apply in the country and state where the web site and mirror sites are located
4. Attribution
Where appropriate, information contained on this site will be supported by clear references to source data and, where possible, have specific HTML links to that data. The date when a clinical page was last modified will be clearly displayed (e.g., at the bottom of the page)
5. Justifiability
Any claims relating to the benefits/performance of a specific treatment, commercial product or service will be supported by appropriate, balanced evidence in the manner outlined above in Principle 4
6. Transparency of authorship
The designers of this web site will seek to provide information in the clearest possible manner and provide contact addresses for visitors that seek further information or support. The Webmaster will display his/her e-mail address clearly throughout the web site
7. Transparency of sponsorship
Support for this web site will be clearly identified, including the identities of commercial and non-commercial organizations that have contributed funding, services, or material for the site
8. Honesty in advertising and editorial policy
If advertising is a source of funding, it will be clearly stated. A brief description of the advertising policy adopted by the web site owners will be displayed on the site. Advertising and other promotional material will be presented to viewers in a manner and context that facilitates differentiation between it and the original material created by the institution operating the site

(Taken From http://www.hon.ch/HONcode/Conduct.html)

on content development and evaluation. Although I learned a lot by comparing packages such as Microsoft FrontPage and Abobe Dreamweaver, these efforts ended up being somewhat peripheral to the goals of the project, and in retrospect I would have been better off deciding to use Homestead directly rather than conducting informal comparison studies. This conclusion not withstanding, the time spent evaluating the various web page authoring packages was hardly time wasted, as I learned a lot that was helpful for other projects.

Like all academic undertakings, time and resource restrictions limit what can reasonably be achieved in any project. It is thus interesting to consider what might be done to extend this project further. My first recommendation in this respect would be to subject the project to a more formal peer-review process, as discussed next.

As noted earlier, the initial version of the site underwent an internal review process by members of our department with an interest in clinical airway management. Following their comments, a number of revisions followed. I also invited members of the Society for Airway Management (www.samhq.com) (the ultimate subject matter experts) to review the site and provide further feedback either in narrative form (a choice that most individuals seem to prefer) or through a suggested structured questionnaire ("rubric"). In future editions it would be nice to have the site reviewed by the Health on the Net Initiative (www.hon.ch, Table 14.2), with the eventual goal of certification by this agency. Another issue is whether another review process focusing on Instructional Design issues would be helpful. Yet another idea for future work is to submit the project for possible registration with MedEd Portal, located online at www.aamc.org/mededportal, a service that seeks to provide high-quality peer-reviewed teaching materials for medical education.

Chapter 15
An Integrated Approach in Medical Decision-Making for Eliciting Knowledge

Harleen Kaur and Siri Krishan Wasan

Abstract Decision-making in healthcare is an important area of research. Knowledge is one of the most significant assets of any organization. Knowledge discovery process consists of an iterative process of data cleaning, Data integration, data selection, data mining, and knowledge presentation. Medical decision-making from diagnosis to patient management is becoming more and more complex. Computer-assisted medical decision-making using data mining techniques is a challenging area of research with the potential to extract useful knowledge for improving the medical decision-making at various levels. Bayesian classifiers based on Bayes theorem of conditional probability fits well into medical diagnosis but has limitations due to its basic assumptions. In this paper, we discuss how Bayesian approach can be used for constructing probabilistic network from medical datasets. We further discuss the need of experience management for better diagnosis and disease management in view of the complexity.

Keywords: Bayesian probablistic frame work · Bayesian classifiers · Bayesian Probability Network (BPN) · Artificial Neural Networks (ANN) · and Knowledge discovery process

15.1 Introduction

Decision-making in healthcare is an important area of research. Patel et al. [1] argued for decision science that broadens the boundaries of traditional decision-making research. Medical databases, if created properly, will be large, complex, heterogeneous, and time-varying. Evolution of stored clinical data can lead to discovery of trends and patterns hidden within the data, which could enhance our understanding of the diseases.

Knowledge is one of the most significant assets of any organization. The role of information technology in healthcare is well established. Knowledge discovery

H. Kaur (✉)
Department of Computer Science, Hamdard University, New Delhi, India
e-mail: harleen_k1@rediffmail.com

A. Lazakidou (ed.), *Web-Based Applications in Healthcare and Biomedicine*, Annals of Information Systems 7, DOI 10.1007/978-1-4419-1274-9_15,

© Springer Science+Business Media, LLC 2010

process consists of an iterative process of data cleaning, data integration, data selection, data mining, pattern recognition, and knowledge presentation. Medical decision-making from diagnosis to patient management is becoming more and more complex due to rapid growth of deadly diseases. Patel et al. [1] indicated the differences between problem-solving and decision-making process. The social implication of healthcare decision-making requires an optimal use of technology with an ultimate aim of providing better healthcare to people in general. We need to create to evolve systems that can improve the medical decision-making process.

Patel et al. [1] focus on the understanding of decision-making process of various participants of healthcare system and made a reveiw of cognitive perspective and empirical research on medical decision-making. Decision-making research is of significant importance in medicine. Healthcare professionals are no doubt expected to be competent and able decision-makers, and their errorneous decisions intentionally or unintentionally will add to patient's suffering including loss of life. Thus medical decision-making must be subjected to public scrutiny, which can be achieved if there is some formal approach for decision-making.

Medical diagnosis is probablistic in nature. Bayesian classifiers on statistical classifiers based on famous Bayes theorem of conditional probability [2]. Thus medical diagnosis fits well into Bayesian probablistic frame work. Long et al. [3] developed a diagnostic capablities of the heart disease program (HDP) based on Bayesian probablity network (BPN). Cooper and Herskovits used Bayesian netwrok to provide insight into the probablistic dependdencies that exists among the case variables. Long et al. [3] have considered the reasoning requirement of heart diseases. There are certain inherent limitations in Bayesian classfication. The major challenge for the application of Bayesian networks for medical decisions/predictions is to represent domain knwoledge in probablistic formalism.

Application of data mining to health databases is no doubt challenging, but shall be rewarding to the society. Knowledge of an organization is an important asset. Unfortunately, knowledge of any health orgnization is confined to only few experts who acquired it through experinces in day-to-day medical practices. Detecting a disease from several factors/symptoms is a many layered problem, and it is resonable to use the experience and knowledge of medical experts alongwith data mining techniques for appropriate decision-making.

15.2 Bayesian Classifiers

Bayesian classifiers are statistical classifiers based on famous Bayes theorem, which can be stated as follows:

If the events $B_1, B_2, \ldots, B_k$ constitute a partition for a sample space S and $P(B_i) \neq 0$, $i = 1, 2, \ldots, k$ for any event A such that $P(A) \neq 0$

$$P(B_r|A) = \frac{P(B_r).P(A|B_r)}{\sum\limits_{j=1}^{k} P(B_i).P(A|B_i)}, \tag{15.1}$$

for $r = 1, 2, 3, \ldots, k$, where $P(X|Y)$ denotes the conditional probability of events X and Y.

Since medical diagnosis is probabilistic in nature, it is well suited for probability theory. Normally, physician asks questions to find patients history performs physical examination and asks for certain pathological and other tests and makes estimate that the patient has a particular disease or not.

Suppose $P(D_i|S)$ is denotes the probability that a patient with a particular syndrome S has a disease $D_{i.}$ then the Bayes theorem will give

$$P(D_i|S) = \frac{P(S|D_i).P(D_i)}{\sum_{j=1}^{k} P(S|D_j)/P(D_j)}, \tag{15.2}$$

where $P(S|D_i)$ denotes the probability of occurrence of the syndrome S in the disease $D_{i.}$, $P(D_j)$ is probability of occurrence of disease D_j. Suppose syndrome S consists of n independent attributes $x_1, x_2, x_3, \ldots, x_n$, then

$$P(S|D_i) = P(X_1|D_i).P(X_2|D_i)...P(X_{n1}D_i). \tag{15.3}$$

Without loss of generality, we can assume that attributes $x_1, x_2, x_3 \ldots, x_n$ take binary values 0 or 1 (i.e., absent or present), then there can be 2^n possible choices for the tuples $(x_1, x_2, x_3, \ldots, x_n)$. If we allow variables $x_1, x_2, x_3, \ldots, x_n$ take q values, then there will be q^n possible choice for $(x_1, x_2, x_3, \ldots, x_n)$.

Bayesian classifiers, also known as naïve Bayesian classifiers, are comparable in performance with decision tree and artificial neural networks (ANN). Bayesian belief networks are graphical models, which can also be used for classification. Computer-based medical diagnosis based on Bayesian techniques was developed for the diagnosis of congenital heart disease. Warner et al. [4] suggested that Bayesian techniques have also been applied for other medical diagnosis such as classification of strokes, ECG stress testing, and coronary heart disease.

Cooper and Herskovits [13] presented a Bayesian method for constructing a probabilistic network from a database of cases and demonstrated that this can provide insight into probabilistic dependences which exist among the case variables. No doubt, probabilistic nature of much of cardiovascular disease fits well into Bayesian probabilistic framework, but the complexity of this disease requires other kind of reasoning.

Long et al. [3], have considered challenges in collecting medical data and its presentation to the physician for appropriate diagnosis. Cardiovascular disease provides a wide range of characteristic and disorders range from acute to chronic. The disease can progress and complicated by additional disease. Long et al. used modified Bayesian Probability Network (BPN) to reason explanation for data and to model casual pathophysiology of the cardiovascular disease. Developing a BPN for diagnosis has many limitations. Bayesian classification assumes that patient's syndrome is disease. It further requires to estimate the probabilistic in relation to all the attributes responsible for a particular disease. Obtaining all the information about a particular patient, at times, may not be possible. Long et al. have explained the problem for modeling heart disease types such as primary aortic regurgitation (AR) can have different etiologies and we may need reasoning for time in the domain. For example, acute myocardial Infarction (MI) could not explain pleural effusion on the same day as pulmonary congestion occasionally causes pleural effusion. One can learn a lot in terms of disease patterns; therefore, it is important to capture experience of experts.

Cooper and Herskovits described a Bayesian approach to learning the qualitative and quantitative dependency relationship among a set of discrete variables and called it as Bayesian Learning of belief network (BLN). Lot of work has been done to develop methods for automated learning from data in the field of statistics and artificial intelligence [5–910]. One can bridge BLN to other AI methods to form a basis for application to ANN and other data mining techniques to evolve medical diagnosis for heart diseases, in particular, and other diseases, in general.

With the advent of sophisticated electronic data repositories, enormous amount of data in medical domain can be stored and useful knowledge can be discovered using data mining methods. We may identify fewer features/attributes responsible for a particular disease using statistical methods, apply Bayesian methods to provide insight into probabilistic dependencies that exist among the features/ attributes. We integrate various classification techniques to determine initial weights for ANN. Modify the weights using captured experiences to ultimately discover rules/algorithms for diagnosis of a particular disease.

Medical decision-making from diagnosis to patient management is becoming more and more complex due to rapid growth of knowledge during the past three decades. It is possible that even with specialization and super specialization, physician may not be able to make an optimal decision [10]. Computer-assisted medical decision-making using data mining techniques may provide a partial solution to the problem. Several Bayesian computer-assisted medical decision-making systems have given better results then senior specialists. Diagnoses of congenital heart disease [4], interpretation of electrocardiogram (ECG) stress testing, classification of strokes [2] are some of the examples where Bayesian systems have been applied.

Bayesian classification is based on certain assumptions which may not be true in real life, for example, many patients may have multiple disorders. Estimation of probabilities of disease by physicians and others may not be satisfactory, and data generated at one location may not applicable at other location. Still, creation of planned clinical databases with an intention of mining and use of Bayesian methods will go a long way in solving problems of diagnoses of various diseases.

Since the medical diagnosis is probabilistic in nature, Bayesian theorem is well suited for medical diagnosis. For a medical dataset, one can describe Bayes's theorem as follows

$$P(D_i|S) = \frac{P(S|D_i)/P(D_i)}{\sum_{j=1}^{n} P(S|D_i)/P(D_j)}, \tag{15.4}$$

where $i = 1, \ldots, n$, and $P(D_i/S)$ is the probability that a patient with a given syndrome S has a disease $D_{i.}$, $P(S|D_i)$ is the probability of occurrence of the syndrome S in the disease D_i, $P(D_i)$ is called the prior prevalence of the disease D_i, we may assume that S consists of independent attributes $S_1, S_2, S_3, \ldots, S_n$, where S_i is binary.

Bayesian networks are increasingly being applied in areas as diverse as the development of probabilistic medical expert systems from databases, information retrieval, and modeling of the human genome. The simple Bayesian method (also called *Naive Bayes* or *Simple Bayesian Probability*) makes an assumption that the data being analyzed are conditionally independent. Bayesian network encodes qualitative and quantitative knowledge. Quantitative knowledge is represented by conditional probability tables (CPTs), while qualitative is encoded by use of directed acyclic graphs (DAG). Such graphs are called Bayesian or probabilistic networks. Bayesian networks can be applied in varieties of medical tasks such as dealing with diagnosis, treatment selection, planning, and prognosis [11]. The basic assumption on Bayesian approaches is that they have the ability to describe, very easily, the influences and probabilistic interactions among variables.

The structure Bayesian model can be applied together with infection disease specialists. The structure of a Bayesian network can be designed using knowledge of known causal dependencies, influences, or correlation; all are derived from the knowledge of domain experts. Bayesian classification is well suited for medical diagnosis. We consider the following example to demonstrate the application of conditional probability in medical problems.

Consider the following table of 50 patients suffering from diabetes. Let S denote the set of these 50 patients given in Table 15.1.

Then $P(G)$ the probability of patients suffering from a heart disease is

$$= 14 + 08/50 = 0.44.$$

Probability $P(G|T)$ of patients suffering from heart disease gives that they are already suffering from diabetes for more than 10 years is as follows:

$$14/20 = 0.70,$$

$$P(G|T) = \frac{n(T \cap G)/n(S)}{n(T)/n(S)}, \tag{15.5}$$

$$= \frac{n(T \cap G)/n(S)}{n(T)/n(S)},$$

$$= \frac{8/50}{8 + 22/50},$$

where T denotes the set of patients.

Table 15.1 Patients records of diabetes and heart disease

	Number of patients with heart disease	Number of patients with no heart disease
Persons suffering from diabetes for 10 years or more than 10 years	14	06
Persons suffering from diabetes for less than 10 years	08	22

Suffering from diabetes for more than or equal to 10 years. Let T' denote the complement of T in S, i.e., persons suffering for diabetes for less than 10 years in Equation (15.6). Then the probability that a person suffering for less than 10 years will have heart disease will be

$$P(G'|T') = \frac{n(T' \cap G')}{P(T')}, \qquad (15.6)$$

$$= \frac{8/50}{8 + 22/50} = 0.266$$

We now demonstrate how Bayesian classifiers can be applied for diagnosis of heart problem. Suppose X_1, X_2, ..., X_n are attributes which have been identified as significant attributes responsible for a particular type of heart disease. Let C_1, C_2, ...,C_n can be in different types of heart disease. Each data sample corresponding to a patient is represented by a vector:

$$X = (x_1,x_2,...,x_n), x_i \in X_i, i = 1,2,...,n. \qquad (15.7)$$

Bayesian classifier will predict that X belongs to the class having the highest posterior probability conditional on X, i.e., Bayesian classifier assigns X to C_i such that $P(C_i\ |X)$ is maximum, i.e., $P(C_i\ |X) > P(C_i\ |X)$ for $1{=}j = m$, $j{\neq}i$. Further $P(C_i\ |X) = P(C_i){=}S_i/S$. Thus $P(C_i|X)$ is maximum if $P(X|C_i)$. $P(C_i)$ is maximum (since $P(X\ )$ is constant). Assuming that types of heart disease are likely, i.e., $P(C_1) = P(C_2)\ \ldots = P(C_m)$, then $P(C_i|X)$ is maximum if $P(C_i|X)$ is maximum. Otherwise, we need to maximize $P(X|C_i)\ P(C_i)$.

Suppose S_i is the number of training sample of C_i, then $P(C_i){=}S_i/S$, where S is the total number of training sample $P(X|C_i)$ by assuming that the attributes X_1, X_2, ..., X_n are independent. Thus $P(X|C_i) = P(X_1|C_i)P(X_2|C_i) \ldots P(X_n|C_i)$.

The naïve Bayesian classifier makes the assumption that the values of the attributes are independent. When this assumption is true, then the Bayesian classifier is the most accurate in comparison with other classifiers [12]. However, in medical problems, particular in respect of heart problem, dependencies can exist between variables. For example, high blood sugar may affect the other attributes responsible for a heart disease.

Bayesian networks are also known as Bayesian belief network or probabilistic networks and can be represented by directed acyclic graphs where nodes represent variables and arcs represent probabilistic dependencies [13]. Artificial Neural Networks (ANN) have potential of applications to biomedical and healthcare systems. ANN is an information paradigm derived from the limited understanding of the functioning of human brain. It is composed of highly interconnected neurons (processes). It solves the problem by breaking them into smaller components and use of massive parallel processing using adaptable interconnections called "weights." ANN can have multiple hidden layers depending on the complexity of the problem. Bayesian classification techniques can provide interaction points for ANN and taken together can provide effective methods for heart disease predictions [10, 14, 15].

Bayesian Networks is a real-world Bayesian analytical tool. Several tasks can make use of such network including prediction of likely causative organisms and the selection of optimal antibiotic therapy. Another application in which Bayesian network can be used is to deal with a variety of medical decision-making tasks under uncertainty. There are many medical databases that make use of Bayesian network such as *MUNIN*, which is a system for obtaining a preliminary diagnosis of neuromuscular diseases on the basis of electromyographic findings. *Child* helps us diagnosing congenital heart diseases. *SWAN* is a system for insulin dose adjustment of diabetes patients.

15.3 Experience Management of Medical Experts

Knowledge Discovery in Database (KDD) is the search for relationship of global patterns that exist but are hidden in large databases [16] and [17]. Medical decision-making from diagnosis to patient management is becoming more and more complex. Errors in physicians' decision or errors in laboratory reports often lead to terrible consequences for a patient. Medical decision-making is based on experience of individual medical expert, which is often not shared. It is possible that even with super specialization, physicians may not be able to make optimal decision. Computer-assisted medical decision (CMD) using data mining techniques may provide a useful solution for better health care. Application of data mining to medical databases is no doubt challenging, but shall be rewarding to the society. Knowledge of any health organization is confined to only few experts who acquired it through their experience. It is important to evolve systems that can capture knowledge and experience from medical databases and through interaction of medical experts [19] and [14]. This can be achieved if medical databases are created with intention of mining. We may make special provisions for recording unexpected events and significant results of any treatment.

With the use of experience of medical experts, we may develop data mining tools/models to discover novel and actionable rules that may provide guidelines for better diagnosis and management of disease. It is possible that there are contradictions between medical-expert diagnostic rules and rules discovered by data mining. Detecting a disease from several factors or symptoms is a many layered problem, and it is reasonable to use knowledge and experience of medical specialists along with data mining techniques for medical diagnosis.

Computers have made significant contribution in basic biomedical research. Simulation of disease process and computer models of biological systems are being manipulated and explored. Medical observations are multivariate, and multivariate analysis of statistics can be applied to classify patients into disease groups. If proper databases are created in respect of patients with heart diseases, multivariate analysis and data mining techniques can be applied in the diagnosis of ischaemic heart disease and myocardial infarction. Simulation of hospital activity can help in solving day-to-day problems faced by hospital management. Classification, an important data mining technique based on a variety of variables, can be of great utility in treatment of patients. Cluster analysis, another important data mining technique, is useful to group together patients who are similar.

In medical sciences, it is important to know what tends to go with what. One would like to develop association rules between smoking and cancer, pre-natal medication and congenital malformation, radiation and leukemia, pollution, and bronchitis.

Association rule mining can find interesting association and connection relationship among large set of medical data items [19]. The discovery of interesting association relationship among huge amount of patient records can help in not only planning proper medicare but also predicting patient condition and recovery [20]. This is possible if proper medical databases are created with intention of mining.

In a healthcare system, predictive modeling for a particular disease is very significant. With medical-expert's opinion, one can identify few attributes about a patient, which are significant in predicting the dangers of patients' chances of getting a particular disease. Data mining can discover large set of rules from medical databases, and medical experts have also evolved some rules in view of their experience. A comparative study of rules discovered by medical experts and rules discovered through data mining can lead to novel and more actionable rules.

Association rule mining can find interesting association or correlation relationship among large set of medical data items. The discovery of interesting association relationship among huge amount of patient records can help in not only planning proper medicare but also in predicting patients' conditions and recovery. The typical market-based analysis can be effectively applied to study the effect of combination of various drugs given to a patients suffering with a particular disease. For example, for patients suffering from typhoid, different combinations of antibiotics are tried. If proper records of treatment of these patients are maintained along with the data of their pathological tests, association rule mining can help the physician in deciding a better course of action for such patients [21].

Market basket analysis may be used to plan marketing of a particular drug. For example, from patient records, one may discover the combination of drugs prescribed for diabetic patients. A proper mining of these records can indicate recovery pattern.

Let U be set of drugs in a medical store. For each patient, we can have a transaction $I \subseteq U$. A transaction T is said to contain A iff $A \subset T$. An association rule is an implication of the form A=> B, $A \subset U$, $B \subset U$, $A \cap B = \Phi$. A rule A=> B hold in transaction set D with support *s* if "*s*" is the percentage of transaction in D that contain both A and B, i.e., $A \cup B$ and it has confidence "*c*" in the transaction set D if *c* is the percentage of transaction in D containing A that also contains B.

We can define a Boolean vector B(I) for a disease I and these Boolean vectors can be analyzed for prescription pattern that reflect the drugs that are frequently prescribed for patients suffering with a particular disease. These patterns can be represented in the form of association rules with certain level of support and confidence. Treatment data of a particular disease can be collected, grouped by medical prescription and association between two sets of medicine can be found. For example, this technique, if applied on patients with coronary artery disease (CAD), will go a long way in determining several categories of these patients. With the experience of heart specialists, one can identify various significant attributes, which will help in the development of a diagnostic model.

Most association rule mining algorithms employ support confidence thresholds to exclude uninteresting rules. But many rules satisfying minimum thresholds and minimum confidence still may not be interesting to medical experts [20]. Ultimately, medical experts can judge if a rule is interesting or not.

In a healthcare system, predictive modeling for a particular disease is significant. With medical experts' opinion based on their experience, we could identify attributes that are significant in predicting the danger of a patent's chances of getting a particular disease [15].

For example, it will be significant for a diabetic patient to know the risk of his/her getting a heart attack or the risk of getting blind. Classification model may be built to categorize critical diabetic patients and predict the risk of his/her getting a heart attack or finding the risk of his/her getting blind. Similarly, using classification technique, one may build a prediction model to categorize cancer patients who could be given radiographic treatment or chemotherapy or both [21]. Basic techniques of classification are decision tree induction, Bayesian classification, and neural network.

15.4 Expert Mining vs. Data Mining

Data mining uses large databases to discover large set rules. Traditional medical expert system extracts knowledge from IF-THEN diagnostic rules whereas machine-learning techniques rely on available databases. Nearest neighbor method, cluster analysis, neural networks, and genetic algorithms can be applied effectively to discover knowledge from medical datasets. However, medical database may have incorrect records and missing records. On the other hand, medical experts may have incorrect rules.

Thus there is a need to have hybrid approach for extracting rules using expert diagnostic techniques and data-driven techniques. We may develop a system which identifies attributes x_1, x_2,x_3, ..., x_n for a particular disease D using expert opinion.

For a particular patient there will be a n-tuple representing values for these attributes. Without loss generality, we may assume that these attributes have binary values so that there are 2^n distinct tuples (x_1, x_2,x_3, ..., x_n).

A brute-force method would require questioning an expert on each of 2^n combinations of X= (x_1, x_2, x_3, ..., x_n). An expert knowledge will be in the form of set of rules say $E = \{R_1, R_2, R_3, \ldots, R_m\}$. On the other hand, data mining techniques results in a set of rules $F = \{S_1, S_2, S_3, \ldots, S_p\}$. We may compare E with F. We may find that some S_i are comparable with some R_j and then may be some S_k, which contradict some R_i. If found that contradicting rules are discovered using misleading cases, we reject them.

Expert mining will require questioning an expert through an interview. We may develop questioning procedure as monotone Boolean function interactively. A rule can be described as a function; $f = X^n \rightarrow A$, where A being a set of predictions. We may define an order in the set of n-tuples $(x_1, x_2, x_3, \ldots, x_n)$ in a simple manner as follows: $(x_1, x_2, x_3, \ldots, x_n) > (y_1, y_2, y_3, \ldots, y_n)$ if and only if $x_i = y_i$. For example, $X = (x_1, x_2, x_3, \ldots, x_n)$ and $Y = (y_1, y_2, y_3, \ldots, y_n)$ represent tuples for two patients in respect of a disease D. We may say that patient Y is more serious than X if $(y_1, y_2, y_3, \ldots, y_n) > (x_1, x_2, x_3, \ldots, x_n)$. Each chain of monotonic values $(x_1, x_2, x_3, \ldots, x_n)$ represents a case. If a subsequent question is determined by answer to previous question, then using Hansel chain [22], number of questions to an expert can be reduced.

Lot of research in data mining is devoted to finding of more and more algorithms. Pazzani [23] states that these algorithms do not have parameters for novelty, utility, and understandability. We want knowledge that is novel, useful, and understandable.

The notions of novelty, utility, interesting, and actionable in terms of discovered rules do not have proper parameters and are not well defined. There is lot of vagueness. We need to evolve a common logical understanding of these parameters by restructuring our parameters. The objective of knowledge discovery cannot be restricted to the satisfaction of expert. Even the satisfaction of medical expert can be enhanced using data mining techniques. Similarly, experience of medical experts if recorded and managed properly will help in evolving proper data mining tools. Pazzani has correctly recognized that KDD must draw on cognitive psychology in addition to database, statistics, and artificial intelligence. Certainly, we will able to increase the usefulness of KDD system by taking human cognitive process into account.

Consistency with prior knowledge should not mean that new knowledge will not be acceptable. Medical experience involves events, problems, and solutions in the context of various diseases and their treatment. It will be useful to have automatic extraction of valid and significant knowledge gained by medical specialists in view of their experience. Experience-based continuous learning combined with knowledge discovery through data mining techniques will go a long way in improving the healthcare services. Every healthcare organization has a responsibility to collect and document the experience gained by various individuals working in the organization. Software engineering approach of Experience Factory (EF) [15, 24] can be used in collecting, documenting, and storing medical experience of a healthcare organization in an Experience Base (EB). Experience Management of medical experts will result in proper decision-making in respect of diagnosis and treatment of diseases. A decision support technology continues to proliferate in medical settings [1]. Medical decisions to treat a patient involve proper diagnosis and a choice of treatment among a set of choices. With the help of data mining techniques applied on properly created medical databases along with the management of medical experience can result in "good decisions," which will choose effectively the best possible alternatives in a given situation. Creation of electronic medical records with the intention of mining and knowledge discovered from the experience of medical experts will generate clinical-practice guidelines. Medical decision-making depends not only on the symptoms (attributes) for a particular disease but also on available alternative. In some situations even the patient has a role to play. For example, if a patient is just informed about his/her having cancer, he/she must decide whether to go for surgery with good survival rate or alternative treatment that carries greater risk. If an automatic system is available, patient himself can find out the result of particular treatment given to patients with similar symptoms. Patel et al. [1] critically review both traditional and recent approach to medical decision-making based on conceptual knowledge in decision-making. Expert mining and data mining with an integrated approach will improve the decision-process, which can result in better patient care and health outcomes.

15.5 Integrated Approach in Medical Decision-Making (A New Paradigm)

There is a need for new approaches for medical decision-making research. Patel et al. reviewed critically the traditional and recent approaches to medical decision-making. We propose a new paradigm in medical decision-making, which involves traditional Bayesian techniques, artificial neural networks, association rule mining and expert mining in the following format.

- create medical databases with the intention of mining
- apply Bayesian techniques identify important attributes responsible for medical decisions at various levels
- use Bayesian techniques to determine user thresholds for specific medical rules and to determine initial weights (in respect of importance) of attributes responsible for a medical decisions
- use association rule mining and artificial neural network (ANN) to determine interesting rules/decisions
- compare the rules so obtained with rules extracted from expert mining
- accept the common matching decisions and review the contradictions if any

The main objective of medical decision-making at various levels should be to reduce patient's suffering and to reduce the cost of the treatment. One may evolve systematic steps for solving urgent and critical medical problems, but for complicated deadly diseases we need a comprehensive approach using data mining techniques on large medical datasets along with experts' experiences. Medical decision-making most involve patient, physician and should take into consideration the economic status of patients.

A decision is characterized by the number of attributes. For example, chronic lung disease, asthma, is characterized by inflammation and spasm in the airway. It can be triggered by environmental factors, infections, allergies, temperature change, etc. Thus to diagnose the disease, we need to consider medical history, physical examination and laboratory tests, emergency indications, and treatment if the physician is helped by automated system of diagnosis. The automated system could be generated using the proposed integrated approach of mining medical datasets of patients already treated with similar diagnosis and extraction of previously known expert knowledge.

Acknowledgments We are grateful to Dr Mrs. Manju Kanga, Associate Specialist, Wycompe Hospital, London, UK, for her valuable comments and suggestions.

References

1. Patel, V. L., Evans D.A., Kaufman, D. R.: Cognitive framework for doctor-patient interaction. In: Evans D. A., Patel V. L., eds. Cognitive Science in Medicine: Biomedical Modeling, MIT Press, Cambridge, MA (1989), 253–308
2. Zagoria, R., Roggia, J.: Transferability of medical support system based Bayesian classification, Med. Decis. Making, 3 (1983), 501–509
3. Long, W. J., Naimi, S., Criscitiello, M. G.: Evaluation of a new method for cardiovascular reasoning, J. Am. Med. Informatics Assoc. 1 (1994), 127–141
4. Warner H., Toronto A., Veasy L., Stepthenson.: A mathematical approach to medical diagnosis – application to congenital heart disease, JAMA (1961), 177–183
5. Blum, R. L.: Discovery, conformation, and incorporation of casual relationships from a large time-oriented clinical database: the RX project, Computers Biomed. Res. 15 (1982), 247–256
6. Carbonell, J. G. (Ed.).: Special volume on machine learning, Artificial Intelligence, 40 (1990), 1–385
7. Hinton, G. E.: Connectionist learning procedures, Artificial Intelligence, 40 (1990), 185–234
8. James, M.: Classification Algorithms, John Wiley & Sons, New York (1985)
9. Michalski, R. S., Carbonell, J. G., Mitchell, T. M.(Ed.).: Machine Learning, Vol. 1, Tioga Press, Palo Alto, CA (1983)
10. Lele, R. D.: Computers in Medicine, Tata Mc Graw Hill Publishing Company diagnosis of coronary-artery disease. The New England Journal of medicine, 300 (1988), 1350–1359
11. Diamond, G. A., Forrester, J. S.: Analysis of Probability as an aid in the clinical diagnosis of coronary-artery disease, The New England Journal of Medicine, 300 (1979), 1350–1359
12. Dagher, A. P., Herskovits, E. H.: Expert refinement of data-derived Bayesian networks for medical diagnosis. American Medical Informatics Association Annual Fall Symposium, Washington, DC (1996)
13. Cooper, G. F., Herskovits, E. H.: A Bayesian Method for the Induction of Probabilistic Networks from Data, Machine Learning, 9 (1992), 309–347
14. Tautz, C., Althoff, K.-D., Nick, M.: Learning from experience–An experience factory case study. In Proceedings of the 13th German Workshop on Machine Learning (FGML 2000), Sankt Augustin, Germany (2000)
15. Scales, R., Embrechts, M.: Computational intelligence techniques for medical diagnostics. In Proceedings of Graduate Research Conference from the world wide web:http://www.cs.rpi.edu/˜bivenj/MRC/proceedings/papers/researchpaper.pdf.2002
16. Han, J., Kamber, M.: Data Mining: Concepts and Techniques, Morgan Kauffmann Publishers, San Francisco (2001)
17. Dunham, M. H.: Data Mining: Introductory and Advanced Topics. 1st Edition Pearson Education (Singapore) Pte. Ltd. (2003)
18. Godin, P., Hubbs, R., et al.: New paradigms for medical decision support and education: the Stanford Health Information Network for Education. Top Health Inf. Manage. 20(2) (1999), 1–14

19. Kaur, H., Wasan, S. K., Al-Hegami, A. S., Bhatnagar, V.: A Unified Approach for Discovery of Interesting Association Rules in Medical Databases, Advances in Data Mining, LNAI-4065 series, 53-63, Springer-Verlag, Berlin, Heidelberg (2006)
20. Wasan, S. K., Bhatnagar, V., Kaur. H.: An Efficient Interestingness based Algorithm for Mining Association Rules in Medical Databases, In: Elleithy K., ed. Advances in Systems, Computing Sciences and Software Engineering, Springer Netherlands (2007)
21. Kaur, H., Wasan, S. K.: Empirical study on applications of data mining techniques in healthcare, J. Comput. Sci. 2(2) (2006), 194–200
22. Cios, K. J., Moore, G. W.: Consistent and complete data and "expert" mining in medicine. Chapter 9. In: Cios K. J. ed. Medical Data Mining and Knowledge Discovery, Springer-Verlag, Heidelberg (2000), 237–278
23. Pazzani, M. J.: Knowledge discovery from data, IEEE Intelligence Systems March–April (2000), 10–13
24. Basili, V. R., Caldiera, G., Rombach, D.: Experience factory. In: Marciniak J. J. ed. Encyclopedia of Software Engineering, John Wiley & Sons, vol. 1 (1994), 469–476

Chapter 16
Using Decision Trees for the Semi-automatic Development of Medical Data Patterns: A Computer-Supported Framework

Aikaterini Fountoulaki, Nikos Karacapilidis, and Manolis Manatakis

Abstract The development of clinical practice guidelines is a difficult task. In most cases, it requires extensive elaboration of medical data repositories and tailoring of the corresponding results according to the medical setting under consideration. This tailoring should account for variations in diverse clinical settings. However, in any case, it has to be based on well-structured medical data patterns that provide experts with the necessary knowledge. Towards facilitating the overall task, this paper presents a computer-supported framework for the semi-automatic development of meaningful medical data patterns. The proposed framework comprises a novel hybrid methodology, which exploits decision trees features, and a web-based system that has been developed to accommodate this methodology. The overall framework pays much attention to the issues of user-friendliness, accuracy of results and visualization of the produced patterns.

Keywords: Decision Trees · Medical Data · Data Patterns · Semi-automatic Development · Web-based System · Machine Learning · Clinical Practice Guidelines

Abbreviations

CPGs	(Clinical Practice Guidelines)
ML	(Machine Learning)
ARFF	(Attribute Relation File Format)
ISS	(Internet Information Server)

16.1 Introduction

Clinical Practice Guidelines (CPGs) have been defined as systematically developed statements to assist physician and patient decisions about appropriate health care for specific clinical circumstances [1]. Numerous CPGs have been developed in diverse

A. Fountoulaki (✉)
Industrial Management and Information Systems Lab, MEAD, University of Patras, 26500 Rion-Patras, Greece
e-mail: fountoul@mech.upatras.gr

A. Lazakidou (ed.), *Web-Based Applications in Healthcare and Biomedicine*, Annals of Information Systems 7, DOI 10.1007/978-1-4419-1274-9_16,
© Springer Science+Business Media, LLC 2010

forms in the past 15 years, while their benefits in the practice of medicine have been reported in many studies (see, for instance, [2]). Much effort is being lately spent in supporting the computerization of the development and utilization of the CPGs. Admittedly, the development of CPGs is a difficult task, which requires input from experts in diverse domains such as clinical medicine, meta-analysis, decision analysis, clinical epidemiology, cost-effectiveness analysis and evidence synthesis. Moreover, their development may follow diverse approaches, such as expert opinion, consensus methods and evidence-based methods [3].

The overall development of CPGs may be split into two equally important phases. The first one concerns the appropriate elaboration of a continuously increasing amount of data, stored in medical data repositories. Data about correct diagnoses are usually stored in the form of medical records in various departments of specialized hospitals. In the majority of cases, it is extremely difficult for physicians to analyse these data in order to make the best diagnosis or to provide the best available treatment for a particular patient. A computer-supported elaboration of this information can lead to the required medical data abstraction, which can be achieved through the development of meaningful medical data patterns. These patterns are abstract representations of a medical decision-making problem. They explore and structure the uncertain, dynamic and complex consequences of a decision, and they assign a value to these consequences [4]. Thus, medical data patterns enable the formal structuring of medical problems, as well as the required support for medical decision-making. They can be used for diagnostic and/or therapeutic purposes.

The second phase concerns the tailoring of these patterns, the ultimate aim being the production of useful CPGs. Usually, medical data patterns have to undergo the judgment of a group of experts, integrate additional parameters in order to account for variation in clinical circumstances and, generally speaking, get customized according to the overall medical setting under consideration. The required transformation of patterns to statements (as CPGs should look like) also needs appropriate textual enrichment of the former.

This paper presents a framework that aims to semi-automate the first of the above two phases. The proposed framework comprises a novel hybrid methodology, which builds on the strengths of existing approaches originally coming from the areas of machine learning, medical informatics and decision-making, and a web-based system that has been especially developed to accommodate this methodology. Much attention has been paid to the issues of user-friendliness, accuracy of results and alternative visualizations of the produced patterns; these issues are critical for both the production of meaningful medical data patterns and their further elaboration towards the development of easily customizable and expressive CPGs. The proposed framework alleviates the burden of handling huge amounts of medical data and does not require from physicians involved in the production of medical data patterns to have any expertise in Machine Learning theory. Moreover, it aids physicians decide about the appropriate treatment of a patient and make the right diagnosis or predictions about a particular health problem.

The remainder of this paper is constructed as follows: Section 2 presents in detail the proposed methodology and sketches the associated implementation issues.

Section 3 demonstrates features and functionalities of the corresponding web-based system through a case concerning the issue of thyroid disease. Section 4 comments on the rationale of the proposed methodology, discusses its limitations and outlines future work directions. Concluding remarks are given in Section 5.

16.2 The Proposed Framework

Our overall framework builds extensively on Machine Learning (ML) theory and approaches. Generally speaking, ML deals with the question of how to construct computer programs that automatically improve with experience [5]. ML methods can be considered as computational procedures that can be trained by a series of input and output data. Once this is completed, they can make estimations and provide outputs for any given data. ML overlaps heavily with statistics, since both fields study the analysis of data. But unlike statistics, ML is concerned with the algorithmic complexity of computational implementations. Today, ML provides several indispensable tools for intelligent data analysis. Upto now, ML techniques have been widely used for many studies in medical prediction, for many different diagnostic problems [6–10]. Patient records with a correct diagnosis provide the required input to ML algorithms. A critical issue to be addressed at this point concerns the proper identification of the parameters to be taken into account by the ML algorithm; this certainly reflects the purpose of elaboration of these data, it affects the results to be obtained, while it has to be done by an expert. This is of course an oversimplification, but in principle, the medical diagnostic knowledge can be automatically derived from the description of cases solved in the past. From the above, it derives that the use of ML techniques for the exploitation of these data can also augment and facilitate the development of medical data patterns.

Various ML techniques, such as decision tree, artificial neural networks, Bayesian learning, and genetic algorithms, have been exploited in the development of CPGs [8, 10–12], each of them having advantages and disadvantages. The proposed methodology exploits a decision tree algorithm to produce a model that will, in turn, be used for the development of medical data patterns. Decision trees offer a supervised approach to classification. They are very popular in ML applications and are also used as prognostic models in medicine. They are attractive because they provide a symbolic representation that allows easy interpretation by the users, even by non-technical people. The representation can also be extended or easily modified when a tree is translated into appropriate rules. Moreover, decision trees are able to handle both categorical and numerical medical data. Besides, they have been proven to be a very good tool towards achieving one of our primary objectives, which is to develop patterns that are easily understood by physicians, both in flowchart and in text form. We want the produced patterns to be meaningful, showing clearly what a physician has to do in order to reach his/her final decision. Decision trees are easy to understand and can be easily converted to a set of production (broadly known as "if-then") rules.

16.2.1 J48 Algorithm

Having decided to follow the decision tree technique, the next step was to select the most appropriate algorithm for our purposes. Towards this, some additional requirements had to be checked. First of all, accuracy in the medical field needs to be as high as possible. Usually, accuracy above a threshold level (chosen by the user) is a necessary prerequisite for a model to be acceptable. Secondly, comprehensibility and stability are very important conditions for the production of medical data patterns, in order for them to be useful [8]. Moreover, because we have medical records to analyse, the chosen ML algorithm has to deal adequately with patient records, which lack certain data. In such kinds of records, there are many errors and uncertainties; the algorithm to be selected has to satisfy this requirement. Reducing the number of tests is another important consideration for cost reduction in cases such as medical diagnosis [11]. Finally, we had to give much attention to the understandability of the model and its ability to produce results that can be easily transformed to a set of "if-then" rules (these rules, together with the decision tree, can then be used for the development of CPGs).

Many decision tree algorithms have been tested for their ability to produce prediction models in the medical field. CART and C4.5 are the most commonly used of them [8, 10, 12]. Our approach adopts the J48 algorithm, which is the release 8 of C4.5 [13]. C4.5 is one of the best known and most widely used learning algorithms, which combines all the characteristics mentioned above. Its accuracy level is high enough, independently of the data volume to be processed. Also, it can handle missing data and can be easily modified into convenient "if-then" rules.

Implementation of J48 was done through Weka, an open-source software, developed at the University of Waikato (http://www.cs.waikato.ac.nz/ml/Weka/). Being a successor of the ID3 algorithm, C4.5 learns decision trees by constructing them in a top-down way, beginning with the question "which attribute should be tested at the root of the tree?". To answer this question, each instance attribute is evaluated using a statistical test to determine how well it classifies the training examples. The important function is the information gain; it measures how well a given attribute separates the training examples according to their target classification. Moreover, C4.5 can easily extract rules from a given set of data, which have a complex correlation with each other. Finally, C4.5 implements a number of improvements to the ID3 algorithm in the areas of missing data, continuous data, pruning rules and splitting criterion.

16.2.2 Data Processing

The proposed methodology processes medical data records to provide the most appropriate solution to a medical problem. It generates decision trees, the nodes of which evaluate the existence or significance of individual features of a problem. The first step of the proposed methodology is to collect the medical data and to load the patients' records that will then be elaborated for the production of the medical data patterns. The patients' records have to be in Attribute

Relation File Format (ARFF). An ARFF file is an ASCII file that describes a list of instances sharing a set of attributes. ARFF files were developed by the Machine Learning Project at the Department of Computer Science of the University of Waikato for use with the Weka ML software (for more details, see http://www.cs.waikato.ac.nz/~ml/weka/arff.html).

Before invoking the J48 model, some critical parameters have to be defined. One of them is the confidence factor that determines the confidence value to be used when pruning the tree (removing branches that are deemed to provide little or no gain in statistical accuracy of the model). Since the default of 25% works reasonably well in most cases, it will likely not have to be modified. However, if the actual error rate on real data (or the error rate on cross-validation) is significantly higher than the error rate on the training data, the decrease of the confidence factor will cause more drastic pruning and a more general model of the data. If a more specific modelling (based on the training data) is needed, the confidence factor can be increased, something that will decrease the amount of pruning that occurs. Another parameter is the minimum number of instances per leaf, which determines the minimum number of instances that must be present in the training data for a new leaf to be created in the decision tree. This parameter can also affect how much generalized or specialized a decision tree is; a higher number will create a more generalized tree and a lower number will create a more specialized tree. Also, if test data is not available, J48 performs a cross-validation using the training data. The number of folds for cross-validation, which depends on the training data set, has to be determined. Extensive tests on numerous data sets have shown that ten-fold cross-validation is one of the best choices for getting the most accurate error estimate. Decreasing the number of folds from the default of ten will likely decrease the amount of time it takes for the decision tree to be generated (while increasing the number of folds will likely increase the amount of time it takes). Of course, increasing the number of folds will create a larger data set for the training data, which may increase accuracy of the decision tree; similarly, decreasing the number of folds will create a smaller data set for the training data, which may decrease the accuracy of the decision tree.

The process of creating the associated datasets (a dataset is an object that can store data and relations) is illustrated in more detail in the sequence diagram appearing in Fig. 16.1. The medical expert has first to select the attributes that he/she wants to analyse. He/she can also select attribute groups. If an attribute group is selected, all the attributes in that group are automatically selected. After the required attributes are selected, their values are extracted from the database and they are stored into a dataset.

The next step for the development of medical data patterns is to add some useful information, known as meta-data, which will further enhance the knowledge embedded in them. These are: title, institution, author, date, validation, purpose-explanation and keywords. Once this is completed, the data are elaborated through Weka, which produces the decision tree in combination with the "if-then" rules and also some statistical information about the accuracy of the produced prediction model. As far as the results of Weka are satisfying, we continue to the next step. The information inputs and the Weka results are combined by a mapping algorithm for the text and flowchart representation of the medical data pattern. The

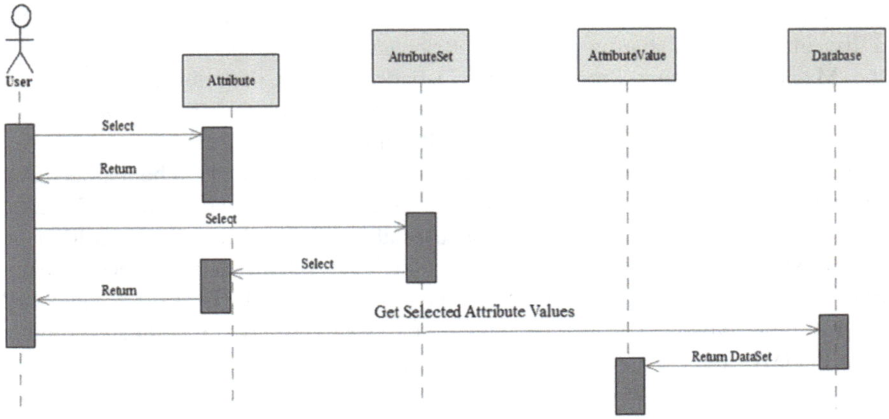

Fig. 16.1 Create DataSet – sequence diagram

final representations of the medical data patterns, both in a text and in a flowchart form, are then produced. Each alternative view of the derived patterns is stored in a medical database accompanied with a set of meta-data.

Figure 16.2 describes the steps that the medical expert should follow in order to develop a medical data pattern. Initially, he/she has to enter the information inputs

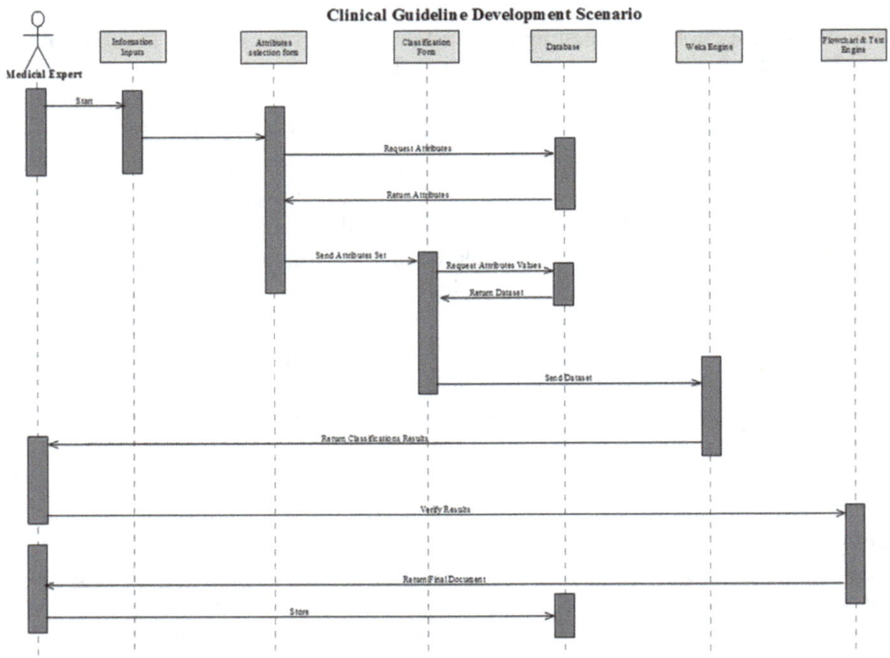

Fig. 16.2 Medical data pattern development – sequence diagram

form. Information inputs are the description of the medical data pattern, the keywords and any other information that are not related with the classification process. After the dataset is ready, it is classified by the Weka engine and the classification results are displayed to the user. The user evaluates the statistical data from the classification process to verify the results. If the results are accepted, they are sent to the "Flowchart and Text Engine", where the final form of the medical data pattern is developed. Finally, the user verifies the pattern and decides whether he/she wants to store it for further use.

16.2.3 Visualization Issues

As mentioned in the introductory section of this paper, the purpose of the proposed methodology is to develop meaningful medical data patterns that will be then elaborated further in order to develop CPGs. It is thus important to take care of the visualization of the derived patterns, taking into consideration their potential usability. Currently existing CPGs are of different types [14–16], each having its own methods of development and dissemination and, therefore, its own strengths and limitations. CPGs can be represented in several different formats, including text, protocol, charts or lists, flowcharts or any combination of the above. Due to the fact that the proposed methodology is based on the decision tree produced by the J48 algorithm, it was difficult to use one of the standard approaches for the CPG representation. We were concentrated on solutions that are represented as clinical algorithms by a combination of already used formats that better suit our approach. Much attention was given to the produced medical data patterns in order for them to be expressive, understandable and usable. We wanted to provide physicians with information that will include all the needed information in an understandable and easily applicable way.

Our text-based representation exploits elements from the Arden Syntax [17], which is an open standard for the procedural representation for modular guidelines. The Arden Syntax for medical logic modules has been designed specifically to share medical knowledge. Our text form, in addition to the "if-then" rules, will include similar information to the maintenance and library categories of the Arden Syntax. This information will be: title of the produced clinical guideline, institution that the data were collected at, author who has developed the medical data pattern, date, validation, purpose-explanation and keywords.

As far as the flowchart-like representation is concerned, we concluded that our proposed methodology must be represented with "successive" check steps, based on the J48 produced decision tree. Physicians will decide what they should do with a specific medical problem by checking in each step the values of the attributes that classify their patient condition better.

16.2.4 Implementation Issues

The proposed methodology is fully supported by an especially developed web-based tool. Its architecture is sketched in Fig. 16.3. As shown, the user's browser connects

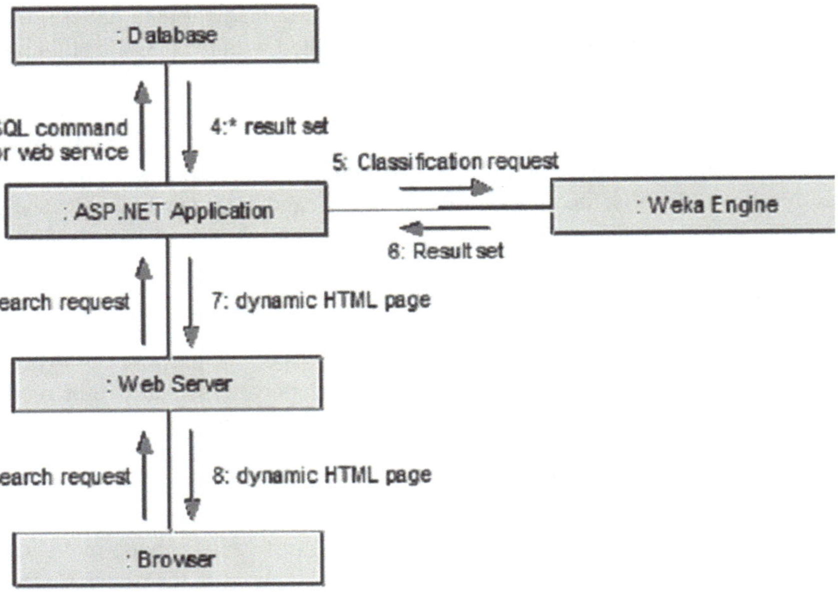

Fig. 16.3 Architecture of the web-based tool (UML collaboration diagram)

to the web server using an HTTP request. The web server hosts the site on the ISS (Internet Information Server), which receives and sends HTTP requests. The ASP.NET application handles these requests. The application data are stored to one or more databases. The application can access the database using SQL commands or a web service. The data analysis is performed through an external classification engine. A request for classification contains the data we want to analyse. The classification engine (Weka) returns the classification results. It contains "if-then" rules, flowchart data and statistical information about the results accuracy. The ASP.NET application dynamically creates HTML pages, which the IIS posts to the users' web browser.

16.3 A Case Study: Thyroid Disease

For the demonstration of the proposed methodology, a case study concerning the issue of the "thyroid disease" is presented. The 3772 records used were supplied by the Caravan Institute and J. Ross Quinlan, New South Wales Institute, Sydney, Australia (these are available online at: http://www.cs.umb.edu/~rickb/files/UCI/hypothyroid.arff). We suppose that a physician has to decide in which of the four classes (primary hypothyroid, compensated hypothyroid, secondary hypothyroid, negative) his/her patient belongs to, before he/she subscribes him a drug. The available information that he/she has are 30 attributes that the four classes depends on. First of all, the dataset had to be loaded in the Weka ARFF file format.

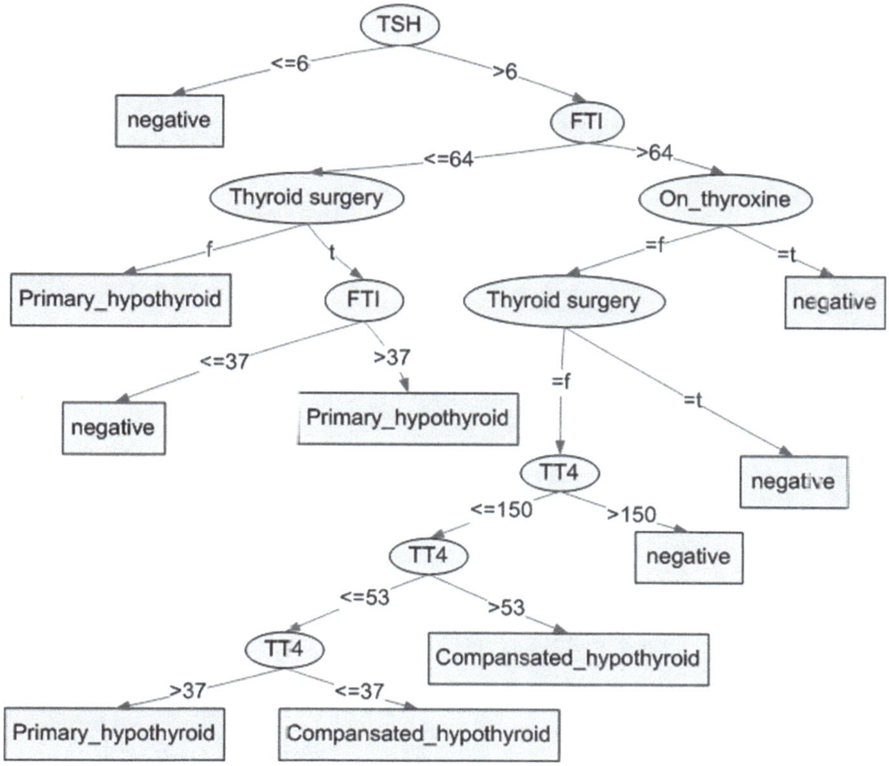

Fig. 16.4 The decision tree for the thyroid disease case

The dataset has 30 attributes, 7 of which are of continuous value (the rest 23 take discrete values). In our study, the dataset was applied to the J48 decision tree algorithm using 10-fold cross-validation. In 10-fold cross-validation, the original sample is partitioned into 10 sub-samples. Of the 10 sub-samples, a single sub-sample is retained as the validation data for testing the model, while the remaining 9 sub-samples are used as training data. The cross-validation process is then repeated 10 times (the folds), with each of the 10 sub-samples used exactly once as the validation data. The 10 results from the folds can then be averaged (or otherwise combined) to produce a single estimation. After the training of J48 through Weka software, we obtain the Weka classifier tree visualizer (see Fig. 16.4), where the different options in each successive step are shown.

The final step of the proposed methodology is to produce meaningful alternative representations of the medical data patterns. For the text-based representation, our methodology enriches the produced "if-then" rules with appropriate meta-data. Figure 16.5 depicts a screenshot of the supporting web-based tool providing such a functionality. The complete text-based representation of the medical data pattern produced for the case under consideration is shown in Fig. 16.6.

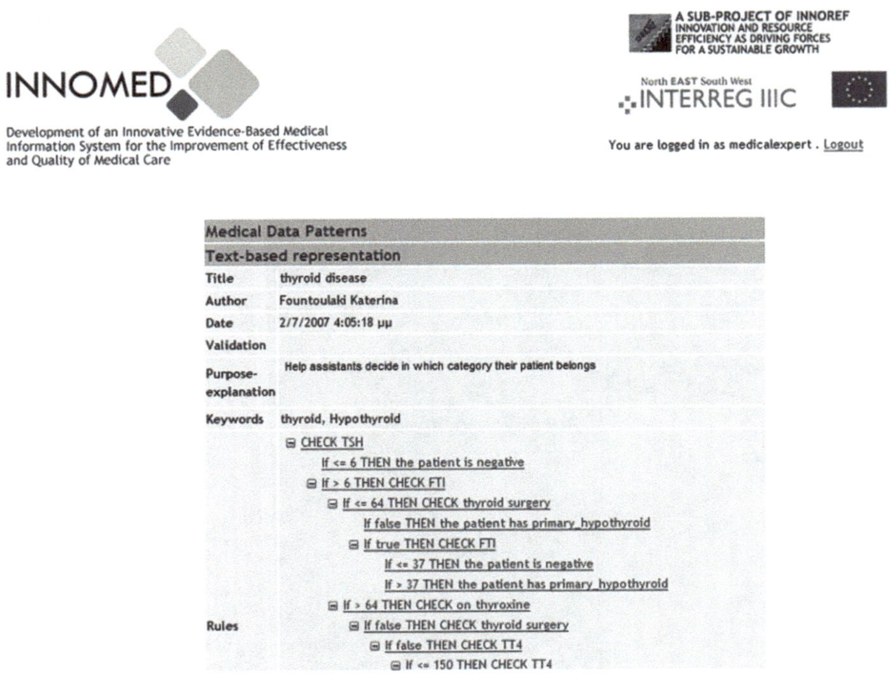

Fig. 16.5 Text-based representation of a medical data pattern for the thyroid disease case

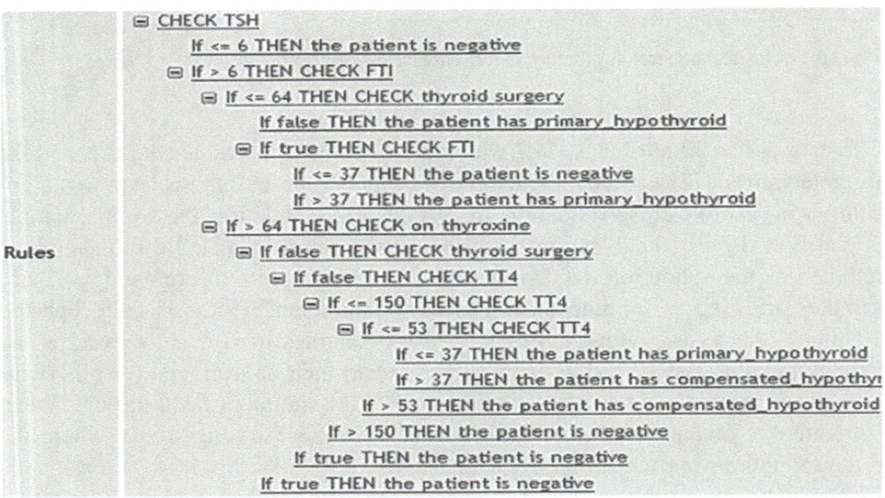

Fig. 16.6 The complete text-based representation of the produced medical data pattern

Based on the Weka classifier tree visualizer, the tool also produces the final flowchart-like medical data pattern (see Fig. 16.7), where ovals represent the successive check steps and parallelograms represent the final advice that is derived in each case. Following a path from the root to the leaves of the diagram, a sequence

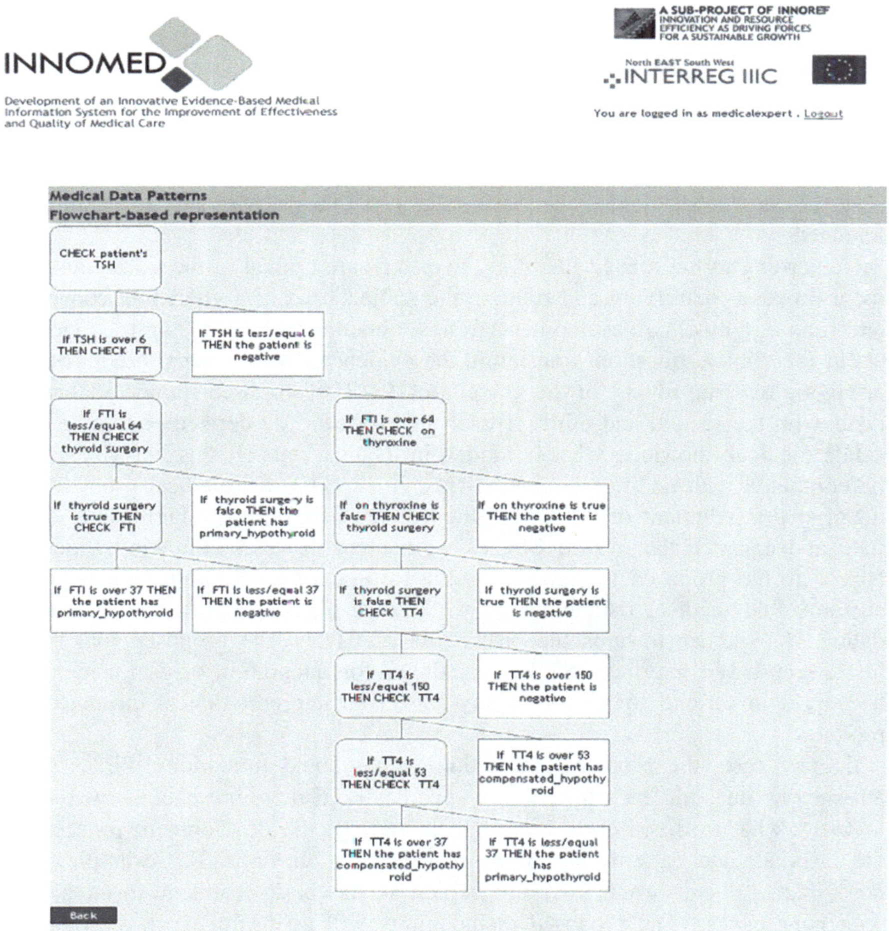

Fig. 16.7 Flowchart-like representation of a medical data pattern for the thyroid disease case

of check tests can be performed, resulting in the classification of a particular patient (or the indication of an advice to be followed).

The alternative or joint consideration of the proposed medical data patterns representations aids physicians obtain a complete picture, thus augmenting the quality of the medical decision-making process they follow. Moreover, the web-based tool developed to support the proposed methodology enables physicians to easily access and explore remote medical data, and to exploit the tool's features and functionalities through just a web browser.

16.4 Discussion

The development of CPGs is a difficult task that highly depends on evergrowing databases of patients data. As argued in [18], "the true value of such data lies in the users' ability to extract useful reports, spot interesting events and trends, support decisions and policy based on statistical analysis and inference, and exploit the data to achieve business, operational, or scientific goals; the problem of knowledge extraction from large databases involves many steps, ranging from data manipulation and retrieval to fundamental mathematical and statistical inference, search, and reasoning". The framework described in this paper has been developed in these lines, aiming to convert the available patients data to meaningful knowledge.

According to the related literature, five steps are critical in the CPGs development process: identifying and refining the subject area of a guideline, convening and running guideline development groups, obtaining and assessing the evidence about the clinical question, translating the evidence into a clinical guideline and arranging external review of the guideline [19]. The proposed framework mainly deals with the second and third steps of the process. The derived patterns encapsulate medical knowledge that is hidden in medical data. If this knowledge will be combined with additional, context-specific aspects of a medical problem and undergo the judgment of an expert, the derived patterns can significantly facilitate and enhance the overall CPGs development process. Following a generic approach, the proposed framework is able to produce easily understandable and customizable medical data patterns, while it also enables the easy accommodation of expertise towards the production of CPGs. The proposed tool is not just a web-based interface to Weka; it allows for integration of useful metadata and, most important, for a more easily conceived interpretation of the outcomes produced.

In any case, the proposed methodology has some limitations. First, it can answer one question each time. More specifically, if there are patients who want to know what to do in each step of their therapy, the development process for the medical data patterns has to be repeated for all steps. For example, suppose that a doctor wants to know which is the best treatment for a patient with bone cancer. The proposed methodology will give him the most appropriate treatment according to his/her patient's attributes, but will not tell him/her what to do after the implementation of the treatment. Second, we assume that the medical records to be processed through our approach do not contain false data that will train the algorithm erroneously and will lead to false medical data patterns. Another restriction concerning the data to be used is that the proposed methodology can only deal with categorical outputs. Being based on Weka software, we will have to choose from the list of attributes the one that we want to predict, but we are able to choose only categorical valued outputs (J48 allows only categorical attributes for output). Predictions, for instance, about what dose of a drug prescription is recommended (real valued output), cannot be handled.

However, we argue that the advantages of the proposed methodology surpass the above limitations. The proposed methodology is able to assist physicians elaborate big volumes of existing medical data (based on real patient records). The developed medical data patterns can help physicians discovering knowledge that is hidden in past cases. Thus, unnecessary tests are avoided, reducing the cost of a therapy and increasing the effectiveness of medical decision-making. Moreover, the developed medical data patterns can be applied to a particular patient, by giving the best individual solution. Besides, it advocates the exploitation of ML techniques in the development of medical data patterns with high accuracy. Issues taken into account during the overall development of the proposed methodology were user-friendliness, accuracy of results and alternative visualization of the outcomes. The semi-automation of the proposed methodology, augmented by the supporting web-based tool, provides physicians with an easy way to manage medical data. They do not need to have any particular ML expertise. The only thing they have to do is to load records and run the learning algorithm. Thereafter, they can use the developed medical data patterns as advisory statements for their decision-making. The criterion for their decision about the adoption of a particular medical data pattern can only be the accuracy level of the produced model.

Future work directions include the exploitation of additional ML algorithms, aiming to eliminate the restrictions of the proposed methodology. Also, the extension of the format currently used for the representation of the medical data patterns in order to deal with data interoperability and integration issues (e.g. data coming from different institutions, stored in different formats or manipulated by different software tools).

16.5 Conclusion

As clinical information is increasingly stored in computer databases, the opportunities for using this information to augment the quality of medical decision-making expand significantly. Current ML algorithms may significantly help practitioners to reveal interesting relationships in their data. This paper has proposed a ML-based hybrid methodology for the semi-automated development of medical data patterns. The proposed methodology is able to elaborate easily and effectively big volumes of data in order to produce advisory clinical knowledge of simple and usable formats, which may help physicians taking the correct actions in medical problems and enable the development of clinical practice guidelines. This methodology is supported by a web-based tool that is being tested in diverse clinical settings. Preliminary results are very positive in terms of ease-of-use and usability. Moreover, these results show that the tool's learning effort is not prohibitive, even for users that are not highly adept in the use of information technologies. In most cases, an introduction of half an hour was sufficient to get users acquainted with the tool's full range of features and functionalities.

Acknowledgments Research carried out in the context of this paper has been partially funded by the "INNO-MED: Development of an Innovative Evidence-Based Medical Information System for the Improvement of Effectiveness and Quality of Medical Care" Research Project (Interreg IIIC – East Zone – RFO INNOREF – INSP09). The authors would also like to thank Stavros Dimopoulos for his help in the development of the tool's interfaces.

References

1. Field M, Lohr K. Clinical Practice Guidelines: Directions for a New Program. , Washington, DC: National Academy Press, 1990.
2. Grimshaw J, Russell I. Effects of clinical guidelines on medical practice: a systematic review of rigorous evaluations. Lancet 1993;342:1317–1322.
3. Brouwers M, Browman G. Development of clinical practice guidelines: surgical perspective. World J Surg 1999;23(12):1236–1241.
4. Owens D, Nease R. Development of outcome-based practice guidelines: a method for structuring problems and synthesizing evidence. Jt Comm J Qual Improvement 1993;19:248–263.
5. Mitchell T. Machine Learning. New York: McGraw-Hill International Editions, 1997.
6. Cooper G, Aliferis C, Ambrosino R, Aronis J, Buchanan B, Caruana R, Fine M, Glymour C, Gordon G, Hanusa B, Janosky J, Meek C, Mitchell T, Richardson T, Spirtes P. An evaluation of machine-learning methods for predicting pneumonia mortality. Artif Intell Med 1997;9(2):107–138.
7. Kukar M, Kononenko I, Silvester T. Machine learning in prognosis of the femoral neck fracture recovery. Artif Intell Med 1996;8:431–451.
8. Mani S, Shankle W, Dick M, Pazzani M. Two-stage machine learning model for guideline development. Artif Intell Med 1999;16(1):51–71.
9. Woolery L, Crzymala-Busse J. Machine learning for an expert system to predict preterm British risk. J Am Inform Assoc 1994;1(6):439–446.
10. Zupan B, Demsar J, Kattan M, Beck J and. Bratko I. Machine learning for survival analysis: a case study on recurrence of prostate cancer. Artif Intell Med 2000;20(1):59–75.
11. Kononenko I. Machine learning for medical diagnosis: history, state of the art and perspective. Artif Intell Med 2001;23(1):89–109.
12. Soman T, Bobbie P. Classification of arrhythmia using machine learning techniques. WSEAS Trans Comput 2005;4(6):548–552.
13. Quinlan R. C4.5: Programs for Machine Learning. San Mateo, CA: Morgan Kaufmann Publishers, 1993.
14. Clercq P, Blom J, Korsten H, Hasman A. Approaches for creating computer-interpretable guidelines that facilitate decision support. Artif Intell Med 2004;31(1):1–27.
15. Peleg M, Tu S, Bury J, Ciccarese P, Fox J, Greenes R, Hall R, Johnson P, Jones N, Kumar A, Miksch S, Quaglini S, Seyfang A, Shortliffe E, Stefanelli M. Comparing computer-interpretable guideline models: a case study approach. J Am Med Inform Assoc 2003;10(1):52–68.
16. Wang D, Peleg M, Tu S, Boxwala A, Greenes R, Patel V, Shortliffe E. Representation primitives, process models and patient data in computer-interpretable clinical practice guidelines: A literature review of guideline representation models. Int J Med Inform 2002;68(1):59–70.
17. Hripcsak G, Clayton P, Pryor T, Haug P, Wigertz O, Van der Lei J. The Arden Syntax for Medical Logic Modules. Proceedings of the 14th Annual Symposium on Computer Applications in Medical Care 1990;200–204.
18. Fayyad U, Piatetsky-Shapiro G, Smyth P. The KDD process for extracting useful knowledge from volumes of data. Commun ACM 1996;39(11):27–34.
19. Shekelle P, Woolf S, Eccles M, Grimshaw J. Clinical guidelines: developing guidelines. Br Med J 1999;318:593–596.

Chapter 17
Telemedicine for the Diabetic Foot: A Model for Improving Medical Care, Developing Decision Support Systems, and Reducing Medical Cost

Adriana Fodor and Eddy Karnieli

Abstract The main purpose of this chapter is to discuss the place of telemedicine in the modern medicine, its present and future application in the clinical medicine. It covers aspects of clinical telemedicine practice, technical advances, principles and practices, health policy and regulation, and health services research dealing with clinical effectiveness, efficacy, and safety of telemedicine and its effects on quality, cost, and accessibility of care. The diabetic foot problem was chosen as a suitable model to examine whether the use of telemedicine technology will improve the quality of medicine and reduce medical costs.

According to the American Telemedicine Association, telemedicine is the exchange of medical information from one site to another using electronic communication, such as telephone, Internet or videoconference to improve patients' health status [1]. Related with telemedicine is the term "telehealth," which covers a quite broader definition of remote healthcare, being more focused on other health-related services that do not always involve direct patient clinical services. Telemedicine practices allow for specialist consultation, direct patient consultation, patient monitoring, and medical education.

Although the term telemedicine is a relatively recent one, since 1970s, medicine has long made use of various communication technologies dating back to 1906. Wilhelm Einthoven, inventor of the electrocardiograph, created the "telecardiogram," which transmitted electrocardiograms via telephone from the clinic to his office, enabling him to monitor his patients' condition at a distance [2]. In the early 1990s, telemedicine experienced a considerable progress due to rapid advancements in information and telecommunications technologies and digital data transmission. Since then, the interest in the use of telemedicine procedures and the number of related publications had rapidly increased. A search of MEDLINE in 1990 found six publications on telemedicine; while by February 2009 there were more than 10,700 entries under the search term "telemedicine."

A. Fodor (✉)
Institute of Endocrinology, Diabetes and Metabolism, Rambam Medical Center, Haifa, Israel; Diabetes, Nutrition and Metabolic Diseases Center, Cluj-Napoca, Romania
e-mail: adifodor@yahoo.com

A. Lazakidou (ed.), *Web-Based Applications in Healthcare and Biomedicine*, Annals of Information Systems 7, DOI 10.1007/978-1-4419-1274-9_17,
© Springer Science+Business Media, LLC 2010

17.1 Clinical Applications of Telemedicine

The potential applications for telemedicine cover the entire field of healthcare, ranging from general practitioners and specialists to hospitals, research and teaching institutions. Telemedicine provides also access to medical care to underserved areas.

The main benefits of telemedicine, as identified by the recent reports, were increased access to health services, cost savings, reduced hospitalizations, enhanced educational opportunities, improved health outcomes, better quality of care, better quality of life and enhanced social support [3–5].

17.1.1 Specialist and Primary Care Consultations

Accordingly to American Telemedicine Association, specialist and primary care consultations may involve a patient "seeing" a health professional over a live video connection or it may use diagnostic images and/or video along with patient data to a specialist for viewing later. This may be used for primary care or for specialist referrals [1]. There is an increasing number of specialty and subspecialty areas that have successfully used telemedicine. Major specialty areas actively using telemedicine include dermatology, ophthalmology, mental health, cardiology, and pathology.

Compensating infrastructural deficits related to geographical location is one of the central goals of telemedicine. Many of the first pilot projects in telemedicine were conducted in remote areas with insufficient healthcare access. Telemedicine enabled people in rural remote areas, conflict and crisis areas, during disasters, the "Third World," and on airplanes, oil platforms, and boats to be cared for and treated by medical facilities located far away [6–10]. In addition to primary diagnosis and treatment planning, telemedicine allows isolated doctors to contact consulting specialists in order to obtain a second opinion and thereby avoiding moving the patient to another location.

Different telemedicine providers have developed networks to provide specialist advice. Some are focused on certain geographical areas like the US army, which provides a web-based teleconsulting service for civil or military hospitals around the Pacific [11]. The RAFT network provides services in nine African countries with a team of specialists based in Geneva [12]. Partners Healthcare, whose specialists are based in the United States and in a tertiary hospital in Phnom Penh, provides support to health workers in northern Cambodia [13]. Other organizations operate globally. The Swinfen Charitable Trust works with more than 100 hospitals around the world, mainly in developing countries and also in some remote areas like the remotest island in the world, Tristan da Cunha. They provide specialist advice from a very large team spread over 13 countries [14].

Telemedicine enables also international exchange of expert opinion. Medical professionals can communicate with colleagues across the globe. Online forums provide doctors with an opportunity to discuss diagnostic and treatment issues, enhancing quality in medicine.

Implementation of telehealth technologies in provider-to-provider care settings had led to a reduction in hospital admissions from emergency departments [15] as well as a reduction in the need for referrals from emergency departments to outside specialists [16]. The use of telehealth technologies to speed the diagnosis in cases where rapid diagnosis is critical for the outcomes was beneficial in the management of acute strokes [17]. Similarly, the use of telehealth technologies in ambulances can also speed the diagnosis and the initiation of important, potentially lifesaving interventions [18].

Telemedicine technology (TMT) at a remote work site offers a convenient alternative to face-to-face visits with providers located at distance from the work site [19]. It is well received by both patients and providers. Patients reported that the telemedicine visit saved them time and the inconvenience in appointment scheduling, travel to and from the clinic visit, absenteeism secondary to the illness and redistribution of work. From the employer's view point, telemedicine services provided a cost-effective medical care [19].

A recent comprehensive analysis undertaken by Center for Information Technology Leadership has found that the potential benefit of implementing telehealth technologies in emergency departments, correctional facilities, nursing homes, and physician offices, far outweighs the costs [20].

Most telemedicine transactions occur within the borders of a single country. In these circumstances, the activity is subject to the laws of that country being mostly regulated. However, telemedicine is also practiced internationally. Extraterritorial jurisdiction is stipulated by US Constitution and requires the states to cooperate with each other when serving process and in the extradition of out-of-state defendants. Unfortunately, in the international arena such cooperation is not assured and the global market for telemedicine services is largely unregulated. It seems unlikely that many foreign countries would extradite their telemedicine providers to the United States or other countries to face trial for unlawful practice, especially if that provider is bringing lots of money into the country through the export of medical services [21].

17.1.2 Imaging Services

Imaging services make the greatest use of telemedicine; thousands of images each year are sent to the specialist over broadband networks and diagnosed with a report sent back. Medical imaging used to be primarily within the domain of radiology; but with the growth in imaging technology, it has been seen in pathology, dermatology, ophthalmology, and cardiology. It is estimated that over 400 hospitals in the United States alone outsource some of their medical imaging services [1]. As telemedicine of remote medical images is not the focus of this chapter, the reader is referred to another review [22].

17.1.3 Home Telehealth

Home telehealth is defined as a service that gives the clinician the ability to remotely monitor and measure patient health data in their home. Remote patient monitoring applications might include telemetry devices to capture a specific vital sign, such as blood glucose or heart ECG or a more sophisticated device to capture a variety of indicators for homebound patients. Such services can be used to supplement the use of visiting nurses [1].

Healthcare professionals are increasingly faced with a rapidly aging population, with an increased prevalence of long-term conditions and preference of elderly people or those with chronic conditions to maintain their independence and continue living in their own homes. At the same time, it is unlikely that in the near future there will be enough nurses to support them adequately and it is also possible that there will be a lack of facilities to accommodate them. One approach to solve the problem is the application of telemedicine in the home environment, i.e. home telecare, also known as home-based e-health or telehomecare.

The number of home telehealth programs implemented and the number of publications detailing positive outcomes for chronic disease management, preventive care, and self-management have increased over the past years. Populations that show the clearest benefits include diabetes, chronic obstructive pulmonary disease, chronic wounds and congestive heart failure [3,4,23,24].

One of the largest telehealth programs is Columbia University's Informatics for Diabetes Education and Telemedicine Project funded by Centers for Medicare & Medicaid Services. This project used a random control trial methodology to select and compare telemedicine case management to usual care, in 1,665 diabetic subjects in New York State, using a home telemedicine unit with videoconference access, remote monitoring of glucose and blood pressure. The project showed improved patient values for glycosylated hemoglobin, blood pressure, and low-density lipoprotein cholesterol [25]. Another example is the Veterans Health Administration (VHA) Care Coordination Services' program. This home telehealth program was implement in 21 integrated service networks of VHA and has served more than 40,000 veterans. The program has demonstrated clear benefits in terms of positive clinical, quality, and financial outcomes for patients with a variety of chronic diseases, since 2003 [26].

As synthesized by Kobb et al. [27], many areas of healthcare could benefit from home telehealth:

- The need to effectively manage the epidemic numbers of people living with chronic diseases.
- The need to improve access to care, increase work efficiency and handle clinician shortages, especially for underserved populations.
- The opportunity to help elders age in place, reducing the costs of institutional care.
- The opportunity to make healthcare a twenty-first-century process by providing seamless, patient-driven care in the right place and at the right time.

A variety of technologies were used for home telecare of the elderly. The main issue is whether these applications meet the needs of elderly people suffering from chronic diseases adequately. The majority of publications reported the use of telecommunication devices for assessing the physical and/or cognitive condition of a patient. They employed videoconference, audio-visual, and telehealth communication units for virtual visits. During these virtual visits the patient was supported, educated on topics related to their status, and consulted for the better management of their disease. The second large category dealt with telemonitoring. The information transmitted was physiological data such as vital signs, symptoms, blood glucose values, blood pressure, and ECGs. This was sent to a central repository via the Internet or a conventional telephone line. The patient's position was monitored using various technologies such as positioning devices with radio frequency identification (RFID) tags, remote video cameras, e-textiles, or sensors.

Studies in patients who were suffering from non-cognitive diseases (hypertension, heart failure, emphysema, coronary artery disease and diabetes) reported that the technology was easy to use and helpful in managing their chronic conditions [26]. Similarly, patients with COPD or chronic heart failure felt comfortable with the videoconference and the other peripheral devices they used [28]. Wilkins et al. [29] indicated that 98% of patients were satisfied when using a web-based teleconsultation system for the care of their chronic wounds. However, home telecare was not always found to be user-friendly for people who had Alzheimer's disease or dementia; due to their learning difficulties they often failed to respond to an established videoconference session [30,31]. As a consequence, the benefit of home telecare in these cognitive diseases over the traditional methods was not significant.

All home telehealth systems should fulfill the following requirements:

- be simple to use;
- operate without interruptions;
- provide computer security and data confidentiality;
- the service should be continuously available.

As long as data confidentiality and security were ensured, there was no major ethical or legal problem with the use of home telehealth in most published studies.

In many studies there were cost reductions in terms of time saving, elimination of traveling expenses, fewer visits to the emergency room, fewer hospitalizations, improved patient compliance with treatment plans, improved patient satisfaction with health services, and improved quality of life [32,33]. These reductions balanced the substantial cost of some home telecare devices. Unfortunately, very few countries have consistent reimbursement policies for home telecare services and most of them are in the public sector [27].

Organizational and societal changes, such as cost reduction policies and an aging population, are the main driving forces for the development of home telecare, especially for elderly patients.

In the future, simple supervision tasks may be handed over by robots. The "Wakamaru" robot (Mitsubishi Heavy Industries, Shinagawa, Japan) is equipped with cameras and can be controlled by voice. The pictures collected by the robot can be transmitted to mobile phones and computers. The Wakamaru robot can monitor elderly patients and their health conditions, report deviation from daily activities, and oversee security in the house [34]. Other robot is "Dr Robot" (InTouch Health, Inc., Santa Barbara, CA, USA), operated by a doctor, which can conduct a ward round and check up on patients [35].

Through the implantation of miniature electronic devices (MEMS – Micro Electro-Mechanical Systems), it is possible to observe various biological functions. The company CardioMEMS (Atlanta, GA, USA) produces MEMS monitoring equipment that can be implanted in the body for transmitting information about blood flow and pressure wirelessly to computer equipment located outside and near the body. Finally, RFID technology offers the possibility of monitoring food, clothes, and the articles that a person uses at home by marking each item with an RFID tag. The RFID tags can be made thin enough to be embedded in labels and tickets, and it is possible to both read and write data to an RFID tag.

The main problems in establishing home telecare systems are the lack of:

- Global guidelines for the practical implementation of home telecare applications. In 1998, the American Telemedicine Association developed the first home telecare clinical guidelines to assist healthcare providers in making decisions about purchasing different technologies and implementing telehealth programs; these guidelines were revised in 2001 [36];
- Consistent reimbursement policies [27];
- Scientific evidence to demonstrate the effectiveness of home telecare applications (random controlled trial [RCT] studies) [27];
- An evaluation framework which considers the legal, ethical, organizational, economical, clinical, usability, quality, and technical aspects [37].

17.1.4 Remote Medical Education and Consumer Information

Remote medical education and consumer information include a number of activities including: continuing medical education credits for health professionals and special medical education seminars for targeted groups in remote locations; the use of call centers and Internet web sites for consumers to obtain specialized health information and on-line discussion groups to provide peer-to-peer support [1].

E-learning has opened up new possibilities in the continuing medical education. Rapid advancements in medical research require that doctors continually be aware of current developments. *E-learning* avoids restrictions imposed by time and location on attending training programs, seminars, and conferences in person [38,39]. Access to medical literature, for example, is made easier by online databases.

17.2 Procedures

Current methods of image and data transmission basically use two main modes of sharing information: store and forward systems and real-time consultations [40,41].

Store-and-forward systems (SAF) transmit digital photographs, video clips, or clinical data. These are initially stored individually on data storage units. The physician can then view the data via e-mail, a web site, or a file on a shared server at her or his convenience. The sender and the recipient could be available at different times. This method also allows a relatively large number of cases to be evaluated in a brief period of time. A disadvantage is that there is no direct communication. Participants are not able to ask questions directly; the physician is thus unable to obtain a more comprehensive patient history. In addition, the recipient only views the selected portion of the image and can thus miss an important secondary diagnosis. In other words, the recipient must rely on the information chosen by the sender. Given the lower requirements in terms of bandwidth for data transmission and technical equipment, SAF is comparatively more affordable than real-time communication. The necessary technical equipment (e.g., digital camera, computer, and modem) is cheaper and widely available. An acceptable transfer delays for store-and-forward procedure (asynchronous) is considered on average less than 24 h [40,41] (Table 17.1).

Table 17.1 Comparison of Advantages and Disadvantages of Real-Time and Store-and-Forward Methods

Real time (synchronous)	Store-and-forward (asynchronous)
Real-time transmission (interactive, delay time less than 1 min)	Delayed transmission (average less than 24 h)
The sender and receiver must be available at the same time for consultation	The sender and receiver could be available at different times for consultation
The recipient may ask the sender for supplementary information	The recipient must rely on the information chosen by the sender
Consultation takes comparatively longer	Consultation takes comparatively less time
Transmission requires higher bandwidth	Transmission requires lower bandwidth (telephone connection is sufficient)
More expensive	Cheaper
Equipment is usually not portable	Equipment is light and portable

Real-time consultations (RT) use systems that enable simultaneous communication between participants, most commonly in the form of videoconferencing between patients and physicians. Real-time telemedicine also covers simple phone calls and tele-surgery procedures. The advantage lies in direct interaction between the sender and the recipient. This requires, however, that all participants be present at the same predetermined time. Individual sessions generally last as long or even longer than traditional face-to-face consultations. The technical requirements and equipment costs as well as technical problems are usually higher than in store-and-forward systems. For real-time transmission (synchronous communication), the acceptable transfer delays is on average less than 1 min [40,41] (Table 17.1). A few systems combine features of both methods, allowing, for example, data to be sent ahead and then discussed in a videoconference.

17.3 Obstacles and Concerns

- One disadvantage of clinical evaluation is lacking findings on palpation, an important diagnostic criteria. The healthcare provider is forced to rely on descriptions.
- A further disadvantage is that the physician only views selected images rather than the entire surface of the skin (as ideally occurs in face-to-face examinations). This can result in missing important information.
- Medicine will become less personal as a result of increasing “mechanization,” and telemedicine consultations will affect important aspects of the physician–patient relationship (such as direct communication and touch).
- Data security is a problem in all information technologies, but it is a particularly important issue in health care. For electronic transmission of patient data, the doctor must ensure that the data are adequately protected, e.g., by means of electronic encoding (cryptography). In addition, data and images should be anonymous so that individual patients cannot be identified. This may be done by using a pseudonym in place of the actual patient name and ensuring that the patient’s face is unrecognizable. Access should be restricted to authorized persons (confidentiality).
- The entire telemedicine consultation should be archived and verifiable, for example, with regard to treatment recommendations made by the physician. There are still legal questions that need to be resolved with regard to responsibility and liability in long-distance diagnoses and treatment. Precise records should be kept during a telemedicine consultation for a later time reconstruction of the data.
- Telemedicine changes the structure of healthcare in such a manner that patients can more readily seek a specialist rather than first consulting a general practitioner and getting a referral. This does not sit well with many doctors who feel threatened by a change in traditional structures.

17.4 Determinants of Telemedicine Implementation

Although it is largely accepted that telemedicine could bring quantitative and qualitative improvement for future healthcare system, many telemedicine initiatives do not survive the research phase or they become a failure in daily practice. Apparently, the implementation of telemedicine initiatives in regular healthcare practice is difficult.

A comprehensive overview of the determinants which influence the success of telemedicine implementations was conducted by Broens et al. [42]. It was shown that *technology* and *acceptance* were the two most reported determinants in the reviewed papers (together 66%) while *organization, financing,* and *policy and legislation*comprised the remaining 34%. The review showed that the major issues for technological acceptance of telemedicine systems were: the availability of support to users, appropriate training for users, usability of the system, and the quality of the devices and network communications. Technology acceptance was also influenced by the patients' and professionals' attitudes towards TMT. Evidence-based medicine was also regarded as a requirement for professional acceptance of TMT.

Costs associated with telemedicine implementation are related to: investments, maintenance and operational costs of the new system. In the research stages of telemedicine, these costs are funded. However, as soon as the projects are ended, there is a lack of financing structure to support the clinical implementation. Most insurance companies do not have standard tariffs for telemedicine services. The implementation and full adoption of telehealth technologies needs a reimbursement model that favors face-to-face visits.

The introduction of telemedicine lead to internal organizational consequences, combined with changes in collaborations with other healthcare organizations. For instance, telemedicine might require changes in collaboration and roles of the teams' members, changes in composition of the personnel, rights, and responsibilities. Thus, a successful telemedicine implementation needs a re-thinking of the internal and external organization [43].

The proper legislation and policy are a prerequisite for telemedicine implementation. Unfortunately, the current legislation and policy do not support many telemedicine applications.

Adequate security mechanisms should be taken into account for successful telemedicine implementations.

It is accepted that proper evaluation framework for telemedicine is needed in order to convince professionals, policy makers, and insurance companies about implementation [37].

17.5 Diabetic FootTMT Model

The purpose of this project was to examine whether the use of TMT will improve quality of medicine and reduce medical costs. The diabetic foot problem was chosen as suitable model to examine this hypothesis, as it is a typical and complex example for a relatively common problem (15% of patients with diabetes suffer from this complication [44]), which requires early diagnosis and treatment by a multi-disciplinary team. This clinical situation eventually results in high medical costs due to the need for expensive antibiotic drugs, multiple and long hospitalization periods, loss of working days, and in many cases, permanent disability due to limb amputation. Therefore, successful implementation of this model will have a distinct beneficial impact on the clinical outcome and will clearly contribute to significant reduction of medical expenses and disabilities.

Brief summary of the main principals of the treatment include:

- Infection treatment – includes disinfection, wide-range antibiotics, and microbial tests.
- Foot care – rest and adjustment of special footwear to prevent pressure.
- Surgical intervention – surgical debridement of the injured area and removal of necrotic tissues; in severe cases – limb amputation.
- Facilitating blood supply to the injured area – meticulous examination of the area applying noninvasive (Doppler, etc.) and/or invasive (angiography) techniques and use of artery by-pass surgery as needed.
- Tight glycemic control – by use of oral hypoglycemic drugs or insulin injections.
- Closure of diabetic wounds – by newer biotechnological ointments (synthetic growth factors) or hyperbaric oxygen therapy or plastic surgery.

Obviously, such diverse therapies require a set of combined and coordinated expertise that is usually unavailable in a single location at the same time. Applying the correct and suitable therapeutic regimen can significantly reduce the need for limb amputation.

Various reasons like Sick Fund policies, transportation problems, and the obvious impaired mobility of diabetic foot patients result in a situation where most of the medical care is handled by the family practitioner. Consultation and referral to specialists take place only once the condition of the patient has severely deteriorated. Practically, the panel of experts needed to treat such complicated cases is remotely located at the medical center. Moreover, seldom are all the specialists concomitantly available for consultation and treatment.

While healthcare has become more complex in general, shared care and frequent communication between primary (family practitioner) and secondary/tertiary care providers (ambulatory/hospital settings) are still unsatisfactory both in Israel and worldwide.

Thereby we examined the hypothesis that by implementing TMT based medical record will virtually bring the consultant to the community clinic and allow multitask and concomitant consultations.

In order to enable medical consultation from a far place using the Internet, a web-based computerized medical patient record software on Oracle data base was established (WebPCR). The web site is located on the hospital web and protected by a fire-wall. Patient data, which include historical details, physical examination, laboratory tests, and relevant digital photos of the diabetic foot, were entered directly into the system from 10 different primary clinics after a short training, with no need for special software implementation. It became apparent that the data accumulated in the current medical record software used at the physicians' office cannot be simply or quickly transferred from the local clinic computerized record to our WebCPR. Thus, the physicians had to fill the data into both systems. Unfortunately, no simple technical solution could be offered probably because of the practitioner clinical record previous design. Lack of time allotted for the examination of the patients in the clinic interfered with entering data into the system in real time. The nursing staff became a significant factor due to their initiative in examining the foot and photographing it and uploading it into WebCPR. Data from 81 patients with diabetic foot from the north of Israel were filed in our WebCPR. All patients had a diagnosis diabetic foot and 54% had evidence of diabetic ulcer. Concomitantly, approximately 35% also suffered from other diabetic debilitating complications (retinopathy and nephropathy). A selected staff of specialists from the Rambam Medical Center, experts in various medical fields (i.e., diabetes, orthopedic surgery, plastic surgery, etc.), gave the telemedicine consultations. The communication and consultation between the practitioners and the experts was executed directly within the WebCPR after sending/receiving an email message. Response time for consultation was between 1 and 24 h. While we first tried to use videoconference with the patient present, it became apparent that timing and slow Internet communications are major impediments.

Access to information was limited to participants in the project. For confidentiality, data input did not include personal identification details of the patients. Patients were identified by a leading number, which was assigned by the secure server application once the on-line record was filed. Thus, in practice, only the family practitioner knew the full personal details of his/her patient. Only participants in the project had access to the database, thus allowing for mutual discussions and analyses of the data available. Data storage, updating and adjusting were secured using a firewall (Fig. 17.1).

Further, in order to increase the quality assurance, we have constructed a computerized decision support system. This novel system uses computer-interpretable guideline modeling language – Guide Line Interchange Format (GLIF3) incorporated with Protégé-2000 tool and based on the clinical guidelines [45] acceptable in the field of diabetic foot. The system has been integrated with the WebPCR. The system on-line examines data entry, the processing, and the decisions taken by the physician and compares them to the existing guidelines. As a result, computer-assisted automatic decision support is presented with warnings and suggestions to the user. Decision support system was tested, run on the actual data base, but has not yet been implemented clinically [46].

Although definitive cost-efficiency analyses are not ready at this time, we believe that improvement in quality and cost reduction of medical care would be achieved by:

- Early and more accurate diagnosis of the "risky diabetic foot" by TMT protocol and pictures revised by the distant consultants and future developed software;
- Improving the inter-communication and consultation among the medical caretakers, i.e., the clinic's nurse, family practitioner, and specialists in their various locations;
- Saving commuting and consultation time to ensure best patient-tailored treatment;
- Eliminating the need for repeated, and sometimes superfluous diagnostic tests;

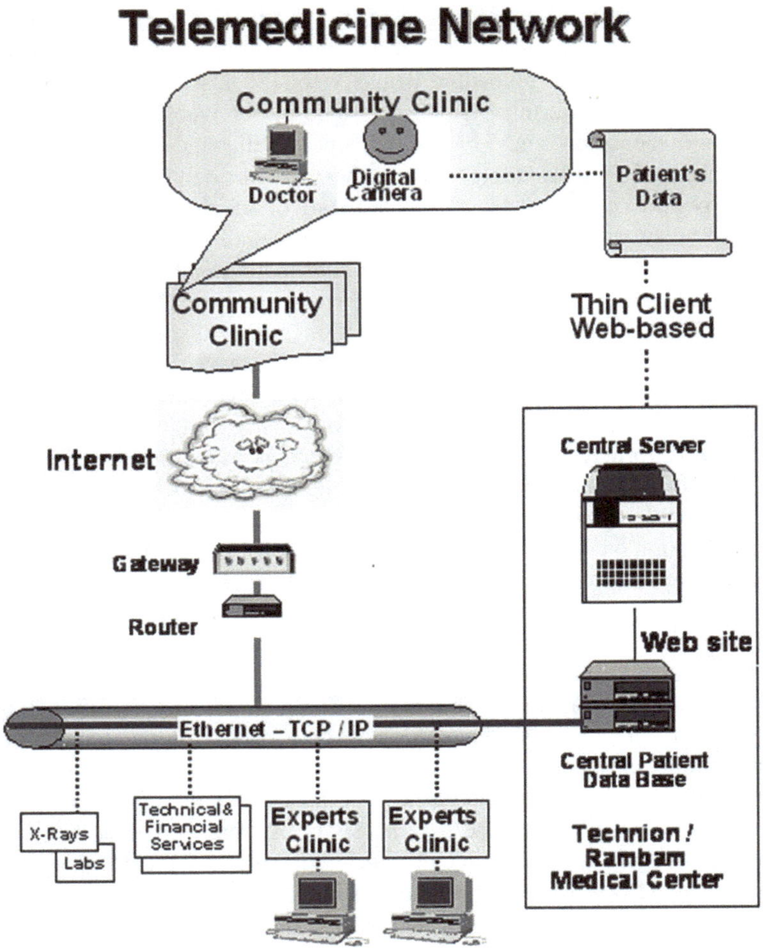

Fig. 17.1 Schematic description of end-user software and database in the TMT network

- Providing early, real-time, multidisciplinary, and high-quality care that could reduce the frequency and the extent of hospitalization as well as disability due to improper treatment;
- Enhancing the quality of treatment and enriching the medical knowledge.
- Applying TMT to implement decision support systems will serve and reinforce all the above-mentioned purposes.
- Transfer protocols from the clinic patient data to WebCPR or similar would make telemedicine consultations more efficient and time-saving.

Thus, web-based computerized medical records are excellent tools for central quality assurance and cost containment procedures. The integration of computerized guideline-based decision support system with the WebCPR as we have developed (or other similar ones) will further improve rapid diagnosis and treatment in diabetic foot and other complex diseases.

Telemedicine based on WebCPR enabled the physician in the community efficient, fast, simultaneous access to the various distant professional consultants in or outside Israel. Good-quality consultations, in a significantly shorter time span than a regular visit in the outpatient clinic, make telemedicine a good alternative for consultation referrals that are impeded by the Sick funds.

Several telecare systems focusing on the diabetic patient have been developed. Most are aimed at home monitoring in order to assist in controlling the patient's blood glucose levels, but only a few are focused on diabetic foot [29,47–50].

In the study of Bangs et al. [47], clinical information and digital photographs were collected from six patients with diabetic ulcers by the home-visiting nurses and sent by email to the vascular surgeon for assessment. Where appropriate, a teleconsultation between the patient and a vascular surgeon was set at the primary care centre. Beneficial effects were reported in terms of patient's satisfaction, travel expenses saving, prioritization of cases, and more rapid care for urgent cases.

In a similar, small pilot study [48,49], five patients were offered three teleconsultations at their homes by a visiting nurse in collaboration with experts at the hospital, through a mobile phone with integrated camera. In spite of many technical problems related to the limited bandwidth of the videophones (connection problems, unsatisfactory quality of live images and audio quality), the patients were satisfied and found the equipment easy to use while the doctors could prescribe treatment at a distance. A difficult task was to schedule the real-time consultation; it requires that visiting nurse, the patient, and the hospital doctor simultaneously select a time to suit all.

Wilbright et al. [50] reported similar rates of ulcer healing between 20 patients treated by a specialist nurse guided by a specialist team through a real-time videoconference, compare with a control group of patients treated face-to-face by the specialist group. While efficient wound healing was obtained, telemedicine allowed overcoming the distance, transportation, and economic barriers of patients from rural locations to visit the specialists.

In other study, a multidisciplinary wound care team located at the regional tertiary care center provided telemedicine consultations for 56 patients with chronic wounds (diabetic and vascular) located in remote VHA outpatient clinics by means of nurse specialists and a store-forward approach. Most of the patients and referring providers indicated a high degree of satisfaction with the teleconsultation system [29].

The rapid and ongoing development of the social and medical uses of information and communication technologies is changing the landscape of health care practice forever. Telemedicine can be seen as a new method of service delivery supported by new technology and existing technology used in new ways. It is likely that in the future every physician will be directly or indirectly confronted with telemedicine; many already have long been using "telemedicine procedures" in the broadest sense. Even the best medical innovation is virtually worthless if it is not accepted by patients and physicians. Large-scale telemedicine implementation implies parallel efforts and a visionary approach: "start small, think big".

References

1. American Telemedicine Association Web site. ATA Defining Telemedicine. http://www.americantelemed.org. Accessed 15 March 2009.
2. Stanberry B. Telemedicine: barriers and opportunities in the 21st century. J Intern Med 2000;247:615–628.
3. Botsis T, Hartvigsen G. Current status and future perspectives in telecare for elderly people suffering from chronic diseases. J Telemed Telecare 2008;14:195–203.
4. Bowles KH, Baugh AC. Applying research evidence to optimize telehomecare. J Cardiovasc Nurs 2007;22:5–15.
5. Jennett PA, Affleck Hall L, Hailey D et al. The socio-economic impact of telehealth: A systematic review. J Telemed Telecare 2003;9:311–320.
6. Mack D, Brantley KM, Bell KG. Mitigating the health effects of disasters for medically underserved populations: Electronic health records, telemedicine, research, screening, and surveillance. J Health Care Poor Underserved 2007;18:432–442.
7. Mair F, Fraser S, Ferguson J et al. Telemedicine via satellite to support offshore oil platforms. J Telemed Telecare 2008;14:129–131.
8. McGee R, Tangalos EG. Delivery of health care to the underserved: Potential contributions of telecommunications technology. Consensus conference entitled "Telemedicine and Access to Care". Mayo Clin Proc 1994;69:1131–1136.
9. Raza T, Joshi M, Schapira RM et al. Pulmonary telemedicine – a model to access the subspecialist services in underserved rural areas. Int J Med Inform 2009;78:53–59.
10. Wootton R. Telemedicine support for the developing world. J Telemed Telecare 2008;14: 109–114.
11. Callahan CW, Malone F, Estroff D et al. Effectiveness of an Internet-based store-and-forward telemedicine system for pediatric subspecialty consultation. Arch Pediatr Adolesc Med 2005;159:389–393.
12. Geissbuhler A, Bagayoko CO, Ly O. The RAFT network: 5 years of distance continuing medical education and tele-consultations over the Internet in French-speaking Africa. Int J Med Inform 2007;76:351–356.
13. Brandling-Bennett HA, Kedar I, Pallin DJ et al. Delivering health care in rural Cambodia via store-and-forward telemedicine: A pilot study. Telemed J E Health 2005;11:56–62.
14. Vassallo DJ, Swinfen P, Swinfen R et al. Experience with a low-cost telemedicine system in three developing countries. J Telemed Telecare 2001;7(pl 1):56–58.
15. Stamford P, Bickford T, Hsiao H et al. The significance of telemedicine in a rural emergency department. IEEE Eng Med Biol Mag 1999;18:45–52.
16. Beach M, Goodall I, Miller P. Evaluating telemedicine for minor injuries units. J Telemed Telecare 2000;6(Suppl 1):S90–S92.
17. Schwamm LH, Rosenthal ES, Hirshberg A et al. Virtual TeleStroke support for the emergency department evaluation of acute stroke. Acad Emerg Med 2004;11:1193–1197.
18. Haskins PA, Ellis DG, Mayrose J. Predicted utilization of emergency medical services telemedicine in decreasing ambulance transports. Prehosp Emerg Care 2002;6:445–448.
19. Varkey P, Schumacher K, Swanton C et al. Telemedicine in the work site: A study of feasibility, and patient and provider satisfaction. J Telemed Telecare 2008;14: 322–325.
20. Pan E, Cusack C, Hook J et al. The value of provider-to-provider telehealth. Telemed J E Health 2008;14:446–453.
21. McLean TR, McLean AB. Hageseth's principle of extraterritorial jurisdiction and international telemedicine. J Telemed Telecare 2008;14:282–284.

22. Krupinski EA, Jiang Y. Anniversary paper: Evaluation of medical imaging systems. Med Phys 2008;35:645–659.
23. Finkelstein SM, Speedie SM, Demiris G et al. Telehomecare: Quality, perception, satisfaction. Telemed J E Health 2004;10:122–128.
24. Hailey D, Roine R, Ohinmaa A. Systematic review of evidence for the benefits of telemedicine. J Telemed Telecare 2002;8(Suppl 1):1–30.
25. Shea S, Weinstock RS, Starren J et al. A randomized trial comparing telemedicine case management with usual care in older, ethnically diverse, medically underserved patients with diabetes mellitus. J Am Med Inform Assoc 2006;13:40–51.
26. Darkins A, Ryan P, Kobb R et al. Care Coordination/Home Telehealth: The systematic implementation of health informatics, home telehealth, and disease management to support the care of veteran patients with chronic conditions. Telemed J E Health 2008;14:1118–1126.
27. Kobb R, Chumbler NR, Brennan DM et al. Home telehealth: Mainstreaming what we do well. Telemed J E Health 2008;14:977–981.
28. Whitten P, Mickus M. Home telecare for COPD/CHF patients: Outcomes and perceptions. J Telemed Telecare 2007;13:69–73.
29. Wilkins EG, Lowery JC, Goldfarb S. Feasibility of virtual wound care: A pilot study. Adv Skin Wound Care 2007;20:275–276, 278.
30. Duke C. The Frail Elderly Community-Based Case Management Project. Geriatr Nurs 2005;26:122–127.
31. mith GE, Lunde AM, Hathaway JC et al. Telehealth home monitoring of solitary persons with mild dementia. Am J Alzheimers Dis Other Demen 2007;22:20–26.
32. Rojas SV, Gagnon MP. A systematic review of the key indicators for assessing telehomecare cost-effectiveness. Telemed J E Health 2008;14:896–904.
33. Seto E. Cost comparison between telemonitoring and usual care of heart failure: A systematic review. Telemed J E Health 2008;14:679–686.
34. Toshiyuri K. The robot designed to "live with humans" 2003. http://www.mhi.co.jp/kobe/wakamaru/english/know/design/index.html. Accessed 15 March 2009.
35. Stephenson G. Dr Robot Tested at Hopkins 2003. http://wwwhopkinsmedicineorg/press/2003/AUGUST/030805HTM. Accessed 15 March 2009.
36. Britton BP. First home telehealth clinical guidelines developed by the American Telemedicine Association. Home Health Nurse 2003;21:703–706.
37. Brown M, Shaw N. Evaluation practices of a major Canadian telehealth provider: Lessons and future directions for the field. Telemed J E Health 2008;14:769–774.
38. Giansanti D, Castrichella L, Giovagnoli MR. New models of e-learning for healthcare professionals: A training course for biomedical laboratory technicians. J Telemed Telecare 2007;13:374–376.
39. Groth K, Olin K, Gran O et al. The role of technology in video-mediated consensus meetings. J Telemed Telecare 2008;14:349–353.
40. Clarke M, Thiyagarajan CA. A systematic review of technical evaluation in telemedicine systems. Telemed J E Health 2008;14:170–183.
41. Lim AC, Egerton IB, Shumack SP. Australian teledermatology: The patient, the doctor and their government. Australas J Dermatol 2000;41:8–13.
42. Broens TH, Huis in't Veld RM, Vollenbroek-Hutten MM et al. Determinants of successful telemedicine implementations: A literature study. J Telemed Telecare 2007;13:303–309.
43. Aas IH. The future of telemedicine – take the organizational challenge! J Telemed Telecare 2007;13:379–381.
44. Boulton AJ. The diabetic foot: A global view. Diabetes Metab Res Rev 2000;16(Suppl 1):S2–S5.
45. Frykberg RG, Zgonis T, Armstrong DG et al. Diabetic foot disorders. A clinical practice guideline (2006 revision). J Foot Ankle Surg 2006;45:S1–S66.

46. Peleg M, Wang D, Fodor A et al. Lessons learned from adapting a generic narrative diabetic-foot guideline to an institutional decision-support system. Stud Health Technol Inform 2008;139:243–252.
47. Bangs I, Clarke M, Hands L et al. An integrated nursing and telemedicine approach to vascular care. J Telemed Telecare 2002;8(Suppl 2):110–112.
48. Clemensen J, Larsen SB, Ejskjaer N. Telemedical treatment at home of diabetic foot ulcers. J Telemed Telecare 2005;11(Suppl 2):S14–S16.
49. Larsen SB, Clemensen J, Ejskjaer N. A feasibility study of UMTS mobile phones for supporting nurses doing home visits to patients with diabetic foot ulcers. J Telemed Telecare 2006;12:358–362.
50. Wilbright WA, Birke JA, Patout CA et al. The use of telemedicine in the management of diabetes-related foot ulceration: a pilot study. Adv Skin Wound Care 2004;17:232–238.

ERRATUM TO:

SOAP/WSDL-Based Web Services for Biomedicine

Thomas Meinel and Ralf Herwig

Max Planck Institute for Molecular Genetics,
Vertebrate Genomics Department,
Bioinformatics Group, Ihnestrasse 63-73,
D-14195 Berlin,
Germany
meinel@molgen.mpg.de, herwig@molgen.mpg.de

A. Lazakidou (ed.), *Web-Based Applications in Healthcare and Biomedicine*,
Annals of Information Systems 7, DOI 10.1007/978-1-4419-1274-9_7,
© Springer Science+Business Media, LLC 2010

DOI 10.1007/978-1-4419-1274-9_18

The original version of this chapter unfortunately contained an incorrect:

a) chapter title
b) name of one of the co-authors

The correct title of the chapter and correct running head on odd pages is:
SOAP/WSDL-Based Web Services for Biomedicine
The correct co-author name is: Ralf Herwig

The original online version of this chapter can be found at
DOI 10.1007/978-1-4419-1274-9_7

Index

Note: The letter "t" and "f" followed by the locators denotes table and figure

A. Lazakidou (ed.), *Web-Based Applications in Health care and Biomedicine,*
Annals of Information Systems 7, DOI 10.1007/978-1-4419-1274-9,

© Springer Science+Business Media, LLC 2010

FSC
www.fsc.org
MIX
Papier | Fördert gute Waldnutzung
FSC® C083411

Kolibri 360 GmbH
Ferdinand-Jühlke-Straße 7
99095 Erfurt, Deutschland
produktsicherheit@kolibri360.de